Praise for *Reflective Organizations: On the Front Lines of QSEN & Reflective Practice Implementation*

"This must-read book, authored by a cadre of health-professions experts, provides testimony that reflective thinking and practice should be the cornerstone of both academic and practice learning environments. Indeed, the argument is made that reflective thinking and practice are the thread transformative organizations use to craft change and innovation. Nurses who read this book will be inspired to be part of interprofessional teams that will transform education and practice in the future."

–*Carol Huston, DPA, MSN, MPA, FAAN*
Director, School of Nursing
California State University, Chico

"Einstein wisely said, 'Insanity is doing the same thing over and over again expecting different results.' We've launched national panels of experts, collected tons of data, published research, and written books. Yet our education and practice have not fundamentally changed. Reflection is not just a skill that can be learned, but a process and way of being that can be translated to our work. Reflection could be the 'glue' that changes the way we work, yet we don't consider it in selection of future nurses and hiring of faculty. And, we don't generally evaluate and reward for reflective practice. Sherwood and Horton-Deutsch present a detailed 'playbook' of reflective strategies and techniques for faculty and practitioners. They present not just the why, but the how. It is a worthy read—a book to study and treasure."

–*Pamela Klauer Triolo, PhD, RN, FAAN*
Author, President, and CEO
Principled Leadership Solutions

"It is highly unlikely that we will or should ever reach a point at which patient care and patient care delivery of tomorrow is the same as it is today. The only way for organizations and healthcare professionals to be successful in this ever-changing healthcare world is to create cultures that value adaptability, flexibility, and continuous learning as paths to quality and safety. The reflective practices described in this new book by Sherwood and Horton-Deutsch are keys to creating and constantly improving successful practices."

–*Beth Ulrich, EdD, RN, FACHE, FAAN*
Professor, University of Texas Health Science Center at Houston School of Nursing
Editor, Nephrology Nursing Journal

Reflective Organizations
On the Front Lines of QSEN & Reflective Practice Implementation

Gwen D. Sherwood, PhD, RN, FAAN, ANEF
Sara Horton-Deutsch, PhD, RN, PMHCNS, FAAN, ANEF

Sigma Theta Tau International
Honor Society of Nursing®

The Honor Society of Nursing, Sigma Theta Tau International (STTI) is a nonprofit organization founded in 1922 whose mission is to support the learning, knowledge, and professional development of nurses committed to making a difference in health worldwide. Members include practicing nurses, instructors, researchers, policymakers, entrepreneurs and others. STTI's 494 chapters are located at 676 institutions of higher education throughout Australia, Botswana, Brazil, Canada, Colombia, Ghana, Hong Kong, Japan, Kenya, Malawi, Mexico, the Netherlands, Pakistan, Portugal, Singapore, South Africa, South Korea, Swaziland, Sweden, Taiwan, Tanzania, United Kingdom, United States, and Wales. More information about STTI can be found online at www.nursingsociety.org.

Sigma Theta Tau International
550 West North Street
Indianapolis, IN, USA 46202

To order additional books, buy in bulk, or order for corporate use, contact Nursing Knowledge International at 888. NKI.4YOU (888.654.4968/US and Canada) or +1.317.634.8171 (outside US and Canada).

To request a review copy for course adoption, email solutions@nursingknowledge.org or call 888.NKI.4YOU (888.654.4968/US and Canada) or +1.317.634.8171 (outside US and Canada).

To request author information, or for speaker or other media requests, contact Marketing, Honor Society of Nursing, Sigma Theta Tau International at 888.634.7575 (US and Canada) or +1.317.634.8171 (outside US and Canada).

ISBN: 9781938835582
EPUB ISBN: 9781938835599
PDF ISBN: 9781938835605
MOBI ISBN: 9781938835612

Library of Congress Cataloging-in-Publication Data

Sherwood, Gwen, author.
 Reflective organizations : on the front lines of QSEN & reflective practice implementation / Gwen Sherwood, Sara Horton-Deutsch.
   p. ; cm.
 Includes bibliographical references and index.
 ISBN 978-1-938835-58-2 (print : alk. paper) -- ISBN 978-1-938835-59-9 (epub) -- ISBN 978-1-938835-60-5 (pdf) -- ISBN 978-1-938835-61-2 (mobi)
 I. Horton-Deutsch, Sara, author. II. Sigma Theta Tau International, issuing body. III. Title.
 [DNLM: 1. Quality and Safety Education for Nurses (Project) 2. Competency-Based Education. 3. Nursing, Practical--education. 4. Leadership. 5. Organizational Innovation. 6. Patient Safety. 7. Quality Improvement. WY 18.8]
 RT76
 610.73071'1--dc23
                     2015014111

First Printing, 2015

Publisher: Dustin Sullivan
Acquisitions Editor: Emily Hatch
Editorial Coordinator: Paula Jeffers
Cover Designer: Rebecca Batchelor
Interior Design/Page Layout: Katy Bodenmiller

Principal Book Editor: Carla Hall
Development and Project Editor: Jennifer Lynn
Copy Editor: Teresa Artman
Proofreader: Todd Lothery
Indexer: Joy Dean Lee

Dedication

We dedicate this book to our families, who help sustain us in our journey, and also to educators and scholars, who are fellow change agents in developing practitioners and organizations engaged in reflective practice and lifelong learning to assure quality safe care of patients.

Acknowledgments

We joyfully acknowledge all those engaged in reflective practices as a way to influence and transform healthcare, who embrace practices that create a culture of inquiry where asking questions and actively involving colleagues, patients, and families in decisions is valued. It is through such practices that quality and safety are attained, organizational cultures are transformed, and viable futures are manifested.

We offer special appreciation and thanks to Emily Hatch and all those at Sigma Theta Tau International who offered patience and perseverance throughout the submission and editing of this work and their encouragement in pursuing this vital topic.

About the Authors

Gwen D. Sherwood, PhD, RN, FAAN, ANEF

Gwen D. Sherwood has a distinguished record in advancing nursing education locally and globally. Professor and Associate Dean for Academic Affairs at the University of North Carolina at Chapel Hill School of Nursing, her work focuses on transforming healthcare environments by expanding relational capacity of healthcare providers. Her studies have examined patient satisfaction with pain management outcomes, the spiritual dimensions of care, and teamwork as a variable in patient safety.

She is Co-Investigator for the award-winning Robert Wood Johnson–funded Quality and Safety Education for Nurses (QSEN) project to transform curricula to prepare nurses for working in and leading quality and safety in redesigned healthcare. Spanning education and practice, the QSEN Steering Team has been recognized with the Sigma Theta Tau International Honor Society Nursing Media Award and the Information Technology Award.

Dr. Sherwood has had a primary influence in the integration of quality and safety in health professions education. She was on the executive team for the UNC at Chapel Hill and Duke University Interprofessional Patient Safety Education Collaborative to measure effectiveness of teaching modalities for interdisciplinary teamwork training for nursing and medical students. She is a senior faculty at the Telluride Science Institute Round Table on Redesigning Health Professions Education to improve patient safety and was an adjunct faculty in the Master's in Patient Safety Leadership Program at the University of Illinois at Chicago School of Medicine. She served on the Research Committee of the National Patient Safety Foundation and the Technical Expert Panel for AHRQ's TeamSTEPPS implementation and as President of the International Association for Human Caring. Widely published, she is co-editor of *International Association for Human Caring; Quality and Safety Education: A Competency Approach in Nursing*, an AJN book of the year; and *Reflective Practice: Transforming Education and Improving Outcomes*.

Dr. Sherwood's distinguished service to the Honor Society for Nursing, Sigma Theta Tau International, includes Distinguished Lecturer, Virginia Henderson Fellow, chair of the global task force for the Scholarship of Reflective Practice position paper, chair of the Research Scholarship Advisory Committee, and two terms as Vice President. Her hospital research team received the 2001 Regional Research Utilization Award for implementing Relationship Centered Care.

Dr. Sherwood's work bridges U.S. and global organizations to expand nursing undergraduate and graduate education capacity to serve developing regions. Formerly Executive Associate Dean at the University of Texas Health Science Center in Houston School of Nursing, she bridged academia and practice through a joint appointment as Co-Director of the Center for Professional Excellence at The Methodist Hospital. She worked with the China Medical Board program in advancing nursing education in China and continues to expand opportunities for faculty development. She participated in advancing nursing in Kazakhstan and Sakhalin with The Methodist Hospital and the American International Health Alliance. She is the External Examiner for Macau Polytechnic Institute in Macau, Visiting Professor with Ramathibodi Hospital School of Nursing in Bangkok, and Team Leader for advancing health professions education in Kenya with IntraHealth International.

Sara Horton-Deutsch, PhD, RN, PMHCNS, FAAN, ANEF

Sara Horton-Deutsch is a Professor and the Jean Watson Caring Science Endowed Chair at the University of Colorado College of Nursing. Dr. Horton-Deutsch is a certified Caritas Coach and an established international leader in the psychiatric mental health nursing community. She has a sound international reputation and is known for her work in leadership development and advancing the art and science of reflective pedagogies in nursing education. She has served as the Division Chair for Education and Research for the International Society of Psychiatric Mental-Health Nurses (ISPN), as a member of the task force for the Scope and Standards of Practice National Review and Revision for psychiatric mental health nursing, and was a member of the Licensure Accreditation Certification and Education network (LACE). Currently, she is president of ISPN and leading the organization through both strategic planning and transformation.

Dr. Horton-Deutsch's work with the national quality and safety work of QSEN has had a significant impact on the quality and care of patients in the psychiatric mental health arena. She influences the teaching/learning mindset of nurse educators around the world through her published scholarship and international, national, and regional presentations. She has been recognized with international, national, and regional awards that attest to her excellence in creative work and leadership skill set.

In 2013, she was named the Jean Watson Endowed Chair in Human Caring Science at the University of Colorado, a role that enables her to continue to influence and impact the development of next generation nursing leaders. In 2015, Dr. Horton-Deutsch will become the director of the regenerated Watson Caring Science Center with the mission of advancing the art and science of human-caring knowledge, ethics, and clinical practice in the fields of nursing and health sciences. The Center will foster research, teaching, and practice of human-caring through an interprofessional PhD program track, Caritas Coach, and other continuing education training programs integrating new knowledge from humanities, arts, cross-cultural spiritual disciplines, and emerging scientific disciplines. The Center will support the development and implementation of innovative approaches to clinical practice and human-caring and healing. It intends to serve as an international and interprofessional resource and clearing house for information related to the theory and practice of human-caring and healing.

Contributing Authors

Gail E. Armstrong, DNP, ACNS-BC, CNE

Associate Professor
University of Colorado College of Nursing

Gail E. Armstrong is an Associate Professor at the University of Colorado College of Nursing, where she has been on faculty for 14 years. Gail has a BA and an MA in literature, an MS in Nursing (with a Clinical Nurse Specialist focus), a Doctorate of Nursing Practice degree, and is finishing a PhD in Nursing

Science at Vanderbilt University. In her PhD research, Gail is studying patient safety and unit-level medication error rates. Along with teaching prelicensure nursing students about quality and safety, Gail teaches interprofessional clinical teams in a 12-month certificate training program in quality, safety, and efficiency. These interprofessional clinical teams apply these concepts to transform the care on their respective units. Gail's scholarship has focused on the integration of updated quality and safety content in nursing curricula.

Amy J. Barton, PhD, RN, FAAN

Professor and Associate Dean for Clinical and Community Affairs
University of Colorado College of Nursing

Amy Barton, Professor, Daniel and Janet Mordecai Endowed Chair in Rural Health Nursing, and Associate Dean for Clinical and Community Affairs at the University of Colorado College of Nursing, is responsible for faculty practice and development of community partnerships. She provided the vision to create Sheridan Health Services, a nurse-managed federally qualified community health center, serving low-income residents in an urban area southwest of Denver, Colorado. Her work in national quality and safety initiatives include the Quality and Safety Education for Nurses initiative and the Institute for Healthcare Improvement/Josiah Macy Jr. Foundation initiative on "Retooling for Quality and Safety." Dr. Barton is a member of the 2005 cohort of the Robert Wood Johnson Executive Nurse Fellows, a Distinguished Practitioner in the National Academies of Practice, a Fellow in the Western Academy of Nursing, and a Fellow in the American Academy of Nursing.

Sheila Blackmur, MSN, RN-BC, CMSRN

Clinical Educator
Southwest General Health Center

Sheila Blackmur received her master's degree in Nursing Education from Regis University. Besides clinical education, her career has included orthopedic, neurosurgical, neurosurgical step-down, out-patient surgery, and patient blood management. She has co-authored "Blood Management: Best-practice

Transfusion Strategies in Nursing 2013." She is board-certified in nursing education and medical surgical nursing, has practiced in the Cleveland Clinic Health System, and is currently a Clinical Educator at Southwest General Health Center in Middleburg Heights, Ohio.

Jan Boller, PhD, RN

Associate Professor and Assistant Dean
Strategic Partnerships/Community Engagement
The Fletcher Jones Endowed Chair for Nursing Safety and Quality
College of Graduate Nursing Western University of Health Sciences

Jan Boller's clinical specialty was in critical care nursing, serving in roles as staff nurse, nurse educator, and critical care clinical nurse specialist. She was President of Health Education International, Inc. and Program Development Director for the American Association of Critical-Care Nursing. After earning her PhD at the University of California, San Francisco, Dr. Boller was Director of Clinical Effectiveness at two Sutter Health facilities in the San Francisco Bay area. Dr. Boller was a consulting project director for the California Institute of Nursing & Health Care 2008 White Paper on Nursing Education Redesign for California. She is co-author of *Daily Miracles: Stories and Practices of Humanity and Excellence in Health Care*, published by Sigma Theta Tau International. The book received an AJN Book of the Year Award. Dr. Boller is on the National Advisory Board for the Quality and Safety Education for Nurses (QSEN) Institute. Her program of interest focuses on cultivating collaborative interprofessional community-focused efforts to improve patient safety and healthcare quality.

Cynthia Sherraden Bradley, MSN, RN

Assistant Professor
University of Central Missouri

Cynthia Sherraden Bradley received a BSN from the University of Kansas and an MSN from the University of Central Missouri, and is currently a doctoral student at Indiana University. As a director of a Kansas City school of nursing program simulation center, she led a task force, resulting in a city-wide collaborative resource for simulation users in the Kansas City metropolitan area called Simulation User Group Across the Region. She has served as a consultant for new simulation programs in Kansas City, in addition integrating simulation into nursing curricula. She is currently an assistant professor at the University of Central Missouri.

Pat Callard, DNP, RN, CNE, CNL

Assistant Professor
College of Graduate Nursing
Course Director, Interprofessional Education
Western University of Health Sciences

Pat Callard received a BSN and an MSN from Kent State University, Kent, Ohio. After working in medical-surgical and critical care, Pat began teaching critical care orientation. That led to a position as a staff educator and ultimately the Director of Educational Services. Following a hospital merger, Pat took responsibility for education across multiple hospitals in a corporate position. Pat has been in academia for the past 10 years and received her DNP. She teaches leadership courses in the College of Graduate Nursing. Pat serves as Course Director for Interprofessional Education at Western University of Health Sciences in Pomona, California. Throughout her career, Pat's interest has focused on critical thinking in nurses and other health professionals.

Mary Ellen Campobasso, MSN, RN, ACNS-BC

Clinical Nurse Educator
Southwest General Health Center

Mary Ellen Campobasso is an ANCC–certified clinical nurse specialist in Adult Health Nursing and also a Gerontological Nurse. She is currently employed as a clinical nurse educator for an acute care hospital, specifically assigned to the following acute care inpatient units: Geriatric and Behavioral-Health Services; Medical-Surgical Pulmonary & Oncology; Dialysis; Maternal-Newborn; and Hospice & Home Health Services. She has expertise in educating adult learners, and in particular, nursing students, nursing assistants, registered nurses, paramedics, and LPNs. She has led discussion groups and debriefed students/nurses about clinical experiences and concerns/issues of interest. She developed QSEN–infused nursing orientation checklists and collaboratively assisted in the redesigning of hospital orientation influenced by QSEN for nursing staff. She organized geriatric and adult health, content-based seminars, and learning modules. She facilitated the implementation of a hospital-wide vascular access program. She has more than 15 years experience as a gerontological nurse in both acute care and long-term care of the older adult. She is a former NICHE coordinator, and she developed a hospital-based Graduate Nurse Resident (GRN) certification program.

Mary A. Dolansky, PhD, RN

Associate Professor
Case Western Reserve University

Mary A. Dolansky is an Associate Professor at the Frances Payne Bolton School of Nursing, Case Western Reserve University and Director of the QSEN Institute (Quality and Safety Education for Nurses). She has co-published two books on quality-improvement education, co-authored several book chapters and articles, and was guest editor on a special quality-improvement education issue in the *Journal of Quality Management in Health Care*. Dr. Dolansky has taught the interdisciplinary course on quality improvement at CWRU for the past 10 years and was chair of the Quality and Safety Task Force at the school of nursing that integrated quality and safety into the undergraduate and graduate curriculum. She is co-director of the VA Transforming Primary care to develop and implement a longitudinal interdisciplinary curriculum that includes integrating teamwork and quality improvement into an academic-clinical medical home model and mentors pre- and post-doctoral nurses in the VA Quality Scholars program. She has published an implementation study on integrating heart failure protocols in a skilled nursing facility.

Kristina Thomas Dreifuerst, PhD, RN, CNE, ANEF

Assistant Professor
Indiana University, Indianapolis, IN

Kristina Thomas Dreifuerst received her bachelor's degree in nursing from Luther College in Decorah, Iowa; her master's degree from the University of Wisconsin in Madison, Wisconsin; and her PhD in nursing from Indiana University, where she is now an Assistant Professor in the School of Nursing at Indianapolis. Dr. Dreifuerst has been a nurse educator for the past 17 years, teaching didactic and clinical courses in traditional and online environments to prelicensure and graduate students. Her research is at the forefront of disciplinary efforts to develop, use, and test innovative teaching methods to improve students' clinical reasoning skills; and investigate how teachers can best be prepared to use evidence-based methods, including simulation and debriefing, to enhance clinical teaching. Her work has been funded by the Robert Wood Johnson Foundation, the National League for Nursing, Sigma Theta Tau International, and Indiana University. She has disseminated her research widely via publications, presentations, and consultantships, nationally and internationally.

Jason Drysdale, MA in ILT

Manager of Instructional Design and E-Learning Technology
University of Colorado Denver

Jason Drysdale is an instructional designer, technologist, and writer/researcher from Denver, Colorado. He has taught and developed online graduate courses in instructional technology, designed courses in a host of other disciplines, and has acted as a consultant on a variety of design-related projects. Jason holds a BA in Christian Ministry from Abilene Christian University, Texas, where he graduated magna cum laude. He graduated with honors from the University of Colorado Denver with an MA in Information and Learning Technologies, with emphases in Adult Learning and Instructional Design. Jason's research interests include games-based learning, collaborative design, online learning, and instructional systems analysis. He lives with his wife, Courtney, on Colorado's Front Range, and enjoys playing guitar, video games, exploring the natural beauty of his home state, and spoiling his Cavalier King Charles Spaniel, Kingsley.

Carol Fowler Durham, EdD, RN, ANEF, FAAN

Clinical Professor and Director, Education-Innovation-Simulation
  Learning Environment (EISLE)
University of North Carolina at Chapel Hill, School of Nursing

Carol Fowler Durham seamlessly integrates excellence in teaching with long experience in practice and scholarship to improve the ways faculties prepare the future nursing workforce. As a member of the RWJF's Quality and Safety Education for Nurses (QSEN) project, Dr. Durham developed simulation-based educational experiences that reflect cutting-edge pedagogy. Dr. Durham has made significant and sustained contributions in interprofessional education (IPE) and is a leader in preparing faculty to integrate quality and safety into their curriculum and their teaching. Disseminating her work widely via publications, presentations, and online modules has extended its impact around the world. Dr. Durham's expertise and innovations in quality and safety education have been widely recognized. She is a fellow in the American Academy of Nursing and the National League for Nursing (NLN) Academy of Nursing Education. Dr. Durham received the 2010 Academic Achievement Award from Western Carolina University. She received the Alumni of the Year award from the University of North Carolina and Western Carolina University in 2008. In 2005, she was awarded the Nurse Educator of the Year from the NC Board of Nursing. She is President of the International Nursing Association for Clinical Simulation & Learning (INACSL).

Linda S. Flores, MSN, RN

Assistant Professor, College of Graduate Nursing
Western University of Health Sciences

Linda Flores is an assistant professor in the MSN-E program at Western University of Health Sciences, College of Graduate Nursing. She teaches throughout the curriculum from health assessment through advanced medical surgical nursing. She has practiced in a variety of nursing settings for more than 15 years, including adult and pediatric emergency nursing, critical care, operative services, vascular access team, ambulatory infusion clinic, and nursing education. Linda received her bachelor's degree in Nursing Science from the University of Virginia, Master of Science-Nurse Educator from California State University, Dominguez Hills. She is certified in emergency nursing, peripherally inserted central catheters, and chemotherapy administration. Linda is a member of the Emergency Nursing Association and Sigma Theta Tau International. She maintains her clinical currency as a relief charge and staff RN at Loma Linda University Medical Center.

Jean Foret Giddens, PhD, RN, FAAN

Dean and Professor
Virginia Commonwealth University, School of Nursing

Jean Giddens is Dean and Professor at the School of Nursing, Virginia Commonwealth University in Richmond, Virginia, and is an alumna of the Robert Wood Johnson Executive Nurse Fellow, 2011 Cohort. Dr. Giddens earned a BSN from the University of Kansas, an MSN from the University of Texas at El Paso, and a PhD in Education and Human Resource Studies from Colorado State University. Dr. Giddens' teaching experience includes associate degree, baccalaureate degree, and graduate degree programs in New Mexico, Texas, Colorado, and Virginia. She is an expert in concept-based curriculum development and evaluation as well as innovative strategies for teaching and learning. Dr. Giddens is the author of multiple journal articles, nursing textbooks, and electronic media, and serves as an education consultant to nursing programs throughout the country.

Katherine Foss, MSN, RN

Supervisor, Clinical Entry Programs and Clinical Scholar
University of Colorado College of Nursing, and University of Colorado
  Hospital, University of Colorado Health

Katherine Foss has 28 years of nursing practice in the acute care setting in a broad range of roles from direct patient care, unit manager, service line clinical nurse specialist, and nursing professional development specialist. Since 2002, her nursing practice and interest has focused primarily in baccalaureate nursing education, specific to exploring, developing, and evaluating new learning environments and opportunities for prelicensure students in the acute care setting. Professional endeavors also include participation in curricular development, guest speaker, and program evaluation, as a subject matter expert, of the Clinical Scholar Workshop, sponsored by the Colorado Center for Nursing Excellence. The workshop is a 40-hour RN professional development course for nurses interested in the clinical instructor role. She is a member of the Association for Nursing Professional Development and Colorado Nurses Association.

Karen Hanford, EdD, MSN, FNP

Founding Dean, College of Graduate Nursing
Western University of Health Sciences

Karen Hanford has more than 30 years of nursing experience, which spans the continuum from critical care nursing to ambulatory care as a family nurse practitioner. As founding dean of CGN, she has been instrumental in curriculum design and achieving Board of Registered Nursing approval and professional accreditation for all graduate programs. The College celebrated its tenth anniversary in 2007 as well as its 10-year re-accreditation from the Commission on Collegiate Nursing Education (CCNE), which is the national accrediting body for the American Association of Colleges of Nursing. Professor Hanford has presented at numerous national meetings in the area of curriculum design and distance teaching. The college is recognized as a leader in distance education. Dean Hanford has more than 20 years of nursing education experience and is an expert in pulmonary nursing. Ms. Hanford has been an advanced practice nurse for 15 years with a special interest in internal medicine.

Marci Luxenburg-Horowitz, DNP, RN, CNL

Assistant Professor, Assistant Director, Health Systems Leadership
College of Graduate Nursing
Western University of Health Sciences

Marci Luxenburg-Horowitz is an assistant professor and assistant director for Health Systems Leadership program within the CGN at Western University of Health Sciences. She has held numerous practice and educational roles throughout her career. Past experiences include working with children and their families in the hospital and community settings, community education, and facilitating the development of community collaboratives to improve health. Current work and interests include improving health system quality and safety through academic-service partnerships, enhancing professional role formation, leadership growth and development of nursing students and professional nurses, transitions into practice of new and experienced nurses, and IPE.

Pamela Ironside, PhD, RN, FAAN, ANEF

Professor and Director of the Center for Research in Nursing Education
Indiana University

Pamela Ironside is a professor and director of the Center for Research in Nursing Education at Indiana University. Her research includes numerous funded investigations of the ways new pedagogies influence the practices of thinking in nursing courses, the ways students' interactions with faculty and preceptors during clinical experiences foster thinking and learning, and the ways in which nursing faculty undertake reform and innovation. She is a member of the National Advisory Council for the Robert Wood Johnson Foundation initiative Evaluating Innovations in Nursing. She is a fellow in the American Academy of Nursing and the Academy of Nursing Education. She is the recipient of the Excellence in Nursing Education Research award from the National League for Nursing, the Scholarship of Teaching and Learning Excellence Award from the American Association of Colleges of Nursing, the Advancing the Science of Nursing award for the Education Section of the Midwest Nursing Research Society, and the Chancellor's Award for Excellence in Teaching at Indiana University-Purdue University Indianapolis.

Benny L. Joyner, Jr., MD, MPH

Assistant Professor
Clinical Co-Director of The Clinical Skills and Patient Simulation Center
Clerkship Director of Fourth-Year Medical Student Critical Care Selective
Director of the Pediatric Critical Care Medicine Fellowship Program
University of North Carolina at Chapel Hill, School of Medicine

Dr. Benny L. Joyner, Jr. is a pediatric intensivist and an Assistant Professor in the Department of Pediatrics. He also serves as the Clinical Co-Director of The Clinical Skills and Patient Simulation Center, which provides simulated experiences to medical, nursing, and pharmacy students. He serves as the Clerkship Director of Fourth year Medical Student Critical Care Selective and Director of the Pediatric Critical Care Medicine Fellowship Program. He received his MD and MPH from UNC at Chapel Hill. He completed a pediatric residency at Albert Einstein College of Medicine in New York and a pediatric critical care fellowship at UNC–Chapel Hill. His areas of interest and research include curriculum development, IPE, simulation, global health, telemedicine, ethics, and patient/family communication.

Mary Jo Krivanek, RN, BSN, MPA

Clinical Nursing Educator
Southwest General Health Center

Mary Jo Krivanek has spent more than 27 years as a Registered Nurse in acute care hospital settings: Neurosurgical Step-Down, Intensive Care Unit Step-Down, Medical Telemetry Unit, and 3 years in clinical management. She has more than 20 years of experience as a preceptor in acute hospital settings and has also been a clinical instructor. Currently she is working in the role of clinical nursing educator for two medical-surgical units, Seidman Cancer Center, agency staff, nursing supervisors, and the Progressive Care Unit in an acute care hospital. Currently she is the chairperson of the Nursing Standards Committee at Southwest General Health Center and the co-chairperson for the Northeast Ohio Nursing Initiative (NEONI) Quality and Safety Division.

Kathryn Kuehn, BA

Executive Director, International Society of Psychiatric-Mental Health Nurses
The Rees Group, Inc.

Kathryn Kuehn holds a BA in journalism from the University of Wisconsin–Madison. She is an award-winning communications and association executive with extensive experience in relationship management, communications strategy, and project management in association, professional society, and business-to-business environments.

Kathy collaborates with and guides nonprofit boards of directors in fulfilling their responsibility to set policy and strategic direction. She manages professional societies' annual business cycles, including budgets, finances, memberships, and conferences, and provides operational support for Executive Committee, standing committee, and task force directives.

Kathy is a results-oriented leader with a proven track record of bringing together teams to identify opportunities, create action plans, and execute strategy. She is a creative visionary who consistently meets organizational goals by working smarter with fewer resources.

Kathy Lay, PhD

Associate Professor
Indiana University School of Social Work

Kathy Lay, PhD completed her doctoral work in social work at University of Louisville, Kent School of Social Work with a minor in women's studies. She has more than 20 years of clinical practice experience with individuals, couples, and families. Currently, her research is focused on recovery processes from substance-use disorders, IPE, and reflective pedagogy.

Angela M. McNelis, PhD, RN, PMHCNS, ANEF, CNE

Professor of Nursing
Indiana University

Angela McNelis received a BSN degree from DePauw University, and MS (Education), MSN (Child/Adolescent Psychiatric Mental Health), and PhD degrees from Indiana University. She is an expert in innovative teaching and/or learning strategies; nursing education research; evaluation; faculty development; academic leadership; and collaborative educational, practice, and community partnerships. She is a fellow of the NLN Academy of Nursing Education, and has been honored numerous times for her excellence in teaching and research both locally and nationally. She is currently funded by the Robert Wood Johnson Foundation to study the nursing faculty shortage and by the Substance Abuse and Mental Health Services Administration to integrate Screening Brief Intervention and Referral to Treatment (SBIRT) into Indiana's healthcare and allied healthcare education systems to improve the health of adolescents and adults at risk for substance-use disorders.

Meg Moorman, PhD, RN, WHNP-BC

Assistant Clinical Professor
Indiana University

Meg Moorman received her BSN from Indiana University and her MSN from Drexel University. As a labor and delivery nurse, she worked in both private practice and in the hospital setting. She completed her Women's Health NP in 1996. She worked for a large healthcare clinic as a Women's Health NP for 14 years. She began teaching at Indiana University in 2007 and completed her PhD in Nursing in 2013. She continues to volunteer as an NP in her community and works as an assistant clinical professor for Indiana University. She currently teaches in the BSN program and focuses her research in the use of the arts and humanities in nursing education.

Karen T. Pardue, PhD, RN, CNE, ANEF

Associate Dean
Associate Professor of Nursing
University of New England

Karen Pardue is the Associate Dean in the Westbrook College of Health Professions at the University of New England (UNE). Her expertise focuses on nursing education and IPE curriculum development and evaluation. Dr. Pardue provided leadership in the design and implementation of UNE's innovative undergraduate IPE coursework. She has diverse experience in nursing education, working in associate, RN-to-BSN, baccalaureate, and master's level programs. For a decade, she provided leadership to a novel international academic partnership involving UNE and Israel College in Tel Aviv. Nationally, she served two terms chairing the NLN Task Group on Innovation in Nursing Education and as a mentor for the Johnson & Johnson/NLN Faculty Mentoring program. She was nominated by the Governor of Maine to serve on the New England Board of Higher Education, and she currently is chair of the Maine delegation. She has published and presented widely on educational innovation and IPE. She was inducted as a Fellow in the Academy of Nursing Education in 2007. She currently has grant funded projects from the Health Resources and Services Administration (HRSA), the Arthur Vining Davis Foundations, and the Josiah Macy Foundation, addressing IPE models and collaborative nursing leadership.

Daniel J. Pesut, PhD, RN, PMHCNS-BC, FAAN

Professor of Nursing, Population Health and Systems Cooperative
  Unit and the Katherine R. and C. Walton Lillehei Chair in Nursing
  Leadership
University of Minnesota School of Nursing

Daniel Pesut is the Director of the Katharine J. Densford International Center for Nursing Leadership at the University of Minnesota School of Nursing, and Professor of Nursing, Population Health and Systems Co-operative Unit. Dr.

Pesut holds the Katherine R. and C. Walton Lillehei Nursing Leadership Chair. Dr. Pesut served on the board of Directors of the Honor Society of Nursing, Sigma Theta Tau International, for 8 years and as President of the Honor Society of Nursing (2003–2005). He is a Fellow in the American Academy of Nursing, and a board-certified clinical nurse specialist in adult psychiatric mental health nursing as well as a Certified Hudson Institute coach. He is an award-winning master teacher. He is a popular author and speaks frequently on a number of topics that include creative and futures-thinking, clinical reasoning, leadership development, and interprofessional health professions education.

Stephen M. Powell, MS

CEO and President
Synensis, LLC

Stephen Powell has been a leader in human factors education, safety, team performance, and communication training for 30 years in the U.S. Navy, the commercial airline industry, and the healthcare industry. He founded Synensis, an evidence-based training and consulting company, in 2004 aimed at improving patient safety and quality of care. Stephen and his wife live in the Atlanta, Georgia metro area. They have two adult children and enjoy traveling, serving others, outdoor sports, and entertaining friends and family. Stephen is a former U.S. Navy pilot and commercial airline captain. He earned his undergraduate degree in mathematics from the University of North Carolina at Chapel Hill and a masters of science in Human Factors from Embry-Riddle University. He is currently pursuing a doctorate in Health Administration at Central Michigan University.

Kelly L. Scolaro, PharmD

Clinical Assistant Professor and Director of Pharmaceutical Care Labs
UNC Eshelman School of Pharmacy, University of North Carolina at Chapel Hill

Kelly L. Scolaro is a clinical assistant professor and director of pharmaceutical care labs in the Division of Practice Advancement and Clinical Education at the University of North Carolina Eshelman School of Pharmacy in Chapel Hill, NC. Kelly received her BS in pharmacy and PharmD from Auburn University. She completed an accredited community pharmacy practice residency at the University of Florida. She has practiced in several areas, including chain community pharmacy; free clinics; and most recently, nonprofit geriatrics clinic. She has published and presented on the topics of nonprescription therapeutics, clinical services in the community pharmacy, distance education, skills lab learning, and IPE. Kelly is an author and reviewer for the American Pharmacists Association's Handbook of Nonprescription Drugs. She is also very active in the American Academy of Colleges of Pharmacy and is serving as the immediate past chair for the Self-Care and Nonprescription Medicines SIG.

Patricia Salazar Shakhshir, PhD, CNS, RN-BC

Assistant Professor, College of Graduate Nursing
Western University of Health Sciences

Patricia (Patti) Shakhshir is an Assistant Professor in the MSN-Entry program and has practiced in the nursing field since 1977. She received an ADN from Loma Linda University, a BSN from Azusa Pacific University, an MSN (Gerontology CNS Option) from Cal State Dominguez Hills, and a PhD in Nursing from Azusa Pacific University. Patti has been a medical-surgical nurse for most of her career, with experience in oncology, orthopedics, gerontology, and pain management.

Patti worked at Pomona Valley Hospital Medical Center for 25 years in various capacities, from staff nurse to pain management/gerontology clinical nurse specialist. She worked at San Antonio Community Hospital as the Pain Management Coordinator (CNS). Experience in academia includes working as adjunct faculty at Azusa Pacific University and full-time at Western University of Health Sciences.

Dawn Salpaka Stone, RN, ANP-BC, COHN-S

Associate Professor, College of Graduate Nursing
Western University of Health Sciences

Dawn Stone teaches MSN and DNP students with a focus on quality and safety in the delivery of interprofessional care to vulnerable groups. She also represents nursing on the design team for interprofessional education at WesternU. Ms. Stone is currently investigating vulnerable populations in workplace settings throughout Los Angeles County, California as a part of her dissertation research study at the University of California, Los Angeles. She is an actively practicing NP with extensive experience in primary care of adults. Ms. Stone's professional activities include service on the American Association of Occupational Health Nurses Practice Committee and as a peer reviewer for Workplace Health and Safety. She has also served as a founding board member for Sigma Theta Tau International's Phi Alpha and Upsilon Beta chapters. In 2014, she was recognized by the California State Association for Occupational Health Nurses as a recipient of the Moore Excellence Award.

Richard Stone, MS

Chief Innovation Officer
Synensis

Richard Stone is a nationally recognized speaker on the power of storytelling. He got his start more than 20 years ago with the creation of the StoryWork Institute, where he developed story-based training programs for team building, leadership development, and diversity training for healthcare institutions, and has worked with hospice volunteers and staff around the country through his program Journey Into the Healing Power of Storytelling. He is also the author of three books: *The Healing Art of Storytelling, Stories: The Family Legacy*, and *The Kingdom of Nowt*, as well as the publisher of the award-winning board game *Pitch-A-Story*. Prior to joining Synensis, he was the StoryAnalytics Master for the IDEAS Innovation team where he co-created StoryCare, an innovative program for driving behavioral change among healthcare staff to improve patient safety and satisfaction, as well as to support the nursing school competencies.

John H. Tegzes, BSN, MA, VMD, Dipl. ABVT

Director of Interprofessional Education
Western University of Health Sciences

As an active member of two health professions (Nursing and Veterinary Medicine), Dr. John Tegzes understands innately what it means to be interprofessional and also how to communicate this in meaningful ways to health profession academics, students, and clinicians. His educational experience includes a BSN in Nursing, an MA in Applied Psychology, and a VMD in Veterinary Medicine. He further specialized in clinical toxicology and has worked interprofessionally as both a nurse and a veterinarian alongside physicians, nurses, and pharmacists at poison centers and diagnostic labs in Oregon and California. Dr. Tegzes is founding faculty member of the College of Veterinary Medicine (CVM) at WesternU, where he was instrumental in the development of the Problem-Based Learning curriculum that is implemented there. His knowledge of small group teaching and learning, and his passion for interprofessional collaborative care, led to his engagement in WesternU's IPE program development, implementation, and evaluation. In July 2012, he assumed the position of Director of IPE for Western University.

Sarah A. Thompson, PhD, RN, FAAN

Dean and Professor
University of Colorado College of Nursing

Sarah Thompson is dean and professor at the University of Colorado College of Nursing. She previously held the position of professor and associate dean of academic programs in the College of Nursing at the University of Nebraska Medical Center. Dr. Thompson is passionate about nursing education, has taught at all levels of nursing education, and has been actively involved in interdisciplinary education both locally and nationally.

Dr. Thompson has actively pursued improving end-of-life care in nursing homes for the past 16 years. Funding from both the Kansas Department on Aging and National Institute of Health have supported her research on the impact of organizational and clinical variables on the quality of nursing home care. Study findings have been widely disseminated in peer-reviewed nursing and interprofessional journals and led to practice changes in nursing homes that include palliative care and falls-prevention programs.

Jean Watson, PhD, RN, AHN-BC, FAAN

Distinguished Professor Emerita
University of Colorado Denver College of Nursing,
  Anschutz Medical Campus
Founder/Director: Watson Caring Science Institute

Jean Watson is known around the world of nursing and healthcare for her scholarship in Caring Science. As the author of Watson Theory of Human Caring, and author of more than 20 books on Caring Science, she is a globally sought-after speaker, consultant, and transformative leader. Her work is studied and used as a guide for nursing education, practice, research, and administration. Caring Science is increasingly the basis for academic-educational curricula and theory-guided professional clinical practices, transforming nursing and healthcare throughout the United States and throughout the world.

Dr. Watson held the nation's first endowed Chair in Caring Science at the University of Colorado for 16 years, where she served as Distinguished Professor, the university's highest recognition for scholarly work. She is the recipient of numerous honors, including a Fulbright Research award in Sweden, a Kellogg Fellowship in Australia, and the Fetzer Institute Norm Cousins Award for her work in relationship-centered caring.

She has been awarded 10 honorary Doctorate Degrees, 7 of which are international. Her books have been translated into 10 languages. In 2008, Dr. Watson established the Watson Caring Science Institute, a nonprofit organization, and the International Caritas Consortium, to extend this work into the world. In 2013, Dr. Watson was designated a Living Legend by the American Academy of Nursing, its highest honor.

Beth M. Weese, MSN, RN, GCNS-BC

Clinical Nursing Educator, Southwest General

Beth Weese is a board certified Geriatric Clinical Nurse Specialist. She received her Bachelor of Science in Nursing from Ohio State University in 1984 and her Masters of Science degree from Kent State University in 1999. She is an active member of the Northeast Ohio Clinical Nurse Specialist Association and is adjunct faculty for Kent State University, along with volunteering as a preceptor for nurse graduate students for both Akron University and Ursuline College. Ms. Weese has had various clinical roles in nursing. She worked in critical care, and has held positions in Nursing Management, Quality Management, and Nursing Informatics. Her present role as clinical educator for Emergency and Critical Care Departments allows her to infuse QSEN into practice.

Donald J. Woodyard, BS

Vice Chair for Finance & Administration
Indiana University School of Medicine, Department of
  Emergency Medicine

Donald J. Woodyard is the Chief Financial Officer for the Department of Emergency Medicine at the Indiana University School of Medicine in Indianapolis, IN. Mr. Woodyard oversees the administrative and financial affairs for a $90 million department with 100 faculty and staff seeing more than 270,000 patient visits annually. He is also the Co-Course Director for the department's CME program. Mr. Woodyard received his BS in biology and graduate certificate in entrepreneurship from the University of North Carolina at Chapel Hill. He served as director of authentic assessment and simulation at the UNC School of Medicine from 2005–2009 and served on the teaching faculty as director of assessment from 2009–2013. During his tenure at UNC, Mr. Woodyard directed several IPE initiatives, including the creation of and first course director for the school's Interprofessional Teamwork Course. He has presented on IPE and teamwork training to national and international audiences across healthcare disciplines. He is the immediate past-Vice President of Finance for the Association of Standardized Patient Educators.

Patricia Kaye Young, PhD, RN

Professor and Graduate Program Coordinator
Minnesota State University, Mankato
School of Nursing

Patricia Young received her bachelor's degree in nursing from the University of Wisconsin–Eau Claire, her master's degree from Marquette University, and her PhD in nursing from the University of Wisconsin–Madison. She has taught graduate and undergraduate nursing courses at Minnesota State University, Mankato since 1986. She served on several NLN committees, including the task force to develop Nurse Educator Competencies, the Healthful Work Environment task group, and the NLN Nurse Educator Workforce Development Advisory Council; she served as Project Director for the NLN Faculty Leadership and Mentoring Program from 2007–2011. Her research contributed to developing the NLN's Healthful Work Environment Tool Kit, Position Statement on Mentoring in Nursing Education, and Mentoring Tool Kit. Dr. Young's research interests include Narrative Pedagogy, the experiences of new teachers in nursing education, teaching family-focused nursing care, faculty mentoring, and the experience of becoming a nurse faculty leader. She has disseminated her research widely via publications and presentations.

Table of Contents

Foreword

Healthcare is in a world of rapid transformation. Social media, TV talk shows and news programs, politicians, healthcare professionals, and consumers all have something to say about this transition. Missing, however, is a clear direction of how to successfully maneuver through the confusion and rapid acceleration of this change in healthcare. Those of us in the healthcare professions and particularly in nursing are charged with a moral imperative to always do our best for our patients and the health of our community. But there is little direction available about how to rapidly adjust to this changing environment.

Gwen D. Sherwood and Sara Horton-Deutsch take this challenge seriously and offer data and evidence-based approaches to facing this rapid transformation with agility, nimbleness, flexibility, and adaptability. This book is based on the premise that nursing must transform education and practice rapidly to meet these new challenges. The creation of learning environments that utilize reflective practice is offered as an effective grounded method from the authors' extensive experience in reflective practice to help organizations continually learn and improve to meet the rapid change. The authors incorporate theory with the novel use of "theory bursts" and compelling data about the effectiveness of reflective practice and reflective learning environments in providing an efficient, structured method to rapidly incorporate new learning. In addition to the exemplary credentials of the authors, the careful selection of contributing authors from divergent backgrounds with extensive experience in reflective practice further strengthens the content.

This book expands the original content of the 2012 book *Reflective Practice: Transforming Education and Improving Outcomes* into reflective learning environments in interprofessional education and practice. Creating resilient organizations using this practice is an important concept for the healthcare of the future. And creating resilient practitioners who utilize reflective practice will be the cornerstone of this future.

Change is difficult for many. The challenge of continually rethinking what we are doing in a rapidly transforming environment can be difficult. In healthcare, we have doers and thinkers. The doers are the people who are task-oriented and believe their work is done when they have effectively checked off the tasks that are indicated in their practice. Checklists are important, but so is the process of continually questioning if this is the best process and if the checklist is the right one. To provide the best care for our healthcare consumers and our communities, it is imperative that we continually challenge ourselves, our practice, and our organizations by critically thinking and utilizing reflection to consider what the latest changes in the transformation of healthcare can mean to our practice. Thinkers automatically incorporate questioning and reflection in their practice to critically evaluate what could be improved tomorrow to enable their practice to produce better clinical and financial outcomes. This is especially important now that paradigms are rapidly changing in healthcare as we move from the sickness/procedure-based model to the prevention/health maintenance model in academia, practice, and policy.

Unfortunately, it is easy to use the filters from past experience and education to view present and future events, which blinds us in recognizing the differences and the truly transformational changes that are beyond traditional thinking. The science (there is enough data and evidence now to think of reflective practice as an emerging science) of reflective practice within an environment of reflection creates the questioning and reflecting needed to develop new models and interventions to create the agility, nimbleness, flexibility, and adaptability the authors note are necessary for this continually transforming healthcare environment.

Sustainable change doesn't happen without a systematic approach to execution. These authors provide a clear structure for developing reflective learning and reflective learning environments for academic nursing and interprofessional practice that are grounded in theory and data. The breakthrough concepts in this text are incredibly valuable for students, leaders, and practitioners to help our profession, organizations, and interprofessional partners achieve excellence.

–Karlene M. Kerfoot, PhD, RN, NEA-BC, FAAN

Introduction

"Without reflection, we go blindly on our way, creating more unintended consequences, and failing to achieve anything useful."–Margaret Wheatley

Most of us prefer operating from established routines so that we know what to expect. We find a way to accomplish something and stick with it. We are in a way comforted by the familiar. However, today's chaotic healthcare environment requires educators and practitioners to be nimble, flexible, and responsive to change. The need for change arises from the awareness that current practices or processes aren't working—that results are not the desired outcomes. Our goal then is to become agile so that we are able to continually adapt, reflect on progress and setbacks, and adjust course along the way; thus, we are able to continually improve through lifelong learning. These are the skills to create, build, and sustain future-oriented healthcare and academic cultures that achieve change.

Catalysts for Changing Paradigms

Faculty working to integrate the Quality and Safety Education for Nurses (QSEN) (Cronenwett et al., 2007; Cronenwett et al., 2009) competencies identified their desire to learn from exemplars of change. These QSEN competencies were based on well-publicized reports from the Institute of Medicine (IOM) that revealed unacceptable outcomes in healthcare (2000) and identified the competencies for health professionals to improve the system (2003). Both faculty and clinicians seek change: Faculty seek pedagogical approaches that are more effective than traditional content-based lectures to enable learners to achieve these competencies, and clinicians seek ways to improve processes, incorporate best practices, and develop safety cultures.

Faculty interest was fueled by the 2010 Carnegie report on transforming nursing education (Benner, Sutphen, Leonard, & Day, 2010) and the IOM task force report on the future of nursing (IOM, 2010). A groundbreaking collaborative report on interprofessional education (IPE) by the Interprofessional Education Collaborative (IPEC, 2011) further stimulated shifting paradigms in nursing and other health professions.

Benner et al. (2010) challenges educators to recognize that pedagogy is as important as content and to develop more active and participatory educational culture to more closely mirror the dynamics of practice. Content-laden curriculum may in fact stifle learner preparation for the realities of the complex clinical environment.

The 2010 IOM report on the future of nursing made bold recommendations for advancing nursing education to better position nurses for a strong advocacy role in which they practice to their full educational capacity. To achieve the aims set forth in this landmark report, nurses need education that prepares them to speak up, participate in interprofessional teams, and lead organizational improvements.

IPEC (2011) identified four competencies now required in all health professions education: communication, teamwork, ethics, and patient-centered care. Evidence increasingly links these four domains to improving healthcare communication, patient-centered care, and quality safe outcomes. And each of these initiatives supports and extends the QSEN and IOM competencies. So how do nurses and other health professionals integrate and sustain these multiple but coordinating calls for change? What are the essential messages driving change?

Changing Paradigms in Health Professions Education

Many educators teach as they were taught, and yet the world has changed; these educators may be preparing graduates for a world that no longer exists. Today's learners have different expectations given that they have lived in a changing environment and had different experiences. Faculty, clinicians, administrators, and other leaders have struggled with organizational culture change in the effort to integrate current knowledge, trends, and technology advances into healthcare. The burden of exploding information that has led to new knowledge compounds the need to rethink traditional content-based teaching methods. We can no longer teach all content; instead, learners require us to provide them with a systematic, reasoned approach so that they can apply what they do know to dynamic situations.

Nurses and other health professionals want to know how to gain traction for change, inspire others to join in, and gain support from organizational leadership. Educators and other health professions leaders themselves need new competencies and mindsets to assist schools and healthcare organizations in grasping the organizational dynamics to change mindsets to include quality and safety as the foundation for nursing practice. Few guidelines or demonstration projects model changes in curriculum revision, classroom design, and teaching modalities.

This book is a response to that gap. Change is more than a series of new activities or tasks. How systems incorporate change into the organization's culture or processes affects sustainability. Systematic change involves a series of carefully crafted steps: clear purpose of the desired change, process steps to lead to desired change, reflective assessment, and evaluation. Systematic change is guided by concepts and models from organizational theories combined with experiential knowledge gained from reflective practices to establish new cultures. Adults learn through experience; applying experiential learning theory can help educators transform approaches to engage learners in seeking change.

Changing organizational culture is complex. The story behind change reveals the subculture and the processes involved in the change. The story may also be the inspiration to enable others to act. Organizations—both clinical delivery sites and academic institutions—struggle to know how to initiate change, develop champions to lead transformation, and implement the many changes in education. Reflective practice is the thread in transforming organizations: hence, creating reflective learning organizations that are nimble, flexible, and adaptive systems.

Reflective Practices in Changing Culture

This book explores ways to address these myriad calls for change. The theme throughout is applying the reflective process of learning from experience to craft future change. Reflection is a systematic way of thinking about actions and responses within a knowledge base; it is learning from experience by considering what you know, believe, and value within the context of current situations, and reframing to develop future responses or actions (Sherwood & Horton-Deutsch, 2012). Reflection applies theory from all ways of knowing and learning as an extension of evidence-based practices and research. Nurses and administrators —in fact, all health professionals—who are seeking to implement new education or practice standards will find the theory bursts and exemplars useful in their work and help expand their leadership capacity in leading the complexities of transformation.

This book is relevant for all nurses, but particularly for interprofessional educators interested in implementing change and wanting to know how to begin, what to expect, and how others have addressed the familiar challenges of the change process. This book provides exemplars in transforming nursing education and practice to achieve new outcomes. It shares how schools of nursing, interprofessional teams, and healthcare delivery settings have sought to address 21st-century healthcare to improve outcomes. It is not an organizational change theory book, but rather intended to inspire those involved in or contemplating change to seek effective solutions by learning from others who have begun the journey. Chapters are developed with a short theory burst, background of the change, and reflective illustrations of how the organization or system embraced change. Reflective questions guide readers to analyze concepts in the stories either individually or in learning groups, so this book can be used by organizational groups, with formal education programs, or as a means of self-development. These questions can also guide readers in applying similar models or examining their own systems for change.

The five parts of this book examine the impetus for change and theories to support change, examples of educational changes, organizational perspectives, interprofessional integration, and future perspectives. Contributors represent an interprofessional cadre of health professions experts from industry, academic, and practice settings. The 2012 Sherwood and Horton-Deutsch book *Reflective Practice: Transforming Education and Improving Outcomes* was about developing reflective practice in education and serves as a companion to this book. This book builds on that theme to examine how educators and others have applied reflective practices to seek change and innovation.

Part I: Call for Transformation

The focus of Part I is the shift from traditional processes and structures to develop transformative, reflective organizations. Change is challenging all healthcare sectors. The chapters in this section will help guide change-seekers by exploring drivers for change in the context of organizational theory, integrate new pedagogical approaches and structures guided by experiential learning, and reflect on exemplars of change.

Chapter 1, "Transforming Education and Practice: The Evidence Base for Change," summarizes the need for transformation from the recent reports that call for change and challenge nurses toward leadership. The IOM reports over the past 15 years have confirmed the urgency of changing the healthcare system (2000) and declared education as the bridge to bring about change (2003). Applying reflective practices can help uncover gaps in the system to move toward improvement and make sense of experience.

Chapter 2, "Transformational Learning: Improving Quality and Safety Through Reflective Pedagogies," examines how the QSEN project has led to a social movement in nursing to transform nursing education. QSEN helped inspire application of reflective, interactive, and innovative pedagogy to engage learners fully in the journey to be a nurse. QSEN's influence is documented in the productivity, publications, and spread accomplished by educators, administrators, and clinicians in leading quality and safety initiatives.

Personal development is the basis of transformative leadership. Whether leading in classroom, clinical, practice, healthcare, or academic settings, effective leaders demonstrate emotional intelligence and the ability to respond thoughtfully to others. Chapter 3, "Practices of Reflective Leaders," examines how reflection on experience helps leaders identify and develop leadership practices. The chapter explores reflective strategies used to develop emotional intelligence and leadership capacity, such as how emerging and experienced leaders monitor feelings, discriminate among emotional reactions, and use the information to guide future responses and actions.

Part II: Reflective Learning Environments in Academic Settings

Part II examines curricula transformation and innovative teaching approaches. Concept-based curricula, debriefing through meaningful learning, interprofessional education in mental health nursing, and Caring Science applied to online teaching help inform new approaches to the teaching-learning paradigm. Case studies are used to analyze care priorities, understand situational context, and process the whole of an event to make sense of practice applications.

Chapter 4, "Developing Concept-Based Curricula," is the personal story from Jean Giddens of the development of concept-based curricula. Concept-based curricula shift from a predominant medical model to the concepts nurses apply in "thinking like a nurse": that is, the concepts that form the basis for decision-making in delivering care. Giddens describes the challenges in creating and leading innovation and ways to manage multiple views and build support for innovation.

Bringing clinical into the classroom and decreasing dependence on content-only presentations helps learners master the art of "thinking like a nurse." In Chapter 5, "Transformation of Teaching and Learning Through Debriefing for Meaningful Learning," Dreifuerst and Bradley describe situated clinical learning using multiple learning contexts. Debriefing for Meaningful Learning (DML) helps learners prepare for the complex clinical environment and gain awareness of how decisions are reached in providing care.

Chapter 6, "The Use of Visual Thinking Strategies in Interprofessional Education," uses Visual Thinking Strategies (VTS) to support development of observational and communication skills. As a teaching technique, VTS helps infuse humanities into healthcare curricula and encourages reflection on attention to detail and nuances of care. It lends itself to interprofessional education by developing teamwork and collaboration.

Chapter 7, "Interprofessional Education in Mental Health: Developing Practitioners Who Work Collaboratively and Provide Patient-Centered Care," applies competencies from QSEN and IPEC in an interprofessional graduate course on treating substance-use disorders that supports improved communication, error reduction, and enhanced delivery of care. Teaching strategies that focus on listening, working collaboratively, and incorporating multiple points of view build mental health practitioners who provide quality care. Helping students develop knowledge of each other's roles and consider what others can do encourages respect, tolerance, and a willingness to work with one another.

Facilitating person-centered care and role-modeling leadership in an online learning environment is challenging. Chapter 8, "An Online Teaching Framework: Using Quality Norms and Caring Science to Build Presence and Engagement in Online Learning Environments," explores the partnership between educators and instructional designers in creating a course that builds authentic presence and engages students in deep transformative learning in an online forum. Horton-Deutsch and Drysdale explore how to adjust the focus of online education to ways of thinking and ways of applying knowledge in building meaningful skills and developing core professional values.

Part III: Reflective Learning Environments Within Healthcare Systems

Healthcare workers want to do their jobs well; they come with a value of contributing to the greater mission of improving health but need the tools and system support. Part III explores how reflection provides the process for asking critical questions that can lead to improvements in quality and safety. It helps open the possibility of change; questions are the first step in the change process. Promoting a spirit of inquiry helps identify potential gaps in the system where errors may occur.

Global nursing leader Jean Watson explores two personal professional reflective leadership experiences in advancing Caring Science in Chapter 9, "Transformational Reflective Organizations: Front-Line Challenges and Changes Guided by Caring Science." Developing the human consciousness of people in an organization shapes how they live organizational values. Integrating a caring model exemplifies how a professional practice model can empower nurses and other healthcare providers to speak up, deliver patient-centered care in interprofessional teams, and develop inquiry-based practice for continuous improvement.

Moving from silo education to interprofessional teaching and learning overcomes system barriers. Chapter 10, "Building Interprofessional Teams," is the story of a patient safety course in teamwork using TeamSTEPPS in simulated learning with nursing, medicine, and pharmacy students that is inspiring academic and healthcare delivery models.

In Chapter 11, "A New Framework for Creating a Resilient Organization Using Reflective Practices," two industry leaders demonstrate how reflection helps define an organization. Using reflective thinking, the QSEN competencies are woven into reflective stories and help caregivers to reexamine their experiences and reconsider actions. Examining experience can ignite passion for safety culture and teamwork behaviors by revealing the impact of actions and attitudes among team members and transform healthcare delivery organizations.

Chapter 12, "QSEN Into Practice at Southwest General Hospital," is a front-line exemplar from Southwest General Hospital in Ohio of integrating the QSEN competencies to reexamine nursing practice and develop new guidelines, standards, and processes that engaged and energized the workforce. Practice settings are interested in how the QSEN competencies fit within the professional practice model of an institution, integrate in performance review, and change practice structure and process.

Part IV: Reflective Learning Environments Expanding Partnerships Across Boundaries

Achieving change is a partnership. Individuals or organizations seldom work alone to accomplish major paradigm shifts. The call for new pedagogies and mindsets to improve outcomes requires partnerships that span boundaries. Collaborative partnerships move away from silo thinking and acting, recognizing that sustaining change results from working together. These chapters share stories of projects and initiatives that involve multiple organizations yet were successful because of the partnerships that resulted.

In Chapter 13, "Colorado QSEN Faculty Workshops—Facilitating Reflection for Curricular Development," faculty at the University of Colorado demonstrate how the QSEN competencies were spread statewide. The faculty led a unified faculty development model across Colorado to assist integration of the competencies and transform care and modeled flexibility and creativity in managing the challenges of facilitating change.

Chapter 14, "Leading Transformation to Learning Organizations: Educating for Patient Safety, Quality, and Interprofessional Practice," offers the stories of three nurse leaders to share how one university transformed to a learning organization to help transform healthcare. Breaking out of traditional structures and process, organization members had to first learn new approaches to bring core values and vision to reality. Their work resulted in an integrated approach to IPE, a story that continues into Chapter 15, "Reflective Organizations: On the Front Lines to Transform Education and Practice." These two chapters illustrate the blending of academic and clinical organizations through the shared tripartite mission of education, practice, and research.

Part V: Sustaining Self and Interprofessional Partnerships: Guiding Transformational Leaders

Reflection is an important self-development strategy. Part V focuses on how to use reflection for continuing growth as a leader, make sense of one's work, and use innovative change methods that support working in partnership with others. This section will explore paths to transforming change including reflective practices, dialogue, circle conversations, appreciative inquiry, and balancing advocacy with inquiry.

Chapter 16, "Building Academic Cultures With Reflective Practice in Mind: Leadership Agility and Transformational Learning," prompts reflection on leadership agility and the skill sets that create, build, and sustain future-oriented academic cultures. Pesut and Thompson examine futures-literacy and futures-thinking to guide and facilitate transformation. Transformation is about responding to a desired future and is supported by futures-literacy. Futures-literacy invites people to create and share stories about the future to inform current practice and realities. Exemplars engage readers in futures-literacy within and across healthcare institutions to create desired futures.

Chapter 17, "Partnering to Create Sustainable Futures: Organizational Leadership Strategies That Invite Engagement, Reflection, and Action," focuses on strategies for leading, advancing, and sustaining professional initiatives, groups, and organizations. Illustrations provide a toolkit for others who are seeking change to examine lessons learned, persevere in the face of uncertainty and challenges, and apply innovative transformation strategies. Professional organizations engaged in transformational work are a critical aspect of advancing and sustaining nursing as they reach other nurses in leadership roles. Together, professional organizations and other areas of nursing can create opportunities for transforming nursing and applying principles of reflective organizations.

Reflective Summary

Contributors for most chapters used the following reflective guide in developing their chapters to describe their project of introduction of change. These reflective questions are adaptable for readers in contemplating change.

Introduction

- Reflect on the need for change. What led you to launch the project?

- What was the goal? What did you hope to achieve?

Background

- What were the driving forces that led to your awareness of the need for change? What was the basis for change/needs assessment/driving forces—anecdotal or data based?

- What theories, experiences, or other ways of knowing guided your work?

- How did you prepare for the implementation of this project? Who participated? How did you decide who to include or exclude and why? What processes did you follow?

The Project

- Describe the project you and your team developed.

- How did you and others facilitate the implementation? Who participated? How was this similar or different from the group who participated initially? What processes were followed? What adjustments were made along the way? Why?

Outcomes

- What was the outcome of your project? Describe the impact.

- What did you experience together as a learning organization? What did you achieve? Where are you now? How did you share the outcomes with stakeholders?

Reflective Response/Recommendations

- What did you learn from this process/project? What surprised you most? In light of this learning, what will you do differently in the future? What will you continue? What did you need to let go of? Why?

- How might this work contribute to transition to practice? What might lead to clinical innovation?

- How did this project help to clarify your values and manage your professional purpose?

- What comes next? How does this exemplar fit into the overall scheme of your future work? How does it fit with your personal/professional development? How will you do your work differently?

Final Reflections

- What are your final thoughts on the main theme of this chapter?

- What would you like readers to take away and consider for the future?

Chapters also include a special feature titled "Reflecting on … ." This feature prompts you with questions that will guide you in thinking reflectively about the various topics being discussed.

References

Benner, P., Sutphen, M., Leonard, V., & Day, L. (2010). *Educating nurses: A call for radical transformation.* San Francisco, CA: Jossey Bass.

Cronenwett, L., Sherwood, G., Barnsteiner, J., Disch, J., Johnson, J., Mitchell, P., … Warren, J. (2007). Quality and safety education for nurses. *Nursing Outlook, 55*(3), 122–131.

Cronenwett, L., Sherwood, G., Pohl, J., Barnsteiner, J., Moore, S., Taylor Sullivan, D., … Warren, J. (2009). Quality and safety education for advanced practice nursing practice. *Nursing Outlook, 57*(6), 338–348.

Institute of Medicine (IOM). (2000). L. T. Kohn, J. M. Corrigan, & M. S. Donaldson (Eds.). *To err is human: Building a safer health system.* Washington, DC: National Academies Press. Retrieved from http://www.iom.edu/Reports/1999/To-Err-is-Human-Building-A-Safer-Health-System.aspx

Institute of Medicine (IOM). (2003). A. C. Greiner, & E. Knebel (Eds.). *Health professions education: A bridge to quality.* Washington, DC: National Academies Press. Retrieved from http://www.iom.edu/Reports/2003/Health-Professions-Education-A-Bridge-to-Quality.aspx

Institute of Medicine (IOM). (2010). *The future of nursing: Leading change, advancing health.* Washington, DC: National Academies Press.

Interprofessional Education Collaborative (IPEC). (2011). *Core competencies for interprofessional collaborative practice.* Retrieved from https://ipecollaborative.org/uploads/IPEC-Core-Competencies.pdf

Sherwood, G., & Horton-Deutsch, S. (Eds.) (2012). *Reflective practice: Transforming education and improving outcomes.* Indianapolis, IN: Sigma Theta Tau International.

Part I
Call for Transformation

Chapter 1

Transforming Education and Practice: The Evidence Base for Change

Gwen D. Sherwood, PhD, RN, FAAN, ANEF
Sara Horton-Deutsch, PhD, RN, PMHCNS, FAAN, ANEF

Faculty, clinicians, administrators, and other leaders have struggled with how to manage organizational culture change to integrate new knowledge, trends, and technology advances into health professions education. This challenge has been particularly true when seeking to improve healthcare outcomes in the wake of the Institute of Medicine (IOM) series of reports on healthcare quality and safety (1999, 2001, 2003). Nurses are uniquely positioned on the front lines of care and leadership to help lead improvement efforts, whether in schools of nursing, clinical settings, or other organizations. Reports of the continuing lack of progress in improving systems of care (Wachter, 2010) demand new approaches: Continuing the same structures and processes are not likely to yield new outcomes.

The IOM issued a clear imperative for health professions schools to become the bridge to quality by transforming health professions education so that all health professionals are able to deliver patient-centered care in interprofessional teams based on evidence-based practice (EBP) with continuous quality improvement in a framework of safety using informatics (IOM, 2003). How does a system, school, team, or other organizational group incorporate new competencies and approaches to create a new culture or way of being? What is the back story of transformation that can inspire and model change for others? The purpose of this chapter is to reflect on how organizations and systems move through change and transformation. This chapter examines the shift from traditional organizations to transformative, reflective learning organizations focused on improvement.

NARRATIVES

The stories of events; the retelling of something that happened. Narratives are the presentation of real-world events that connect them in a story-like way. Narrative meaning is created by establishing that something is part of a whole and connected to other events and meanings that help inform and teach lessons (Ironside & Cerbie, 2012).

From Reflection to Transformation

Narrative, as told through stories and exemplars, has been a powerful and effective tool for creating change. With any change, it is the back story that shares how that change came to be and its impact on the culture; the story weaves organization theory and experience through a reflective process that shares the transformative process (Powell & Stone, 2015). Changing organizational culture is complex, but the story behind the change can inspire others to act. Organizations—both clinical delivery sites and academic institutions—struggle to know how to initiate change, develop champions to lead transformation, and implement the many advances in education. Reflective practice is the thread in transforming organizations: As group members in the organization act, reflect, and reframe into new ways of being, they create in essence a reflective organization focused on continuous learning and improvement.

Health professionals in all settings have asked:

- How do we make sense of new standards and engage faculty and clinicians in the changes required?

- What are ways to integrate quality and safety to transform organizations?

The purpose of this book is to explore ways to integrate the myriad influences on the future of healthcare education and delivery by sharing real-world stories of change and transformation. Chapters offer a short theory burst or background to begin, followed by an unfolding case of organizational change that illustrates how the project emerged and came to life. To guide others interested in implementing change, exemplars tell the story of how nurses and other leaders in schools and healthcare settings have sought to address the challenges of 21st-century healthcare to improve outcomes; several exemplars also illustrate the transition to an interprofessional framework. The book is not an organizational change theory textbook, but is rather intended to inspire those involved in or contemplating change to seek effective solutions by learning from others who have begun the journey.

Effective change is a complicated process that involves a series of carefully crafted steps:

1. Focus on a clear purpose of the desired change.

2. Manage challenges.

3. Sustain change.

4. Use reflective assessment and evaluation of change to tell the story of managing the complexities of change and transformation.

The purpose is examining how to shift from traditional organizations to transformative, reflective learning organizations focused on improvement. The goal is to help change-seekers with integration of new competencies and concepts and address regulatory changes by sharing unfolding organizational stories using reflective practices.

Background: Inspiring Change

Several catalysts over the past decade have inspired innovations in nursing. The response to the 2012 *Reflective Practice: Transforming Education and Improving Outcomes* (Sherwood & Horton-Deutsch, 2012a) indicated that as educators were engaged in implementing reflective practices into education as they shared their experiences, they asked for additional resources. Further, the Quality and Safety Education for Nurses (QSEN) project (Cronenwett et al., 2007) and several key publications were fueling integration and spread of innovation across nursing and the health professions. These reports provided additional support for the call for change that earlier IOM reports (2001, 2003) initiated. The Carnegie report on transforming nursing education (Benner, Sutphen, Leonard, & Day, 2010), the IOM task force report on the future of nursing (IOM, 2010), and a groundbreaking collaborative report on interprofessional education helped stimulate shifting paradigms in nursing and other health professions (IPEC, 2011). These groundbreaking initiatives (respectively, Cronenwett et al., 2007; Benner et al., 2010; IOM, 2010; and IPEC, 2011) ignited the enthusiasm and commitment of educators and clinicians to reconsider traditional approaches to open dialogue to reframe mindsets.

Questions arose from all areas of nursing to know more about how to implement the essential messages from these signature projects that held promise for advancing nursing. Faculty sought pedagogical approaches that could be more effective than traditional content-based lectures to enable learners to achieve new competencies. Clinicians sought ways to improve processes, incorporate best practices, and develop safety cultures. This search proved the inspiration for this book: how to take advantage of these initiatives to change and transform nursing and healthcare. Applying reflective practices to the change process, early adopters engaged in reflective practices on the stories behind integration of the QSEN competencies and responded to the challenges the reports presented.

Quality and Safety Education for Nurses

The QSEN project helped inspire a renaissance in nursing education. QSEN established behavioral objectives as the knowledge, skills, and attitudes needed to achieve the six IOM competencies for all health professionals to improve healthcare from a system perspective (Cronenwett et al., 2007, 2009):

- **Patient-centered care:** Value the patient or designee in planning and decision-making to coordinate and provide compassion based on respect for a patient's preferences, values, and needs.

- **Teamwork and collaboration:** Work effectively across nursing and healthcare disciplines for effective teamwork with open communication, mutual respect, and shared decision-making to achieve quality patient care.

- **Evidence-based practice:** Integrate best current evidence with clinical expertise and patient/family preferences and values for delivery of optimal healthcare.

- **Quality improvement:** Measure and use data to monitor the outcomes of care processes and design and test changes to continuously improve the quality and safety of healthcare systems.

- **Safety:** Minimize risk of harm to patients and providers through both system effectiveness and individual performance.

- **Informatics:** Use information and technology to communicate, manage knowledge, mitigate error, and support decision-making.

These competencies are embedded in nursing education standards at both prelicensure and graduate levels so that all nurses have opportunities for achieving the competencies. The QSEN Pilot School Learning Collaborative (Cronenwett, Sherwood,

QSEN PROJECT (THE QUALITY AND SAFETY EDUCATION FOR NURSES PROJECT)

The national response for nursing to the Institute of Medicine (IOM) series of reports on improving the healthcare system, including six competencies needed by all health professionals if we are to improve healthcare quality and safety: patient-centered care, teamwork and collaboration, quality improvement, evidence-based practice, safety, and informatics. Funded by the Robert Wood Johnson Foundation, QSEN was led by an expert panel and an advisory board to name the knowledge, skills, and attitudes for each competency so that quality and safety are part of the professional identity and formation of nurses. The competencies have been incorporated into nursing accreditation standards to assure integration in all nursing curricula and spread to nursing practice (www.QSEN.org).

& Gelmon, 2009) demonstrated the need for faculty development to assist schools and healthcare organizations in grasping the organizational dynamics in changing mindsets to include quality and safety as the foundation for nursing practice. Faculty and students have been energized by the opportunity to do good work by improving healthcare systems and integrating safety practices. However, few guidelines or demonstration projects are available from which to guide changes in curriculum revision, classroom design, and teaching modalities.

The Carnegie Report on Nursing

Benner et al. (2010) reported an extensive analysis of nursing education in the United States and called for sweeping transformation in educating nurses to better prepare graduates for the realities of the changing clinical environment. Noting a lack of a major paradigm shift in nursing education over the past 40 years, the report challenges educators to recognize that pedagogy is as important as content. Many nursing curricula are content-laden, which may in fact stifle learner preparation for the realities of the complex clinical environment. Graduates may have difficulty transitioning from carefully created didactic learning to the dynamics of acute care; developing a more active and participatory educational culture may better mirror the dynamics of practice and impact new graduate retention. With more than one-half of new graduates changing jobs in the first year of practice, the smooth transition from academia to practice is a major and costly issue. To make adjustments, some schools are replacing curricula based on disease taxonomies in the medical model with other frameworks, such as concept-based curricula (Giddens, 2015), and replacing traditional lectures with more active pedagogies, such as unfolding case studies.

The Future of Nursing

The 2010 IOM report *The Future of Nursing* underscores the imperative to help nurses develop leadership capacity for helping transform healthcare. This report on the future of nursing provided detailed aspirations for advancing nursing to help improve the healthcare delivery system. The report added recommendations for new educational and clinical approaches in nursing to better position nurses for a strong advocacy role in which they practice to their full educational capacity. To achieve the aims set forth in this landmark report, nurses need advances in education to be better prepared to speak up, participate in interprofessional teams, and lead organizational improvements. The report recommended new educational and clinical approaches in nursing to better position nurses for a strong advocacy role in which they practice to their full educational capacity.

Interprofessional Education Collaborative

Last, representatives from the health professions reached consensus on four domains of interprofessional practice for all health professions education, which are now embedded in accreditation standards (Interprofessional Education Collaborative, 2011):

- **Values/ethics:** Maintain a climate of mutual respect and shared values.

- **Roles and responsibilities:** Work within roles and responsibilities for all team members to meet healthcare needs of those served.

- **Communication:** Communicate with all team members with respect to support a team approach in providing care.

- **Teamwork and team-based care:** Build team dynamics and relationships to effectively deliver patient-centered care that is safe, timely, efficient, effective, and equitable.

Increasingly, interprofessional education and practice are linked to improving healthcare communication, patient-centered care, and quality safe outcomes. Although these reports support and extend the QSEN and IOM competencies, with a plethora of innovations, how do nurses and other health professionals integrate and sustain these multiple yet coordinating calls for change?

REFLECTING ON ... CHANGE

- *How do the preceding reports and initiatives challenge your view of nursing education?*

- *How are you incorporating the QSEN competencies into your teaching and practice?*

- *How would you initiate a new discussion about the new competencies identified by the QSEN and IPEC initiatives?*

Reflective Practice: Foundation for Change

The goal of this book is to guide you in how to apply the reflective process of learning from experience to craft desired change that can be applied individually or in organizations or systems (Sherwood & Horton-Deutsch, 2012b). *Reflection* is a systematic way of thinking about actions and responses using knowledge; it is learning from experience by considering what one knows, believes, and values within the context of current situations, and then reframing to develop future responses or actions. This process applies theory from all ways of knowing so that learning is applied and integrated into future decision-making: thus, an extension of evidence-based practices and research.

Challenges in Changing Organizational Culture

In spite of costly orientations and staff development opportunities, organizational group members are rarely educated on organizational practices and culture. *Organizational culture* is the collective values, beliefs, and norms held by group members (Triolo, 2012). Organizational culture is important when assessing an organization's ability to change and implement new practices (Bellot, 2011). Effective organizations are those that learn and adapt to changing environments to achieve best outcomes, sometimes referred to as learning organizations.

Perspectives on Organizational Culture

Organizational culture is difficult to explain and capture. Theories about organizations help illuminate and understand culture by explaining concepts and enhancing cultural elements important to the organization. Theories also note enhancing and dysfunctional patterns; thus, in studying organizations, it is often helpful to do so in the context of a particular theoretical model. To begin to understand organizational change and transformation, this section examines major concepts in organizational theories that become evident in the stories and cases that are included throughout the remainder of the book.

Three fundamental cultural elements define organizations and their culture (Schein, 2010):

- **Artifacts** are evidences visible to those inside and outside the organization, such as standard dress codes, policies and organizational structures, emotional climate, and the way in which work is accomplished.

- **Espoused values** are the organization's mission and philosophy, goals, and strategies displayed by the organization's leaders.

- **Assumptions** are the beliefs and assumed concepts that underlie the organization's culture that may not be visible to those in or outside the organization.

These three elements may rarely be discussed within the organization but are significant factors in the organization's operations and outcomes. For instance, what behaviors are tolerated? Is patient safety just a policy, or does an open and just error-reporting system exist?

Understanding the interactions of each element helps you understand and describe the whole of an organization's culture. A lack of congruence among the three elements creates dissonance within the organization as members become confused about goals, mission, and actions, resulting in inefficiency and low morale (Schein, 2010). As an open system, organizations are subject to continuous internal and external pressures, making it difficult to sustain culture.

Culture is the interplay of structure, reward systems, the people themselves, information systems, leadership, and processes by which the organization operates (Triolo, 2012). Organization members exhibit facets of motivation, trust, and communication in how they interact and accomplish the work of the organization (Schein, 2010). Culture is a learned experience that takes place within groups and is established and reinforced by the behaviors members observe as successful or that is tolerated by the group. Culture is shaped by how work is accomplished and problems are resolved. You may learn about culture in formal education—experienced and enforced from witnessing behavior in critical events and behavior modeled by the culture's leader. Members assume that these behaviors work, and therefore become part of the assumptions underlying the organization's culture. Alternative groups may establish their own identity to meet the needs of their group and coexist within the larger culture, such as departments, units, or committees.

CULTURE

The interplay of structure, reward systems, the people themselves, information systems, leadership, and processes by which the organization operates (Triolo, 2012). It is based on the shared experiences and communicated through the social interactions of group members encompassing values, beliefs, and norms that shape how group members treat each other (Bellot, 2011).

Culture is based on shared experiences and is expressed through the social interactions of group members (Bellot, 2011). For example, organizational culture encompasses informal values, beliefs, and norms that shape how staff provide patient care and build relationships up and down the organization. Group members engage in multiple ways to learn new processes and behaviors to create change. A distinguishing characteristic of healthy organizations is the capacity to constantly adapt to change and innovation, thus continuously improving. Learning organizations examine beliefs, analyze systems and workflow, and consider how culture impacts organizational goals to achieve better outcomes. However, organizations must be prepared to help sustain newly learned behaviors to prevent reversion to previous behaviors (Schein, 2010).

Communication is an essential organizational process and shapes culture; culture and communication are intertwined such that culture is lived through the interactions of its members (Bellot, 2011). Group members receive, interpret, and evaluate input through continuous communication from and by the organization using multiple approaches.

Organizations are changed and sustained through the way culture manages change processes, shares stories, resolves problems and conflict, and approaches teaching and learning (Singer, Falwell, Gaba, Meterko, Rosen, Hartman, & Baker, 2009).

Shaping Culture: Shared Mental Models

Shared mental models are the overlapping concepts held by group members and include the thought processes about how something works in the real world. These shared explanations serve to get everyone on the same page and lessen ambiguity about organizational culture through shared representations of events and concepts. Shared mental models provide a framework to assess and explain what happens in the organization's environment (Van den Bossche, Gijselaers, Segers, Woltjer, & Kirschner, 2011). Group members develop shared mental models through explanation of thought processes and working relationships. Shared mental models enhance team communication and effectiveness in completing complex tasks; therefore, closely held shared mental models enable the system to learn and adapt to rapidly changing environments to achieve best outcomes.

REFLECTING ON ... MENTAL MODELS

- *What firmly held mental models exist within your organization?*
- *How do these mental models shape behavior and influence approaches to problem-solving?*
- *How can members of your organization explore these models to enhance team communication?*

Learning Through Experience and Story

Understanding how culture is formed and reinforced throughout the organization is a key to effective change. Assumptions are deeply held and are not often apparent, yet they serve as the starting point for successful change in culture.

Assumptions often surface according to the congruency of shared mental models across the organization. The beliefs, values, and expectations of organization members affect organization change. Learning from experience involves action and reflection. Through reflection, concrete experiences are assimilated and transformed into abstract concepts and become the basis for actions that are tested in new experiences (Kolb, 1984); learners experience, reflect, apply, and evaluate. The impact of learning is deepened by having adequate time for reflection and discussion (Oxendine, Robinson, & Wilson, 2004). See Figure 1.1.

FIGURE 1.1

Learning is nonlinear, occurring in a cyclic process.
Source: Kolb, 1984.

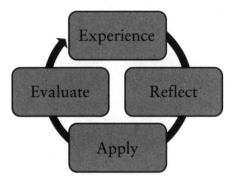

Experiential learning theory is a cyclical process of (Oxendine et al., 2004):

- Introducing and engaging in a realistic experience
- Discussing and reflecting on the experience to understand and grasp abstract concepts and emotional aspects
- Experimenting with new concepts through discussion
- Connecting experience to real-life applications

Learning is not a destination but rather a process that is unending. That is, learners experience an activity, reflect on that activity, apply it to real-life situations, and evaluate the impact of the activity for future actions. Experiential learning is differentiated from cognitive theories of learning that focus on acquisition and manipulation of information and behavioral theories that do not account for learners' subjective experiences (Kolb, 1984). Cognitive and behavioral theories focus on the ability to repeat what is learned. In experiential learning, thoughts and ideas change according to experiences (Kolb, 1984). Experiential learning helps to explain and understand the cases, stories, and exemplars presented in later chapters.

> **REFLECTING ON … EXPERIENTIAL LEARNING THEORY**
>
> - *How can experiential learning theory guide needed changes within your organization?*

Culture as a Critical Component of Quality and Safety

Reason (1997) linked organizational culture with safety culture. *Patient safety* is the integrated pattern of individual and organizational behavior based upon shared beliefs and values in seeking to minimize patient harm that may occur from the care delivery process. Learning organizations promote a culture of continuous learning with the goal of improving patient care (Firth-Cozens, 2001). Organizational culture is an important consideration in an organization's ability to change and successfully implement new practices.

Creating and improving patient safety culture within healthcare organizations is essential to improving patient care outcomes. It happens through enhanced team communication, open reporting of errors, and learning from mistakes (Bowie, 2010). To develop a safety culture, group members need ways to develop trust, improve communication, and share knowledge. Communication failures (written, oral, and electronic) erode patient care and are at the root of most sentinel events (The Joint Commission, 2012). Patient care outcomes are negatively affected by communication lapses when employees are uninformed, have poor handoff processes, or make decisions out of fear. Communication failures often result from the interplay among cultural norms, complex care, and individual factors (Bowie, 2010). To improve safety, organizations must first attend to culture.

Safety is closely linked to attitudes and behavior. Prevailing mindsets across the care team are integral to culture at both the unit and organizational level; however, attitudes and behaviors are difficult to change. The slow change marked over the past 15 years since the release of the IOM report indicates new approaches to accomplish system change are imperative to improve care outcomes (Wachter, 2010).

Patient safety culture reflects the ability of both individuals and the organization to deal with risks and hazards in avoiding errors and achieving their goals (Reason, 1997; Armstrong & Sherwood, 2012). Organizations with a positive safety culture are founded on mutual trust, shared perceptions (mental models) of the importance of safety, and confidence in the efficacy of preventive measures (Onge, Hodges, McBride, & Parnell, 2013). Social learning theory is embedded in the concept of patient safety culture to encompass how staff learn and share attitudes and behaviors. Each unit or microsystem within the organization is defined by a set of accepted norms of behavior and attitudes reinforced by leadership as well as by co-workers. The nuances within each unit's culture are manifested in the behavior and attitudes of both front-line nurses and their unit managers. Interactions are an important part of safety culture developed through shared values and productive communication among nurses, patients, and the entire system (Onge et al., 2013).

Transforming Systems

The ultimate goal of education is *transformation*—a change in behavior, attitudes, and ways of being and doing. Nurses and other health professionals who engage in continuous learning through a process of self-assessment and integration of knowledge are prepared to help lead and transform systems of care that can improve patient care outcomes. Educational approaches that include open, interactive dialogue between learners and educators—whether in academic or clinical settings—foster a learning environment that helps build the characteristics and skill set to improve organizations. Learner-centered education built on the principles of experiential learning co-creates learning in partnership with educators and learners (Horton-Deutsch, Sherwood, & Armstrong, 2012) and prepares nurses to work in organizations that continuously attend to their culture and work to improve their systems.

New Approaches to Creating the Future

We do what is familiar. New terrain seems bumpy and scary. It is challenging to break habits to form new practices and engage others in change. Leadership approaches that may have served well in the past may need to change if we are to generate the outcomes demanded by the current work environment. Reports of inefficiencies and challenging outcomes throughout healthcare and health professions education demand new responses. Creating an organizational culture that renews and energizes group members and provides for safety or an educational program that prepares practitioners for futuristic practice is the 21st-century challenge for educators and clinicians. How will we take advantage of opportunity and apply a new lens to create an exciting future (Pesut & Thompson, 2015)?

To prepare for a future of collaborative practice and effective organizational culture means letting go of worn-out processes, checking assumptions, and examining values and beliefs for relevancy. Creating new structures and approaches does not come all at once: It is a time-consuming process of persistence, diligence, and open leadership. Creative approaches and strategies do not emerge as a lightning bolt yet come in tiny steps, bits of insight, and incremental changes (Sawyer, 2013). Creativity is a part of effective learning, not from rote memorization but from building on knowledge to find fresh solutions to persistent problems, making decisions, and creating change. Change agents can adopt the principles and practices of creativity to explore and manage change in their organization or system (see Table 1.1). Creativity among leaders contributes to transformation through open attitudes, flexibility, and using setbacks and challenges as opportunities to move forward. Creative leaders are continuous learners and may utilize leadership development from multiple sources (Sawyer, 2013).

This book shares exceptional experiences and practices that are creating change and transformation. Emotionally intelligent leaders (Horton-Deutsch & Sherwood, 2008) are generative reflective leaders who capture opportunities to address culture and resolve problems so that group members build and sustain

GENERATIVE LEADERS

Transformational leaders who motivate engagement, active participation, and mindful practice.

trust, motivation, and communication (Disch, 2012). Generative leaders are transformational leaders who motivate engagement, active participation, and mindful practice. Reflective leaders continually examine their own experience within what they know to continually develop a professional practice model by identifying patterns that influence decisions and enable others to do so as well. These are traits and strategies that come to life in the chapters that follow.

Table 1.1: Levels of Reflection (Freshwater, 2008)

LEVEL OF REFLECTION	MODEL OF REFLECTION	STAGE OF DEVELOPMENT
Descriptive	Reflective journals, reporting incidents, reflection-on-action	Practice becomes conscious
Dialogic	Discourse with peers in various arenas including clinical supervision	Practice becomes deliberative
Critical	Able to provide reasoning for actions by engaging in critical conversation about practice with self and others	Transformative practice, practice improvement, move to innovation

Final Reflections

Organizational culture is difficult to understand and analyze yet critical to improve healthcare systems and schools of nursing. Understanding how culture influences organizations as well as taking the time to identify and explore shared mental models provides the foundation for completing complex tasks. Sharing stories is one way to understand an organization's culture and then uncover assumptions that serve as a starting point for change. Through reflecting on experiences together, nurse leaders and organizational members learn to assimilate and transform abstract concepts into new ideas for approaching change. Using experiential learning theory, members engage in new activities wherein they test ideas, reflect, apply, and evaluate the impact for future actions. Nurses and other health professionals who engage in this form of continuous learning through reflection are prepared to lead and transform systems of care that result in improved patient care and organizational cultures that embody quality and safety outcomes.

References

Armstrong, G., & Sherwood, G. (2012). Reflection and mindful practice: A means to quality and safety. In G. Sherwood, & S. Horton-Deutsch (Eds.), *Reflective practice: Transforming education and improving outcomes* (pp. 21–40). Indianapolis, IN: Sigma Theta Tau International.

Bellot, J. (2011). Defining and assessing organizational culture. *Nursing Forum, 46*(1), 29–37. doi:10.1111/j.1744-6198.2010.00207.x

Benner, P., Sutphen, M., Leonard, V., & Day, L. (2010). *Educating nurses: A call for radical transformation.* San Francisco, CA: Jossey-Bass.

Bowie, P. (2010). Leadership and implementing a safety culture. *Practice Nurse, 40*(10) 32–35.

Cronenwett, L., Sherwood, G., Barnsteiner, J., Disch, J., Johnson, J., Mitchell, P., … Warren, J. (2007). Quality and safety education for nurses. *Nursing Outlook, 55*(3), 122–131.

Cronenwett, L., Sherwood, G., & Gelmon, S. (2009). Improving quality and safety education: The QSEN learning collaborative. *Nursing Outlook, 57*(6), 304–312.

Cronenwett, L., Sherwood, G., Pohl, J., Barnsteiner, J., Moore, S., Disch, J., Johnson, … Warren, J. (2009). Quality and safety education for advanced nursing practice. *Nursing Outlook, 57*(6), 338–348.

Disch, J. (2012). Leadership to create change. In G. Sherwood, & J. Barnsteiner (Eds.), *Quality and safety in nursing: A competency approach to improving outcomes* (pp. 289–304). Hoboken, NJ: Wiley-Blackwell.

Firth-Cozens, J. (2001). Cultures for improving patient safety through learning: The role of teamwork. *Quality in Health Care, 10*(2), 26–31. doi:10.1136/qhc.0100026

Giddens, J. (2015). Developing concept-based curricula. In G. Sherwood, & S. Horton-Deutsch (Eds.), *Reflective Organizations: On the Front Lines of QSEN & Reflective Practice Implementation* (pp. 71–84). Indianapolis, IN: Sigma Theta Tau International.

Horton-Deutsch, S., & Sherwood, G. (2008). Reflection: An educational strategy to develop emotionally competent nurse leaders. *Journal of Nursing Management, 16*(8), 946–954.

Horton-Deutsch, S., Sherwood, G., & Armstrong, G. (2012). Reflection in class room and clinical contexts: Assessment and evaluation. In G. Sherwood, & S. Horton-Deutsch (Eds.), *Reflective practice: Transforming education and improving outcomes* (pp. 169–186). Indianapolis, IN: Sigma Theta Tau International.

Institute of Medicine. (1999). *To err is human: Building a safer health system.* Washington, DC: National Academies Press.

Institute of Medicine. (2001). *Crossing the quality chasm: A new health system for the 21st century.* Washington, DC: National Academies Press.

Institute of Medicine. (2003). *Health professions education: A bridge to quality.* Washington, DC: National Academies Press.

Institute of Medicine. (2010). *The future of nursing: Leading change, advancing health.* Washington DC: National Academies Press.

Interprofessional Education Collaborative. (2011). *Core competencies for interprofessional collaborative practice.* Interprofessional Education Collaborative (IPEC). Retrieved from https://ipecollaborative.org/uploads/IPEC-Core-Competencies.pdf

The Joint Commission. (2012). *Sentinel event data.* Retrieved from http://www.jointcommission.org/assets/1/18/root_causes_event_type_2004_2Q2012.pdf

Kolb, D. A. (1984). *Experiential learning: Experience as the source of learning and development.* Englewood Cliffs, NJ: Prentice-Hall.

Onge, J., Hodges, T., McBride, M., & Parnell, R. (2013). An innovative tool for experiential learning of nursing quality and safety competencies. *Nurse Educator, 38*(2), 71–75. doi:10.1097/NNE.0b013e3182829c7d

Oxendine, C., Robinson, J., & Wilson, G. (2004). Experiential learning. In M. Orey (Ed.), *Emerging perspectives on learning, teaching, and technology.* Retrieved from http://projects.coe.uga.edu/epltt/

Pesut, D., & Thompson, S. (2015). Building academic cultures with reflective practice in mind: Leadership agility and transformational learning. In G. Sherwood, & S. Horton-Deutsch (Eds.), *Reflective Organizations: On the Front Lines of QSEN & Reflective Practice Implementation* (pp. 339–359). Indianapolis, IN: Sigma Theta Tau International.

Powell, S., & Stone, R. A. (2015). A new framework for creating a resilient organization using reflective practices. In G. Sherwood, & S. Horton-Deutsch (Eds.), *Reflective Organizations: On the Front Lines of QSEN & Reflective Practice Implementation* (215–241). Indianapolis, IN: Sigma Theta Tau International.

Reason, J. (1997). *Managing the risks of organizational accidents.* Aldershot, UK: Ashgate.

Sawyer, K. (2013). *Zigzag: The surprising path to greater creativity.* San Francisco, CA: Jossey-Bass.

Schein, E. (2010). *Organizational culture and leadership.* San Francisco, CA: Jossey-Bass.

Sherwood, G., & Horton-Deutsch, S. (Eds.) (2012a). *Reflective practice: Transforming education and improving outcomes.* Indianapolis, IN: Sigma Theta Tau International.

Sherwood, G., & Horton-Deutsch, S. (2012b). Turning vision into action: Reflection to build a spirit of inquiry. In G. Sherwood, & S. Horton-Deutsch (Eds.), *Reflective practice: Transforming education and improving outcomes* (pp. 3–20). Indianapolis, IN: Sigma Theta Tau International.

Singer, S. J., Falwell, A., Gaba, D., Meterko, M., Rosen, A., Hartmann, C., & Baker, L. (2009). Identifying organizational cultures that promote patient safety. *Healthcare Management Review, 34*(4), 300–311.

Swenson, M., & Sims, S. (2012). Reflective ways of working together: Using liberating structures. In G. Sherwood, & S. Horton-Deutsch (Eds.), *Reflective practice: Transforming education and improving outcomes* (pp. 229–234). Indianapolis, IN: Sigma Theta Tau International.

Triolo, P. (2012). Creating cultures of excellence: Transforming organizations. In G. Sherwood, & J. Barnsteiner (Eds.), *Quality and safety in nursing: A competency approach to improving outcomes* (pp. 305–322). Hoboken, NJ: Wiley-Blackwell.

Van den Bossche, P., Gijselaers, W., Segers, M., Woltjer, G., & Kirschner, P. (2011). Team learning: Building shared mental models. *Instructional Science, 39*(3), 283–301. doi:10.1007/s11251-010-9128-3

Wachter, R. M. (2010). Patient safety at ten: Unmistakable progress, troubling gaps. *Health Affairs, 29*(1), 165–173.

Chapter 2
Transformational Learning: Improving Quality and Safety Through Reflective Pedagogies

Gwen D. Sherwood, PhD, RN, FAAN, ANEF
Sara Horton-Deutsch, PhD, RN, PMHCNS, FAAN, ANEF
Pamela Ironside, PhD, RN, FAAN, ANEF

In 2005, at the genesis of what became the Quality and Safety Education for Nurses (QSEN) project, the goal was to develop a plan for integrating the six competencies that the Institute of Medicine (IOM, 2003) identified for improving healthcare quality and safety outcomes into nursing education. In the end, the QSEN project has contributed to a transformation of nursing education by engaging faculty in integrating quality and safety across educational settings. Integration of the competencies continues to spread, and the synergy of QSEN continues to lead changes throughout nursing education and now practice (Cronenwett, Sherwood, & Gelmon, 2009; Cronenwett et al., 2007). What dynamics converged to generate such a rapid spread in creating such change?

This chapter traces how that stalwart beginning led to a social movement among nurses who realized the impact the quality and safety competencies could have on improving how nurses were prepared for practice. The chapter examines the outcomes of QSEN and explores the work of educators in preparing new graduates—work that is now inspiring practice changes to improve patient care outcomes. With funding for four phases of grants from the Robert Wood Johnson Foundation, the unfolding of QSEN over 7 years has been eloquently described by thought leader Linda Cronenwett (Cronenwett, 2012). Since that time, the QSEN story has continued to unfold, transitioning as the QSEN Institute (http://qsen.org/) of the Case Western Reserve University Frances Payne Bolton School of Nursing, directed by Mary Dolansky, who describes the transition later in the chapter.

QSEN was developed through four phases so that each phase could be planned based on the results of the preceding phase. The need for faculty development was a consistent revelation throughout each of the four project phases. Educators consistently identified the needed additional preparation to be able to develop and integrate both content and new pedagogical strategies to prepare graduates who viewed quality and safety as integral to their professional practice. From the outset, pedagogical experts have been leaders in the work of QSEN, and they have helped spread reflective, interactive, and innovative pedagogies to engage learners in developing mindful practice in which they ask questions about the outcomes of their work and continually seek improvement. To address this need, phases III and IV supported faculty development in a train-the-trainer approach, using interactive teaching approaches for the competencies. These phases are described later in this chapter.

Faculty engaged in implementing the QSEN competencies embraced the opportunity to advance nursing education and recognized the role that nurses can have in improving systems throughout healthcare. The timing of two key publications by Benner, Sutphen, Leonard, and Day (2010) and a new IOM report on nursing (2010) spurred these efforts (see Chapter 1). These reports helped provide road maps for transforming nursing education to address the needs of 21st-century healthcare. Embraced by these resources, nurse educators enthusiastically began to integrate new ideas and concepts into curricula, embrace new pedagogies, and create new experiential and reflective learning environments.

QSEN: Transforming Education as the Bridge to Quality

Reports from the IOM over the past 15 years described the need for system changes as the key to improve healthcare outcomes (2000, 2003). The 2003 report cited education as the bridge for improving healthcare; transforming health professions education with integration of critical competencies is essential to address the startling gaps identified in the 2000 report. In 2005, the QSEN project (Cronenwett et al., 2007) adopted the IOM (2003) framework that all health professionals must be prepared with quality and safety competencies defined in Chapter 1:

- Patient-centered care

- Teamwork and collaboration

- Evidence-based practice (EBP)

- Quality improvement

- Safety

- Informatics

The 2003 IOM report also discussed the need for educational changes to include the competencies as well as address changes in how to teach health professionals. The report cited reflection as a primary learning method to engage health professionals in expanding capacity to lead system redesigns in their work. Improving quality and safety derives from a culture of inquiry that values asking questions and seeking best evidence to determine what actions are needed and why, as well as to determine how to improve system processes.

REFLECTING ON ... NURSING EDUCATION

- *What values guide your work as a health professional?*

- *What assumptions about nursing curricula, student learning experiences, and partnerships between academia and clinical settings should be questioned?*

- *How can reflective practice help clarify values and assumptions that influence your professional development?*

Engaging faculty and students in reflective practice is an approach to positive change that can help uncover gaps in the system and instigate quality-improvement strategies. This represented a change in mindset from accepting dysfunction and ineffective processes in the system. Improvement is a two-step process: first, recognizing gaps; and second, having a mindset to then report the inadequacy in providing good care so that gaps can be addressed. Improvement is not being satisfied with the status quo, but rather, seeking ways to improve and repair system processes. Reflective practice is engaging in practice with a mindful presence with a mindset for asking questions about practice and seeking ways to improve outcomes of care. This chapter, then, examines both the impact of QSEN in nursing education and practice and the role of reflective practices in preparing nurses with the skills for system improvements.

Quality and Safety as Core Values: Creating a Safety Mindset

Quality and safety are core values in nursing and healthcare. Healthcare providers typically choose a health professions career based on an ethical framework of contributing to the greater good; as professionals, they want to do good work and take pride in doing things right and in doing the right thing. Doing work well contributes to higher satisfaction, which in turn increases retention as part of a healthy work environment (Aiken, Clarke, & Sloane, 2012). Providing quality care helps build trust between provider and patient/

family as well as among providers (Simmons & Sherwood, 2010). Engaged nurses reflect on what they do and ask critical questions to continually improve their work. This spirit of inquiry leads to a system perspective beyond individual performance to investigate gaps in care outcomes and common process breakdowns, the very foundation of a culture of safety (Sherwood & Zomorodi, 2013).

The QSEN project team of competency and pedagogical experts, librarian, webmaster, clinical and organizational leaders, and interprofessional representatives (see Cronenwett, 2012, for a complete list) immediately recognized a gap in systems thinking about quality and safety among educators and clinicians. The team viewed safety from the individual's performance perspective—and, therefore, when mistakes happened, the focus was on assigning individual blame. The question was how learners move from focusing only on individual perspectives to consider quality and safety from a system perspective. In addition, there was considerable discussion in the first year among the QSEN Steering Team that many nursing graduates were not prepared to meet growing expectations in practice to address gaps in quality and safety (Sherwood & Drenkard, 2007). Regulatory pressures were driving rapid change in practice to improve outcomes, yet nursing curricula and faculty development had not caught up with the changes.

Even though a majority of schools of nursing reported in a national survey that they included most of the IOM competencies in their curriculum, subsequent focus groups revealed a significant need for faculty development to accommodate the full scope of the knowledge, skills, and attitudes (KSAs) needed to achieve the QSEN competencies (Cronenwett et al., 2007; Smith, Cronenwett, & Sherwood, 2007). Educators represented in the focus groups disclosed a lack of expertise and the need to adopt a change in mindset to be prepared to lead transformation of curricula and teaching strategies to assure learners would achieve the quality and safety competencies needed to improve systems of care. Many analogies and paradigm cases have been used from aviation and other high-reliability organizations to help shape how concepts related to quality and safety are understood and applied in healthcare (Armstrong & Sherwood, 2012a).

REFLECTING ON ... THE IMPACT OF QSEN

- *How has QSEN impacted your work as a nurse, whether in academic or clinical settings?*

- *In trying to introduce the QSEN competencies in your workplace, whether a clinical or academic setting, what strategies have helped to inspire others to help integrate?*

The Four Phases of QSEN: From Idea to Transformation

The overarching goal of QSEN was to reshape nursing professional identity formation to include a commitment to developing quality and safety competencies as part of nurses' daily work: That is, quality and safety are embedded in the framework of a good nurse. Based on previous evidence of nurses' motivation for quality work, impact on retention, and contribution to a healthy work environment (Aiken, Clarke, & Sloane, 2012), the underlying assumptions for developing the QSEN model derived from Will, Idea, and Execution (Cronenwett, 2012):

- **Will:** Nurses want to do good work.

- **Idea:** Nurses will do good work when provided the tools.

- **Execution:** Nurses will do good work when provided the tools and the environment to support good work; therefore, organizational leadership is vital to improve quality and safety.

QSEN unfolded in four phases (see the following sidebar). The focus of phase I was to identify the KSAs for the six competencies that the IOM identified in the 2003 Health Professions Education report. There are 162 KSA objective statements for the six competencies to guide educators in integrating KSAs into curricula (Cronenwett et al., 2007). Phase II developed a Pilot School Learning Collaborative in which 15 schools, with a partner from a practice organization, were selected as early adopters (Cronenwett, Sherwood, & Gelmon, 2009). Each school completed a yearlong demonstration project to illustrate integration of at least one competency (reported on http://qsen.org/). As schools reported their outcomes in the final Collaborative Workshop, it was again clear that faculty development was an imperative.

OVERVIEW OF QSEN PHASES I–IV WITH OUTCOMES

Phase I, 2005–2007: Prelicensure Competency Development

- *Expert panel and Advisory Board defined the IOM competencies with objectives for the KSAs required (Cronenwett et al., 2007)*
- *Adopted by nursing education credentialing and licensing agencies (AACN, 2009; NLN, 2010; Spector, Ulrich, & Barnsteiner, 2012)*
- *Established robust website with annotated bibliography, teaching strategies, videos, and modules (http://qsen.org/)*

Phase II, 2007–2009: Pilot School Learning Collaborative

- *Developed Initial Graduate Education KSAs (Cronenwett et al., 2009); updated by AACN (2012)*
- *Piloted 15 School Learning Collaborative (Cronenwett, Sherwood, & Gelmon, 2009)*
- *Examined placement of KSAs for beginner, intermediate, and advanced across curriculum (Barton et al., 2009)*
- *Surveyed graduating student competency (Sullivan, Hirst, & Cronenwett, 2009)*
- *Established VA Scholars Quality Program (Moore, Dolansky, & Singh, 2012)*
- *Named 40 experts as QSEN Facilitators on the QSEN website (http://qsen.org/)*

Phase III, 2009–2011: Faculty Development to Achieve Curriculum Integration (partnership with University of North Carolina–Chapel Hill and American Association of Colleges of Nursing)

- *Integrated QSEN in nursing textbooks and journal articles*
- *Posted 18 learning modules on the website*
- *AACN team led Regional Faculty Development Workshops*
- *UNC–CH initiated annual QSEN National Forums*

continues

Phase IV, 2011–2012: Faculty Development

- *AACN team continued Regional Faculty Development Workshops*
- *Fully subscribed QSEN National Forum*
- *Published landmark textbook as comprehensive reference (Sherwood & Barnsteiner, 2012)*

Schools reported that the competencies rarely occur as a standalone competency; the competencies integrate one to the other. For example, patient-centered care is very much a part of teamwork and collaboration as patients and their families become active members of the team; EBPs also respect patient preferences; and, patients and families are valuable safety allies. Barton et al. (2009) led a Delphi study to help educators recognize basic to advanced KSAs to help educators effectively integrate competencies across a curriculum. To prepare nurses for the growing interprofessional environment, Dr. Shirley Moore at Case Western Reserve University led the Veteran's Administration (VA) Quality Scholars program that advanced capacity of nurses to lead quality improvement initiatives (Moore, Dolansky, & Singh, 2012).

INTEGRATING QSEN INTO A LARGE HOSPITAL SYSTEM: ON THE FRONT LINES

Cecelia L. Crawford, DNP, RN;
Lori Hamilton, BSN, RN;
and Yolanda Ramirez, MPH, RN
Southern California Patient Care Services Kaiser Permanente, Pasadena, CA

The QSEN competencies define accountabilities the American public can expect of registered nurses. These competencies, initially outlined for prelicensure nursing students, readily translate into the acute care setting with great promise for assessing and prompting quality improvement in the healthcare setting. The following is an example of how a large integrated healthcare system utilized the QSEN model to assess some of its quality programs.

The Quality and Patient Safety Program within the Kaiser Permanente Southern California (SCAL) Regional Patient Care Services (PCS) Department has provided safe and high-quality nursing care in the acute care setting for many years. It is imperative that quality and patient safety programs function at optimal levels using successful practices, the best evidence, high-quality data, and sustainable structures and processes. In order to determine the current state and components of this patient-focused program, a comprehensive evaluation was conducted from September 2014 to January 2015. The evaluation examined five core quality and patient safety programs at both a regional and medical center level. These programs included Falls Prevention, Hospital Acquired Pressure Ulcer Prevention, Medication Safety, Mobility/Ambulation, and Safe Patient Handling. All five of these patient-centric programs drive multiple Kaiser Permanente organizational initiatives involving nurse-sensitive indicators. The evaluation goal was to determine the current structures, processes, outcomes, and best practices for each individual program and the Regional PCS program as a whole.

The examination included quality and patient safety programs within Kaiser Permanente Northern and Southern California Regions and select SCAL Medical Centers and Safety Net Hospitals. This evaluation was accomplished by conducting interviews with various healthcare providers, clinicians, and nonclinicians. In addition, a questionnaire based on the structured interview questions was sent upon request. Preexisting internal and external tools, models, processes, charters, minutes, best practices, and other resources were reviewed in detail. The information gathered was then compiled, analyzed, and reorganized within a QSEN model specific to each program, as well as an overarching model for the regional PCS program. Although QSEN was originally designed for the academic environment, the individual QSEN models emphasize the organizational system focus needed for improvement in each program using best practices. In addition, each QSEN model has potential as a gap-analysis tool at the medical center level.

Using the data and information results from the program evaluation, as well as evidence-based models, tools, and other resources, the Kaiser Permanente SCAL Regional Quality and Patient Safety Program can continue the trend of optimal patient outcomes and satisfaction. The QSEN model ensures that safe and high-quality patient care is matched to 21st-century nursing practice.

Faculty Development: Early Adopters as Change Agents

Throughout the project, faculty development prevailed as a major need, both for didactic and clinical learning (Armstrong, Sherwood, & Tagliareni, 2009) and pedagogical approaches. In phases III and IV, the American Association of Colleges of Nursing (AACN) developed a project team to lead a series of highly successful regional faculty development workshops that allowed schools to send a faculty member for training so that person could return to the school as the trainer of other faculty (Barnsteiner et al., 2013). The 11 workshops were oversubscribed, with faculty wanting to participate. As part of the Steering Team, Pamela Ironside added another faculty development strategy by developing a series of 18 modules (available on the website) to address pedagogy, managing the learning environment, and development as an educator. Simultaneously, the Steering Team at the University of North Carolina worked on developing educational resources that included integrating QSEN competencies into nursing textbooks, spearheading several special topic professional journal issues, and initiating an annual QSEN National Forum for sharing ideas across nursing (Cronenwett, 2012; Sherwood, 2011).

Faculty who were early adopters became engaged in the work, recruited others to the work, and recognized that how they teach is as important as what they teach. Faculty recognized that they lacked knowledge and skills to lead quality improvement; there is a language and toolset involved in moving from recognizing a gap in care to knowing how to lead an improvement process. Faculty needed knowledge and skills in the next step from recognizing a near-miss or an adverse event to how to address a system change to prevent recurrence. In other words, they needed to know the science: the background of knowledge supporting quality and safety.

And, as faculty worked on strategies to incorporate the QSEN competencies, they considered redesigning classrooms to be less reliant on content lectures. They asked questions on how to create clinically focused teaching, prepare unfolding case studies, lead reflective analytical discussions on cases so learners apply what they know to determine actions in planning care, and refocus clinical learning with a safety focus. Faculty recognized new meanings for familiar terms; safety no longer meant just checking for bedrails and making sure that medications were administered on time.

The science emerging around safety was more complex: Safety depends on a transparent safety culture in which nurses report and analyze mistakes as well as near-misses so that processes are instilled to prevent future mistakes (Armstrong & Sherwood, 2012b). They monitor actions and decisions to be open to alternatives and self-correct. Maintaining an open questioning perspective is important to avoid premature closure on actions and also to consider alternatives. Safety comprises treating the patient and family as safety allies and partners in their care. As nurses embraced new perspectives of safety science, they recognized that variations in outcomes may be more than an individual response but, instead, a need for changes in systems of care.

The 162 objective statements for the KSAs for each competency are extensive, and faculty readily saw the need for additional preparation to engage in the changes required. QSEN brought the drivers for change to the forefront and encouraged work already being done. Most importantly, QSEN, through the annual National Forum and the website, provided a platform to widely share emerging strategies in education and practice. It is typical in approaching change to worry that outcomes will not improve—that what we are currently doing with a measure of success must be the best way—and so we resist change. Faculty who already felt that their graduates were respected and achieving noteworthy passing rates on the licensing exam wanted evidence that these changes would yield the outcomes desired. Evidence came in the dissemination from the Pilot Learning Collaborative (Cronenwett, Sherwood, & Gelmon, 2009), the Self-Assessment of New Graduates (Sullivan, Hirst, & Cronenwett, 2009), adoption of QSEN as the framework for transition to practice (Spector, Ulrich, & Barnsteiner, 2012), presentations and discussions at the annual National Forum, and a mixture of key publications referencing QSEN integration. The QSEN team created an attitude of willingness to spread ideas generously, which propelled the acceptance of change. The following sidebar illustrates how the spread of QSEN was adapted to address graduate learning needs in a specialty practice, and applied reflective practice.

WHAT QSEN MEANS TO ME: QSEN APPLICATION IN PSYCHIATRIC MENTAL HEALTH

Sara Horton-Deutsch, PhD, RN, PMHCNS, FAAN, ANEF
Professor and Watson Human Caring Science Endowed Chair
University of Colorado Anschutz Medical Campus

Over a period of 5 years (2006–2011), colleagues and I incorporated principles and practices of reflection into traditional approaches of psychiatric–mental health nursing education, including case study analysis and mini lectures (Horton-Deutsch, McNelis, & O'Haver Day, 2012). This approach engaged students through experiential learning activities with guided reflective questions. We saw the value in using these reflective practice pedagogies build through time as our students adjusted to this more active approach and recognized how it aligned with their clinical practice.

Enthusiastic about our discovery, we began speaking to other colleagues at conferences about how reflection was adding depth to teaching in both academic and practice environments, and through this process, students develop their own sense of commitment and identify as advanced practice psychiatric nurses. We dialogued about how providing feedback on these learning activities can be challenging because of their abstractness and sought ways to more accurately assess students' learning, including professional development, critical reflection, and skill development.

Through dialogue with others, we recognized that by connecting reflective practice pedagogies to the QSEN competencies, we had a method of assessment that guided students' learning. QSEN served as a bridge, spanning the obstacle of assessment and evaluation. It was a more structured guide providing concrete evidence of student learning through the assessment of attainment of knowledge, skills, and attitudes (KSAs). We were able to gather further interest in using this pedagogical approach from colleagues across the country within undergraduate and graduate nursing education.

As interest gathered and colleagues began to link reflective practice pedagogies to the QSEN competencies, we asked them to contribute their scholarly endeavors to a special issue in the Archives of Psychiatric Nursing. The issue was published in October 2012 and led by an introductory article titled "Taking Charge of Our Future: Curricular Approaches to Improving Quality and Safety in Psychiatric Nursing Practice and Health Care." Since that time the QSEN competencies

> *have continued to serve as a framework to guide educational transformation that aims to continuously improve the quality and safety of patient care and our healthcare systems through the development of patient-centered care, teamwork and collaboration, evidence-based practice, quality improvement, safety, and informatics.*

For many faculty, it was through the QSEN sessions that they began a journey of improving pedagogical literacy and overcame fears that changes would reduce student outcomes. QSEN innovators and early adopters demonstrated that the competencies, including all the KSAs, could be integrated into nursing curricula with even stronger results. The impact of QSEN was demonstrated in practice through integration into professional practice models. This confirmed the project team's belief that nurses have the will—and when given the ideas and an environment that supports execution, substantive changes could occur.

REFLECTING ON ... NURSING EDUCATION

- *How are the QSEN competencies applied in population-specific settings or groups of patients?*

- *As new graduates enter practice having been prepared with the QSEN competencies, what challenges confront them in practice?*

- *What is your response to the QSEN application of Will, Idea, and Execution? What evidence do you see that nurses have the will to make changes?*

QSEN Impact: Signs of Success

The inclusion of a librarian and webmaster in the QSEN team help direct information management and distribution, which proved to be a key success strategy. A user-friendly website (http://qsen.org/), with its expansive peer-reviewed teaching strategies, teaching videos, learning modules, annotated bibliography for the competencies, and other resources, became the signature of QSEN. The website was a popular, highly accessed resource. As usage rose, between November 2009 and November 2010, the website had 5,148,515 hits with an average of 14,105 per day. As the project continued, authors and publishers of nursing textbooks began to include QSEN competencies and learning activities; by the start of phase IV, 20 textbooks had integrated the QSEN competencies. For example, learning exercises were added to Riley's communication text (Sherwood, 2012a), and chapters in texts (Sherwood, 2012b) and instructor manuals for several fundamental textbooks included QSEN applications. By the conclusion of phase IV funding in 2012, more than 1,200 nursing faculty had participated in the AACN's regional faculty development workshops, and more than 2,100 had participated in the annual QSEN National Forums. Graduates of nursing schools that used the QSEN framework reported that they inquired in job interviews how the agency approached quality and safety. National nursing leaders noted QSEN was more than just developing quality and safety competencies but referred to the synergy that emerged from the integration across nursing as a social movement and one of the most significant paradigm shifts in nursing's history.

In 2014, Science Direct reported the original 2007 article describing that QSEN had been cited almost 200 times and was ranked in the top 1% of health-related publications. A Google search on December 31, 2014, showed more than 400 citations for QSEN. The QSEN team published a best-selling, award-winning textbook titled *Quality and Safety in Nursing: A Competency Approach to Improving Outcomes* (Sherwood & Barnsteiner, 2012), now translated in three languages, with more in development—evidence that the work is now recognized globally. Professional journals have published a number of special topic issues on quality and safety and the QSEN project, including:

- *Nursing Outlook:* May–June 2007; November–December 2009
- *Journal of Urologic Nursing:* December 2008
- *Journal of Nursing Education:* December 2009
- *Nursing Clinics of North America:* September–October 2012
- *Archives of Psychiatric Nursing:* October 2012
- *Journal of Professional Nursing:* March–April 2013

> ## REFLECTING ON ... FULLY INTEGRATING QSEN
>
> - *What are strategies for continuing to integrate QSEN competencies in all of nursing, particularly outpatient or ambulatory care settings?*
> - *What is the future of QSEN, given that the goal is to assure integration in all curricula?*

Innovations in Transforming the Educational Paradigm

Benner, Sutphen, Leonard, and Day (2010) issued a call for an educational awakening to develop active learning rather than passive learning focused on acquiring content. The timing was ideal in fueling faculty interest in implementing the QSEN competencies (see Chapter 1). In advocating educational transformation, Benner and her colleagues encouraged faculty to use situated coaching and experiential learning activities to assist students to reach a deeper understanding of concepts and application to real-world situations. Transformational learning is more than acquiring new knowledge; it includes critical reflection to question assumptions, values, and perspectives in making decisions and choices in daily work (Sherwood & Horton-Deutsch, 2012). Transformational learning recognizes and evaluates knowledge utilization in practice with clinical judgment to continually assess how to address ever-changing situations in patient care.

The QSEN work stimulated interest in transforming education and has been in the forefront of leading integration of the quality and safety competencies as well as changes in pedagogical

SITUATED COACHING

Meaningful learning takes place only when embedded in the social and physical context in which it will be used (Benner et al., 2010).

EXPERIENTIAL LEARNING ACTIVITIES

Involves action and reflection; learners assimilate concrete experiences, transform them into abstract concepts, and use this as the basis for actions tested in new situations (Kolb, 1984).

approaches (Ironside & Cerbie, 2012). As faculty developed strategies to teach the competencies, they recognized that it was not just what is taught (content) but also how it is taught (pedagogy) that helps learners sustain behavior and attitude change. Traditional content-based lectures may achieve surface learning only, which limits ability to translate to the complexities of patient care in actual practice; lecture as an example of passive learning rarely achieves behavior change (Benner et al., 2010). Educators who focus on deep learning integrate application opportunities, such as case study analysis, in which learners apply knowledge and think critically about care priorities and decisions.

For some schools, quality and safety became the organizing framework and was infused into the educational philosophy and mission (Sherwood, LaFramboise, Miller, & Robertson, 2012). To reinforce a safety mindset, educators may thread the KSAs throughout the curriculum using a variety of instructional strategies. Questions may be added to existing assignments that help learners reflect on safety implications, sections added to analysis papers that explore quality and safety, and discussions in post-clinical briefings. Unfolding case studies that simulate clinical experiences may be used in didactic discussions (Durham & Sherwood, 2008) or as the basis for simulated learning with high-fidelity human patient simulators (Durham & Alden, 2012). Throughout the four phases of the QSEN project, educators who began to let go of old assumptions became more engaged in shifting the educational paradigm and helped move QSEN to a tipping point that has contributed to re-energizing nursing education (Barnsteiner et al., 2013).

Reflective Practice: Driving Change

QSEN leaders developed multiple strategies in achieving change and integrating the competencies. Early on, reflective practice emerged as an important learning strategy in helping learners achieve the quality and safety competencies. Throughout the following sections, we explore application of reflective practice used by QSEN facilitators. Reflective practice was not new to nursing education; it was more fully developed as educators recognized a more systematic and guided approach to reflection-enhanced learning (Armstrong & Sherwood,

2012b). Many faculty had employed a general assignment for students to write a reflection in their clinical journal; however, these lacked deep analysis on what happened and how the learner engaged, responded, and reconsidered actions. Using guided reflection as a systematic approach to learning, learners are more able to develop reasoned action (Johns, 2006). Reflective practice fosters mindful engagement in work that helps make sense of events, improves practice, and builds professional maturity (Sherwood & Horton-Deutsch, 2012), essential skills, and attitudes for practice development.

QSEN facilitators recognized that to improve practice, nurses must develop a new mindset about safety and quality that recognizes practice issues and advocates for and leads to improvements to the system. By helping learners develop reflective practice within their academic study, they reinforce systematic thinking about experience. Reflective practice helps develop a new mindset by raising questions about assumptions, values, and current knowledge. Reflective practice is based on inquiry and engaged purpose; it is characterized by openness to improvement, analysis of what happened in a situation, and incorporating what you know. Experience is an important part of learning by reflecting on practice and moving from content-based surface learning toward deeper learning. Kolb's experiential learning theory helps explain a cycle of learning in which the learner experiences the activity, reflects on the activity, applies it to a real-life situation, and then evaluates the impact for future actions (Kolb, 1984). Experience is the key part of transformational learning, which separates experiential learning (flexible, no end point) from cognitive learning (acquiring and manipulating knowledge). The role of the educator is to help learners analyze their ideas through the cycle of experience and reflection in which they continually move toward professional maturity.

Learner-Centered Approaches to Transforming Education

In considering pedagogical approaches as educators integrated the QSEN competencies, the educators became concerned with a learner-centered environment to create space and intentionality to promote deliberate practice, develop critical thinking, and apply clinical reasoning (O'Haver Day & McNelis, 2012). A reflective approach to teaching and learning begins with a focus on purpose:

- Why am I here?

- What do I want from this experience?

- What am I willing to invest to achieve my purpose?

Engaging learners in purposeful reflective practice requires educators to remain open to inquiry and shifts control from educator to learner. Learners are encouraged to be creative and innovative, be comfortable with uncertainty and change, feel safe to ask challenging questions, and monitor reactions to confirm responses are consistent with intentions. Educators encourage open dialogue with learners to reflect on their actions so they examine outcomes in a manner that can lead to better choices in the future, thus enhancing tacit learning (Horton-Deutsch, Drew, & Beck-Coon, 2012).

Helping learners master the KSAs in the six competencies promoted systematic thinking that ingrained habits of the mind for constant improvement. Learning through reflection advances professional knowledge and skill through two active learning processes: reflection-in-action (reflecting during the encounter) and reflection-on-action (reflecting after the experience). Mezirow (1981) described reflection as moving from consciousness (the way we think about something) to critical consciousness (where we analyze our thinking process). In learning from experience, reflection guides learners to construct, deconstruct, and reconstruct experience (Gibbs, 1988):

1. Describe what happened.

2. How would you respond to similar experiences in the future?

3. During this experience, what were you thinking or feeling?

4. What alternatives were there? What else could you have done?

5. In considering this experience, what went well and what concerned you?

6. How do you make sense of the experience?

Providing a format for learners to develop a systematic way of reviewing experiences encourages thoughtful practice based on a spirit of inquiry.

Narrative Pedagogies: Case-Based Learning

Educators increasingly applied narrative pedagogies as effective in developing safety awareness by learning from stories and front-line paradigm cases. Narrative learning helps students examine the possibilities for acting in various encounters by collectively interpreting their experiences and challenging prevailing responses (Ironside & Cerbie, 2012). Whether writing their own experiences or listening to others' stories, learners can consider both the strengths and limitations that they bring to a situation and collectively share insights and illuminate each other's blind spots or oversights. Collectively sharing and interpreting experiences fosters cycles of interpretation so that multiple perspectives can be explored. Reflection is a key aspect of interpretation within narrative learning and involves thinking, listening, reflecting, and analyzing responses. To guide this reflection, educators often ask students to write from prompts: "Today in clinical, my values were challenged when ...," "Today I did not know what to do when ...," or "I was surprised to find that ..." (Armstrong & Sherwood, 2012b; Ironside & Cerbie, 2012).

Narrative pedagogy, through cycles of interpretation, helps uncover attitudes that may not have yet surfaced to consciousness but pose barriers in delivering patient-centered care. Discussing cases in class before encountering the actual experience in clinical settings helps learners dissect their thinking and feelings about ethical frameworks in care delivery as well as their values that affect responses to care needs, and then reconsider holistic approaches to patients and their families.

Reflective Educators: Key to Change

Educators, too, become more aware of their own reinforcing behaviors for self-sealing and self-correcting. Openness to new ideas in developing their teaching style and creating learning environments affects how they integrate course content with clinical or rethinking such sacred traditions as nursing fundamentals

(Armstrong & Barton, 2013; Armstrong et al., 2009). Safety-conscious educators themselves develop presence and attention and facilitate engaged, spirited inquiry of active learning; deepen self-awareness of themselves and relationships with learners; and build mutually respectful relationships with peers, learners, and patients. As reflective educators, they model awareness in relation to self and others and address the role of human factors in creating safe practice.

Final Reflections

Achieving the QSEN goal of transforming nurse identity to include quality and safety competencies as a core part of daily work requires education. As educators engaged in implementing the quality and safety competencies and adopted innovative instructional approaches, they expressed renewed energy and motivation. Reflective practice was earlier identified by the IOM to foster professional practice based on quality and safety, and became a primary pedagogical approach. Providing a structured approach helped learners and clinicians recognize cues to access the depth and breadth for learning through experience. Cues offer systematic mode of reflective inquiry. Flexible, iterative, and occurring in a back-and-forth manner, learners continuously deepen reflective capacity. Over time with practice, cues are internalized and constantly refined in helping develop professional maturity.

We salute the Robert Wood Johnson Foundation for the four phases of funding that provided a launching pad with a systematic yet dynamic approach to improve quality and safety through nursing education that will reverberate for decades to come. The QSEN story lives on through the QSEN Institute and through evolving adoption in practice settings. Integration for education and practice continues to spread to yet-unknown impact nationally and internationally. Quality and safety are universal themes in nursing and all of healthcare. It will be told as individuals and organizations reflect, learn, and grow toward continual transformation. Transformation is dynamic, never static, and demands continual change. We must each continually reflect and ask: What am I learning today, and how will this improve my work?

We conclude this chapter with a description of the transition to the QSEN Institute written by Director Mary Dolansky. The following sidebar summarizes the continuing impact of QSEN in transforming nursing to include a focus on quality and safety.

TRANSITIONING FROM QSEN TO THE QSEN INSTITUTE

Mary A. Dolansky, RN, PhD, Director, QSEN Institute
Frances Payne Bolton School of Nursing, Case Western Reserve University

The Quality and Safety Education for Nurses started in 2005 as nursing leaders responded to the Institute of Medicine's reports of the need to improve the quality of healthcare. During the 7 years of funding from the Robert Wood Johnson Foundation, competencies were developed, a resource-rich website (QSEN.org) was launched, and three conferences were held for nurses across the country. The mission of QSEN is to address the challenge of assuring that nurses have the knowledge, skills, and attitudes necessary to continuously improve the quality and safety of the healthcare systems in which they work.

The impact that QSEN had on the nursing profession was impressive, as after only 7 years, QSEN competencies were the foundation of nurse residency programs, the Future of Nursing Action Coalitions, integrated into professional organizations' standards, and integrated into textbooks and the NCLEX exam. In 2012, QSEN transitioned to the Frances Payne Bolton School of Nursing at Case Western Reserve University to ensure that the QSEN work continued and expanded.

Now the QSEN Institute, the enduring philosophy is that it "takes a village"— that is, the QSEN Institute represents the voices of nurses across the world who are engaged in QSEN's important work of weaving contemporary quality and safety concepts into the fabric of the nursing profession. The QSEN.org website is a virtual resource center that is created by nurses from across the world as they contribute their teaching strategies, share their expertise, and network. Nurses in doctoral programs contribute to the virtual resource center by using practicum hours to enhance components. The virtual resource center's dynamic nature relies on nurses' contributions from across the world. The QSEN Institute's virtual resource center and annual conference provide an opportunity for nurses to reflect on their work from the lens of quality and safety and learn from this ways to impact the quality and safety of healthcare.

References

Aiken, L. H., Clarke, S. P., & Sloane, D. M. (2012). Hospital staffing, organization, and quality of care; Cross-national findings. *International Journal for Quality in Health Care, 14*(1), 5–13.

American Association of Colleges of Nursing. (2009). *The essentials of baccalaureate education for professional nursing practice.* Washington, DC: American Association of Colleges of Nursing.

American Association of Colleges of Nursing. (2012). *QSEN education consortium: Graduate-level QSEN competencies, knowledge, skills and attitudes.* Retrieved from http://www.aacn.nche.edu/faculty/qsen/competencies.pdf

Armstrong, G., & Barton, A. (2013). Fundamentally updating fundamentals. *Journal of Professional Nursing, 29*(2), 82–87.

Armstrong, G., & Sherwood, G. (2012a). Patient safety. In J. Giddens (Ed.), *Concepts in nursing practice* (pp. 434–442). St. Louis, MO: Elsevier.

Armstrong, G., & Sherwood, G. (2012b). Reflection and mindful practice: A means to quality and safety. In G. Sherwood, & S. Horton-Deutsch (Eds.), *Reflective practice: Transforming education and improving outcomes* (pp. 21–40). Indianapolis, IN: Sigma Theta Tau International.

Armstrong, G., Sherwood, G., & Tagliareni, E. (2009). Quality and Safety Education in Nursing (QSEN): Integrating recommendations from IOM into clinical nursing education. In T. Valiga, & N. Ard (Eds.), *Clinical nursing education: Critical reflections* (pp. 207–226). New York, NY: National League for Nursing Press.

Barnsteiner, J., Disch, J., Johnson, J., McGuinn, K., Chappell, K., & Swartwout, E. (2013). Diffusing QSEN competencies across schools of nursing: The AACN/RWJF Faculty Development Institutes. *Journal of Professional Nursing, 29*(2), 68–74.

Barton, A. J., Armstrong, G., Preheim, G., Gelmon, S. B., & Andrus, L. C. (2009). A national Delphi to determine developmental progression of quality and safety competencies in nursing education. *Nursing Outlook, 57*(6), 313–322.

Benner, P., Sutphen, M., Leonard, V., & Day, L. (2010). *Educating nurses: A call for radical transformation.* San Francisco, CA: Jossey-Bass.

Cronenwett, L. (2012). A national initiative: Quality and Safety Education for Nurses (QSEN). In G. Sherwood, & J. Barnsteiner (Eds.), *Quality and safety in nursing: A competency approach to improving outcomes* (pp. 49–64). Hoboken, NJ: Wiley-Blackwell.

Cronenwett, L., Sherwood, G., Barnsteiner, J., Disch, J., Johnson, J., Mitchell, P., ... Warren, J. (2007). Quality and safety education for nurses. *Nursing Outlook, 55*(3), 122–131.

Cronenwett, L., Sherwood, G., & Gelmon, S. (2009). Improving quality and safety education: The QSEN Learning Collaborative. *Nursing Outlook, 57*(6), 304–312.

Cronenwett, L., Sherwood, G., Pohl, J., Barnsteiner, J., Moore, S., Taylor Sullivan, D., ... Warren, J. (2009). Quality and safety education for advanced practice nursing practice. *Nursing Outlook, 57*(6), 338–348.

Durham, C., & Sherwood, G. (2008). Education to bridge the quality gap: A case study approach. *Journal of Urologic Nursing*, Special Topic Issue on Quality, *28*(6), 431–438.

Durham, C., & Alden, K. (2012). *Integrating quality and safety competencies in simulation*. In G. Sherwood, & J. Barnsteiner (Eds.), *Quality and safety in nursing: A competency approach to improving outcomes* (pp. 227–250). Hoboken, NJ: Wiley-Blackwell.

Gibbs, G. (1988). *Learning by doing: A guide to teaching and learning methods.* Further Education Unit, Oxford Polytechnic, Now Oxford Brookes University. Retrieved from http://www2.glos.ac.uk/offload/tli/lets/lathe/issue1/issue1/pdf#oage=5

Horton-Deutsch, S., Drew, B. L., & Beck-Coon, K. (2012). Mindful learners. In G. Sherwood, & S. Horton-Deutsch (Eds.), *Reflective practice: Transforming education and improving outcomes* (pp. 79–96). Indianapolis, IN: Sigma Theta Tau International.

Horton-Deutsch, S., McNelis, A., & O'Haver Day, P. (2012). Developing a reflection-centered curriculum for graduate psychiatric nursing education. *Archives of Psychiatric Nursing, 26*(5), 341–349.

Institute of Medicine (IOM). (2000). L.T. Kohn, J.M. Corrigan, & M.S. Donaldson (Eds.), *To err is human: Building a safer health system.* Washington, DC: National Academies Press. Retrieved from http://www.iom.edu/Reports/1999/To-Err-is-Human-Building-A-Safer-Health-System.aspx

Institute of Medicine (IOM). (2003). A.C. Greiner, & E. Knebel (Eds.), *Health professions education: A bridge to quality.* Washington, DC: National Academies Press. Retrieved from http://www.iom.edu/Reports/2003/Health-Professions-Education-A-Bridge-to-Quality.aspx

Institute of Medicine (IOM). (2010). *The future of nursing: Leading change, advancing health.* Washington DC: National Academies Press.

Ironside, P., & Cerbie, E. (2012). *Narrative teaching strategies to foster quality and safety.* In G. Sherwood, & J. Barnsteiner (Eds.), *Quality and safety in nursing: A competency approach to improving outcomes* (pp. 211–225). Hoboken, NJ: Wiley-Blackwell.

Johns, C. (2006). *Engaging in reflective practice: A narrative approach.* Oxford, UK: Blackwell.

Kolb, D. A. (1984). *Experiential Learning: Experience as the source of learning and development.* Englewood Cliffs, NJ: Prentice-Hall.

McNelis, A., & Horton-Deutsch, S. (2012). Taking charge of our future: Curricular approaches that improve quality and safety in psychiatric nursing practice and health care. *Archives of Psychiatric Nursing, 256*(5), 339–340.

Mezirow, J. (1981). Critical theory of adult learning and education. *Adult Education, 3*(1), 3–24.

Moore, S., Dolansky, M., & Singh, M. (2012). Interprofessional approaches to quality and safety education. In G. Sherwood, & J. Barnsteiner (Eds.), *Quality and safety in nursing: A competency approach to improving outcomes* (pp. 251–266). Hoboken, NJ: Wiley-Blackwell.

National League for Nursing. (2010). *Outcomes and competencies for graduates of practical/vocational, diploma, associate degree, baccalaureate, masters, doctoral and research doctorate programs in nursing.* New York, NY: National League for Nursing.

O'Haver Day, P., & McNelis, A. (2012). The mindful educator. In G. Sherwood, & S. Horton-Deutsch (Eds.), *Reflective practice: Transforming education and improving outcomes* (pp. 63–77). Indianapolis, IN: Sigma Theta Tau International.

Sherwood, G., & Drenkard, K. (2007). Quality and safety curricula in nursing education: Matching practice realities. *Nursing Outlook, 55*(3), 151–155.

Sherwood, G., & Barnsteiner, J. (Eds). (2012). *Quality and safety in nursing: A competency approach to improving outcomes.* Ames, Iowa: Wiley-Blackwell.

Sherwood, G., & Horton-Deutsch, S. (2012). Turning vision into action: Reflection to build a spirit of inquiry. In G. Sherwood, & S. Horton-Deutsch (Eds.), *Reflective practice: Transforming education and improving outcomes* (pp. 3–20). Indianapolis, IN: Sigma Theta Tau International.

Sherwood, G., & Zomorodi, M. (2013). A new mindset for quality and safety: The QSEN competencies redefine nurses' roles in practice. *Journal of Nephrology Nursing, 419*(1), 15–24.

Sherwood, G. (2011). Integrating quality and safety science in nursing education and practice. *Journal of Research in Nursing, 16*(3), 226–240. doi:10:1177/1744987111400960

Sherwood, G. (2012a). QSEN teaching textboxes. In J. Riley (Ed.). *Communication in nursing* (pp. 29, 79, 80, 99, 141, 152, 201, 220, 252, 253, 262, 325). New York, NY: Elsevier.

Sherwood, G. (2012b). Quality and Safety in Nursing Education (QSEN). In B. Cherry, & S. Jacobs (Eds.), *Contemporary nursing: Issues, trends and management* (6th ed.) (pp. 393–404). New York, NY: Elsevier.

Sherwood, G., LaFramboise, L., Miller, C., & Robertson, B. (2012). Quality and Safety Education for Nurses: Integrating quality and safety competencies into nursing education. In B. Youngberg (Ed.), *Patient safety* (2nd ed.) (pp. 381–392). Sudbury, MA: Jones and Bartlett Learning.

Simmons, D., & Sherwood, G. (2010). Neonatal intensive care unit and emergency department nurses' descriptions of working together: Building team relationships to improve safety. *Critical Care Nursing Clinics of North America, 22*(2), 253–260.

Smith E., Cronenwett L., & Sherwood G., (2007). Quality and safety education: Prelicensure nursing educator views. *Nursing Outlook, 55*(3), 132–137.

Spector, N., Ulrich, B., & Barnsteiner, J. (2012). New graduate transition into practice: Improving quality and safety. In G. Sherwood, & J. Barnsteiner (Eds.), *Quality and safety in nursing: A competency approach to improving outcomes* (pp. 267–288). Hoboken, NJ: Wiley-Blackwell.

Sullivan, D. T., Hirst, D., & Cronenwett, L. (2009). Assessing quality and safety competencies of graduating prelicensure nursing students. *Nursing Outlook, 57*(6), 323–331.

Chapter 3
Practices of Reflective Leaders

Patricia K. Young, PhD, RN
Karen T. Pardue, PhD, RN, CNE, ANEF
Sara Horton-Deutsch, PhD, RN, PMHCNS, FAAN, ANEF

Whether leading in classrooms, clinical practice, healthcare delivery, or academic administrative settings, effective leaders draw upon lessons learned from experiences—their own and others—thoughtfully responding to the everyday challenges that occur in our increasingly complex organizational systems. This chapter examines how reflection on experience helps leaders identify *leadership practices*—particular ways of leading that they may want to continue to enact, extend, challenge, or overcome. Through gathering one's thoughts, reflective leadership calls forth personal development and creates a space for organizational transformation.

Background

The authors of this chapter—Patricia Young, Karen Pardue, and Sara Horton-Deutsch—met through their involvement in the National League for Nursing/ Johnson & Johnson (NLN/J&J) Faculty Leadership and Mentoring Program.

This program paired experienced faculty leaders—*mentors*—with less-experienced educators who demonstrated potential for leadership—*protégés*. Five mentor/protégé pairs worked for 1 year to attain leadership goals that the protégés set, and the group of 10 worked with the program director on a project aimed to transform nursing education. Pardue was a mentor, and Horton-Deutsch was a protégé (although they were not a matched pair), and Young was the program director during the first year (2007–2008) of the 4-year run of the program.

For their group project, the 2007/2008 cohort conducted an interpretive phenomenological study of the lived experiences of becoming a nurse faculty leader. As part of this study, members of the cohort interviewed 23 self-identified faculty leaders in attendance at the 2008 NLN Faculty Leadership Conference. They identified whether the faculty participants were formal or informal leaders in the classroom, among their peers, at their institution, or more broadly in academe. Cohort members then recorded the participants' stories about how they became leaders, transcribed the recorded stories, and analyzed the written texts for recurring themes and patterns. Publication of the cohort's initial findings occurred in 2011 (Young, Pearsall, Stiles, Nelson, & Horton-Deutsch, 2011); two subgroups of the cohort then published themes that they interpreted in-depth (Horton-Deutsch, Young, & Nelson, 2010[*]; Stiles, Pardue, Young, & Morales, 2011).

One theme—namely, taking risks—was further explored through data obtained in 2010–2011 when seven researchers from the cohort re-interviewed six of the original faculty participants and conducted two focus group discussions, focusing on the experience of taking risks as a nurse faculty leader. The findings from this in-depth review of the data were presented as three subthemes focusing on how leaders take risks (Horton-Deutsch et al., 2014; Pardue, Young, Horton-Deutsch, Pearsall, & Halstead, manuscript in preparation; Pearsall et al., 2014).

---

[*]*It might appear that the publication date of the subgroup's findings would be the same year as the initial findings. The cohort's initial findings were submitted for publication in 2009 but did not appear in publication until 2011. The Horton-Deutsch, Young, & Nelson manuscript was submitted months later in 2009 but was actually published in 2010, which was earlier than the initial findings.*

Underpinning the totality of this collective work is the practice of reflecting on one's experience. Reflection was necessary as both a participant and as a researcher, and participants revealed reflection as a distinct practice of leadership. Specifically, reflecting—along with persevering and learning to relate with others in new ways—was illuminated as to how nurse faculty leaders faced challenges (Horton-Deutsch et al., 2010). *Reflection*—a deliberate process of introspection or focused self-awareness—was internalized and described as a part of who leaders were. That is, "[R]eflection is a passive practice of thinking that leads to thoughtful action; one must be deliberate about creating the pause or the space for thinking" (Horton-Deutsch et al., 2010, p. 491).

REFLECTION

A passive practice of thinking that leads to thoughtful action (Horton-Deutsch et al., 2010, p. 491).

HERMENEUTICS

Interpretation; in this context, interpretation to understand the meaning of human experience.

The authors understood the significance of cultivating reflective practices for leadership development early in this work. We challenged ourselves to think of a time where we believed that reflection really mattered in our decision-making. We formed a focus group and shared our stories, recorded and transcribed them, and analyzed them hermeneutically. This final study prepared us to write this chapter and affirmed our belief in the significance of leadership reflection in practice. Figure 3.1 presents the themes and subthemes that we explicate throughout this collective body of work and that we will refer to throughout this chapter.

This chapter presents cumulative findings from this series of studies on the practices of becoming a nurse faculty leader. This research illuminates the importance of reflective skills for leaders and encourages development of reflective practice. Sharing the journeys of more than 35 nurse faculty leaders, this collective work presents practical knowledge about developing as a leader within and outside nursing education. Herein lie the ways of leadership needed to sustain academic and healthcare settings—wherever nurse educators lead. We offer questions designed for personal reflection on your own leadership practices to encourage introspection and also challenge you to consider your own leadership practices and areas for growth.

FIGURE 3.1
*Practices of
Becoming a Nurse
Faculty Leader*

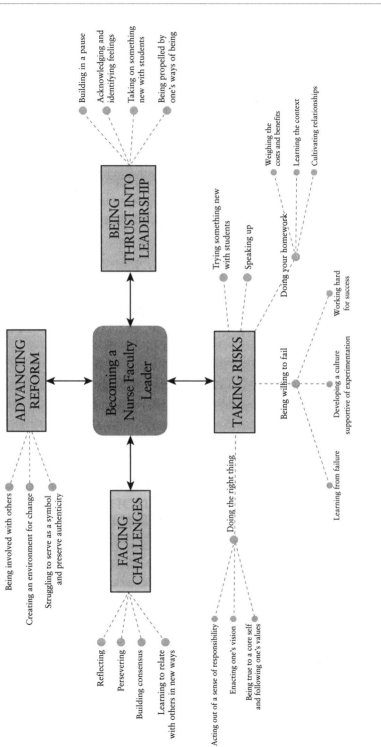

Leadership Practices

The practice of reflecting interwove throughout the authors' experiences as participants in the NLN/ J&J Faculty Leadership and Mentoring Program. *Interpretive research* (hermeneutic analysis) is a reiterative process of reading the text (data), writing an interpretation, and then rereading and rewriting as continued reflective dwelling in the narrative data reshapes understanding. We engaged in reflection through reading the data, writing interpretations, and then reading the interpretations generated by research team members and having a dialogue with the team. Furthermore, participants engaged in reflection on their experiences when they told us their stories, which eventually revealed to us how they became leaders, and their practices of leading. Thus, reflection underpins this study and identification of leadership practices.

LEADERSHIP PRACTICES

Common, everyday, habitual experiences that shape becoming and being a nurse faculty leader.

INTERPRETIVE PHENOMENOLOGICAL RESEARCH

The study of the experience of a particular phenomenon and the interpretation of that experience for its meaning and significance.

Being Thrust Into Leadership

Nurse educators with advanced or specialty education may be thrust into leadership when "taking on something new and succeeding" or simply by "enacting their ways of being" (Young et al., 2011). Whether they are called upon by others to lead in a last-minute situation or responding to their own internal drive to make decisions, take risks, or advocate for change, educators who do not see themselves as leaders do not anticipate leadership and often feel unprepared (Young et al., 2011). Educators can ask themselves how they can develop their identity as leaders. Leaders can ask themselves in whom do they see unacknowledged leadership practices, and also how they can help that person see himself or herself as a leader (Young et al., 2011).

 Pausing for reflection. Building in a pause for reflection is one effective practice that educators can use when they find themselves facing the situation of being asked to take on a new assignment and feeling that leadership is being thrust upon them. When being asked to lead, the idea is not to commit initially—that is, don't say "yes" or "no" immediately—but instead say, "I'll think about it and get back to you." Thinking about an offer and getting more information about it may actually allow you to say yes to an opportunity to grow and learn. This benefit is especially true when saying yes to a request that feels risky: It is often the risky nature of a request to take the lead that gives you pause and makes you take one step back to think about it further. Letting a request "marinate" in this way enables leaders to do the homework of outlining the pros and cons of taking on something new and gauging whether you have the capacity to lead in the particular situation or the energy to learn a new role.

Giving yourself time to reflect on the ramifications of a decision, such as identifying the worst-case scenario or what could be gained or lost by a course of action, is a small but significant practice of leadership. As an intentional practice, leaders might automatically respond to all requests with, "Let me think about that" so as to be thoughtful about what they do. One aspect of this reflection may involve talking to others—not so that you can hear others' viewpoints about what should be done, but to be able to hear yourself saying it out loud. Leaders look for someone to listen to their thinking so that they can listen to themselves. A leader may not know what he or she thinks until it is said out loud; listening to yourself think aloud can guide your decision-making.

Another significant aspect of taking time to reflect is being *transparent* about it—letting others know you are doing it. When others know that you put intentional thought into something, they might understand and accept it better. Being transparent about building in a pause lets other people know that you are dedicating time and thought to them. In the process of building in a pause for inner exploration, leaders consider the following:

- What do I bring to the current situation?
- What skills do I have?
- What do others bring to the current situation?
- What skills do they have?
- What does this situation call for or demand of me and of others?

- What constraints do I see?

- What am I feeling right now?

- What are my expectations?

Acknowledging and identifying feelings. Acknowledging and identifying your feelings in response to a situation is another small but significant act of being thrust into leadership. Being asked to step into a leadership role commonly evokes an emotional response—one that you can use to trigger reflective thinking. Thoughtful reflection may reveal expectations that you didn't know you held and also help to dissipate anger or disappointment in a situation.

REFLECTING ON ... EXPERIENCING ANGER AS A LEADER

- *What are my expectations in this situation that have not been met?*

Leaders find it helpful to reflect whenever they experience feeling overwhelmed, angry, disappointed, fearful, or uncertain. On the other hand, do feelings of joy, elation, or excitement trigger reflective thinking? Thoughts of gratitude and appreciation may transform thinking and how you approach leadership situations. For instance, keeping a gratitude journal is an intentional practice that focuses thinking on what is right with things rather than what is wrong. Journaling is a reflective practice to make meaning of experiences and recognize a person's growth and development—that those who feel thrust into leadership might welcome.

Facing Challenges

Facing challenges is a common experience for many nurse leaders seeking to advance their careers by taking on new positions and responsibilities. Reflecting, persevering through difficulties, and learning to relate to others in new ways represent how nurse faculty face challenges while becoming a leader (Horton-Deutsch et al., 2010). These practices support leadership development by facilitating self-exploration, thoughtful interactions with self and others, and values clarification.

SELF-AWARENESS

The capacity for self-examination and the ability to see oneself as separate from another and the environment.

OTHER-AWARENESS

The capacity to observe and interpret the emotions of others.

Self-discovery occurs when leaders reflect on their own strengths and how they can put those strengths to use to make the greatest impact. For instance, when leaders thoughtfully consider their contributions to a difficult interaction, own their part in it, and model the way for others through honest expression, their actions open dialogue and pave the way for successful outcomes. The practice of reflecting helps leaders to develop self- and other-awareness and leads to more caring relational interactions where people are open to learning from one another (Kouzes & Posner, 2007). Reflecting allows leaders to not only consider their own strengths but also recognize and build on the strengths of others.

Listening attentively is an important part of nursing leadership and helps the leader to persevere while facing challenges. Key aspects of building relational capacity is to listen, encourage others to recognize each person's point of view, and ask questions in order to cultivate a deeper dialogue and understanding. These approaches facilitate working together while vicariously building relationships and empowering others to work toward successful outcomes.

Reflecting and persevering while facing challenges leads to a transformation where leaders ultimately learn to relate to others in new ways. A key activity that helps leaders to make this transformation is to actively pause, wait and encourage members to listen, and acknowledge each other's point of view. Pausing involves actively listening and remaining engaged while waiting: It is a way of persevering that allows everyone to be heard before making a decision. Learning to relate to others in new ways takes time and perseverance: It requires being silent and deeply listening for the essence of what is being said until a new way can be found to come together.

Building consensus is one specific way leaders learn to connect with others and garner support for their goals (Young et al., 2011). It takes a lot of behind-the-scenes work to get everyone to talk until all agree on the same course of action, requiring persistence as well as resiliency for the ongoing nature of facing challenges. In some instances, leaders may realize that building consensus can feel like a political process.

REFLECTING ON ... CONSENSUS BUILDING

- *How do I build consensus when I face a divisive issue?*
- *What can I do to stay resilient when facing challenges?*

Patterson, Grenny, McMillan, and Switzler (2012) provide some helpful hints for engaging in consensus-driven decision-making (see the following sidebar).

TIPS FOR DECISION-MAKING BY CONSENSUS

Remember that consensus is not meant for all decisions. To determine whether a decision is best made by consensus, consider the following: Who cares? Who knows? Who must agree? How many people is it worth involving? Consensus is applicable when issues are high-stakes and complex, or when everyone must support the final decision. Not everyone has to agree on the decision, but everyone must be able to live with it.

Consider the following tips:

- *Consensus isn't about getting your way: It's about doing what is best for everyone involved. Thus, consensus involves compromise and acceptance that you might get your second or third choice.*
- *Building consensus involves healthy dialogue. People need to be able to say what they can live with and what they can't live with.*
- *Decisions need to be made on the basis of which proposal has the best merit, not on whose turn it is to get their way.*

continues

- *Decisions need to be out in the open and made by the entire group. Reservations need to be aired before a decision is reached, not afterward.*

- *If the decision fails, own the failure as a group rather than pointing fingers and saying, "I told you so."*

Source: Adapted from Patterson, Grenny, McMillan, and Switzler (2012), pp. 166–173.

Taking Risks

The stories of leaders reveal many ways they engage in the practice of taking risks. This is not to say that nurse leaders are risky about what they do, but to acknowledge that risk-taking is an everyday experience in leadership. The stories helped us to understand and identify the art of taking risks as a leader. Several themes illuminate practices of risk-taking.

Trying something new. Nurse educators identify themselves as leaders when they take risks with their teaching by trying something new with students. Whether teachers are motivated by boredom, the need for curricular reform, or a desire to exercise creativity, moving out of the comfort zone of a familiar approach to teaching feels risky because by doing something they have never done before, they open themselves to failure (Young, 2004). Moreover, teachers who lead educational change may be perceived by other faculty as disrupting the status quo and may face resistance to their ideas (Young et al., 2011). Implementing change in one's teaching despite the feelings of risk and pushback from colleagues is one hallmark of a faculty leader.

REFLECTING ON ... HOW TO FACILITATE THE ACCEPTANCE OF NEW TEACHING TECHNIQUES

- *What barriers do I or the larger system present to educators wanting to try something new in the classroom?*

- *What can I do to facilitate faculty who take risks in the classroom so they have the freedom to be creative and try new things?*

Source: Young et al., 2011.

Speaking up. Nurse leaders speak up when challenging the status quo, advocating for change, promoting their vision for the future, or defending those who have little voice. The practice of speaking up is *mindful*—that is, it requires a leader to reflect, gather information, and determine the best time and place and to whom to speak for best outcomes. It means knowing when not to speak up as well (Young et al., 2011). Reflection is important for leaders to come to understand *how* to speak up. Asking oneself, "How can I best advocate for what I believe in?" is one way to begin reflecting and preparing to speak up. Kouzes and Posner (2012) note that leaders build credibility with followers by challenging processes when they know what they stand for and then act on it.

Doing your homework. Risk-taking manifests itself in many forms, including making unpopular decisions, embarking on innovation, or addressing difficult budgetary issues (Pearsall et al., 2014). An everyday leadership practice associated with risk-taking involves doing your homework. Homework entails a self-organizing, self-regulating activity (Corno, 2000); the purpose of homework is to enhance knowledge, make connections, and increase future preparedness (Horowitz, 2006). Doing one's homework assists nurse faculty leaders in executing measured approaches to risk-taking—and in so doing, enhances the likelihood for success.

Weighing the costs and the benefits is a deliberate practice of doing homework. This balancing involves careful and methodical consideration as to the pros and cons of a given situation. In this instance, doing homework might initially involve gathering any missing or needed information. The leader then steps back to reflect, taking thorough stock of the situation. Through personal introspection and thoughtful deliberation, leaders gain greater understanding and avoid potential perils in the risk-taking process. Consider a time when you weighed the costs and benefits of a situation—how did you approach this activity?

Learning the context is another deliberate practice of doing homework. Leaders gain a greater understanding of the environment through networking, asking questions, and gathering additional perspectives unique to the institution. These deliberate steps help the leader to fully appreciate the nuances embedded within the organizational climate. Gaining this enhanced understanding is essential for maximizing leadership success when embarking on risky or uncertain decisions.

Bringing people together and *cultivating relationships* offers another homework practice supportive of leadership risk-taking. Enhancing collaboration and building community serves to unite people, thus promoting teamwork and commitment among the collective. This cooperative action serves to mitigate risk (Pearsall et al., 2014) because liability is subsequently distributed across members of the organization.

REFLECTING ON ... HOMEWORK PRACTICES

- *What homework practices do I commonly enact when facing a risky decision?*
- *What additional measured approaches might I consider?*
- *What methods have I used to learn the nuances of the organizational context?*
- *What is my approach for cultivating relationships across the institution?*

Doing the right thing. One aspect of risk-taking that stands out among nurse leaders is how they go about doing the right thing. Leaders often drive practices of doing the right thing through their sense of professional responsibility, vision for the future, and/or being true to both their values and self (Horton-Deutsch et al., 2014). These practices help faculty assess their comfort with risk, explore ways to engage in risk, and use the knowledge gained for professional growth to further develop as a leaders.

Doing the right thing as *originating from a sense of responsibility* is often seen as an action congruent to either a current role or professional goals. For example, a director of a nursing program often expresses an obligation to ensure that students receive a quality education. Balancing this goal with the needs of faculty, the institution, and the wider community is a complicated task. At times, leaders must make decisions that do not please every constituent; however, a sense of responsibility to follow particular policies or procedures to ensure program quality ultimately guides the decision. Making decisions that are not popular can be risky; therefore, attending to how one goes about doing the right thing through careful and thoughtful interactions, deliberately attending to others perspectives, and honoring relationships all serve to help minimize risk (Horton-Deutsch et al., 2010; Pearsall et al., 2014; Stiles, Horton-Deustch, & Andrews, 2014).

Doing the right thing is predicated on the ability to envision what is right. This ability means being able to see the bigger picture or forecast a preferred future for a program or institution (Horton-Deutsch et al., 2014). Imagination, ingenuity, and a firm belief in one's own vision all support this practice. This way of leading not only requires having the vision but also *enacting the vision* through discerning a course of action, speaking up, and building consensus. Kouzes and Posner (2012) add that personal passion occupies the core of doing what is right. Passion inspires vision, igniting the energy and motivation for leadership. The passionate leader is compelled to act based upon an unwavering commitment to a course of action (Young, 2011). Thus, doing the right thing means being self-aware, thinking strategically, and engaging in risk-taking action in order to achieve one's goals.

Remaining true to yourself and your values. While informed by vision, doing the right thing is additionally grounded in being true to a core self and following your values. Impactful leaders are in touch with their own moral compass and describe the internal conflict that they experience when facing situations that clash with their values (Horton-Deutsch et al., 2014). This moral distress, coupled with a deep inner sense of personal responsibility, commonly propels leaders to take action despite possible adverse consequences. For instance, in the case of a perceived prejudice experienced by a faculty member, a leader may speak up on behalf of the faculty member despite concern of not being supported by the institution. Being true to one's core and having the courage to take this type of risk is the mark of a leader. Significant for this practice is knowing your values: Self-awareness provides a strong foundation for leadership. Kouzes and Posner (2007) describe a values clarification exercise that may help leaders to identify their fundamental beliefs to gain clarity about what doing the right thing means to them (see the following sidebar).

WRITE A TRIBUTE TO YOURSELF

Imagine that you will be the guest of honor at a dinner hosted by your national nursing organization, and you are being honored as Leader of the Year. What would you most like others to say about you? How would you like to be remembered? What would make you proud? Before you begin writing your tribute, it may be helpful to reflect on the following questions:

- *What do you stand for? Why?*

- *What do you believe in? Why?*

- *What are you discontented about? Why?*

- *What brings you suffering? Why?*

- *What makes you weep and wail? Why?*

- *What brings you joy? Why?*

- *What are you passionate about? Why?*

- *What keeps you awake at night? Why?*

- *What thought has grabbed hold and won't let go? Why?*

- *What do you want for your life? Why?*

- *What is it that you really care about? Why?*

Source: Adapted from Kouzes and Posner, 2007, pp. 69–70.

Accepting the possibility of failure. The process of taking risks and facing challenges may result in failure. Being willing to fail reveals a less-explored aspect of nursing leadership. Willingness to fail describes the disposition of being open to the possibilities that are realized through failure. This practice is an intentional one that facilitates addressing challenges, taking risks, and embarking upon reform (Pardue, Young, Horton-Deutsch, Pearsall, & Halstead, manuscript in preparation).

Developing a culture supportive of experimentation is an essential practice of being willing to fail. The notion of experimentation conveys a methodical investigation as well as receptivity to testing possible problem-solving approaches. As with any experiment, some outcomes will be successful, and others will not. A climate of experimentation is defined by curiosity, placing greater value and emphasis on the testing process itself and less on the actual outcome. This results in failure being reframed from negative to positive given that something new is learned and gained from this inquisitive posture.

Learning lessons from failure reveals a visible and important leadership practice. Examining adversity provides a unique opportunity for personal, professional, and organizational growth as well as the development of new insights. Embracing all that can be learned from failure—as opposed to renouncing it—is an invaluable mindset, ultimately serving to inform future leadership success. As a reflective exercise, leaders might consider their level of commitment to experimentation and also the tangible ways in which they advance inquisitiveness within their organization. Leaders might also contemplate their own personal response to failure.

REFLECTING ON ... FAILURE

- *Does failure invoke a negative reaction? Why is this so?*
- *How are failures thoughtfully dissected in order to learn potential lessons from the experience?*

The experience of failure commonly results in the leadership practice of *engaging in hard work.* Consider a time when one of your decisions resulted in failure. Did you feel that you needed more time or support to "work out the kinks" or determine how best to "stretch" your colleagues as a result of the experience (Pardue et al., manuscript in preparation)? It is not uncommon for failure to engender additional leadership work; navigating the hard work of failure ultimately leads to organizational success. Such work might be conceptualized as rehearsal, as a process of slow achievements incrementally work toward success (Pardue et al., manuscript in preparation).

REFLECTING ON ... WHAT IT TAKES TO ACHIEVE SUCCESS

- *How receptive are you as a leader to embracing additional work?*

- *Do you shy away from extra labor, or do you affirm this as a potential learning opportunity?*

Advancing Reform

The process of facing challenges and taking risks actively engages nurse leaders in advancing reform. Shepherding change can be demanding, yet through self-examination and reflection on the experience, leaders grow and affirm their capacity to lead (Stiles et al., 2011). A number of intentional practices favorably support leadership development for advancing reform.

Engaging with others. Being involved with others cultivates relationships and generates energy in discovering new and unconventional ways for nurse educators to work together. Engaging with others stimulates a genuine give and take, providing an opportunity to think through diverse viewpoints and perspectives. Advancing reform rarely signifies individual work, but rather relies on an earnest engagement of the whole.

REFLECTING ON ... BEING INVOLVED WITH OTHERS

- *In what ways do I reach out to others in the change process?*

- *Do I listen carefully and seek feedback?*

- *Is my approach inclusive?*

- *What is my response to change?*

During this process of being involved with others, it is important for leaders to *remain authentic* or true to their core values and beliefs (Stiles et al., 2011). The position of leader may inherently exert a level of influence on group dynamics, thus impacting the everyday exchange of ideas. Leaders need to consider their ways of being with others and also reflect upon how they understand and present themselves in the context of their leadership role.

Cultivating environments for change. Reform is additionally supported by the leadership practice of creating *environments for change*. This means cultivating climates receptive to fresh ideas and innovative approaches, and then adopting change in small, manageable steps (Stiles et al., 2011). For example, an academic dean challenges a nursing program to consider new approaches to the curriculum. Creative ideas are exchanged, and faculty members are then encouraged to adopt one small component as a starting point. The dean realizes that partitioning a large change into incremental, achievable portions builds collective confidence and energy around the change process (Kouzes & Posner, 2003; Stiles et al., 2011). Consider a time when your organization embarked on a change and ask yourself the following:

ENVIRONMENT FOR CHANGE

A workplace culture characterized by openness to innovation, working collaboratively, and where people feel safe trying out new ideas (Stiles et al., 2011).

REFLECTING ON ... CHANGE

- *How accepting is your institution to change and reform?*
- *What approach do you use in working with others throughout the change process?*
- *In what ways do your practices inhibit reform?*
- *Are you open to taking baby steps in support of future larger steps? If not, what would it take for you to become open to change?*

Final Reflections

This chapter provides an examination of leadership practices as described by emerging and established nurse faculty leaders, highlighting the value of reflection as an intentional strategy for leadership development. Stories from more than 35 nurse faculty leaders illuminate how being thrust into leadership, taking risks, facing challenges, and advancing reform are common everyday leadership experiences that require thoughtful examination. Reflection on these leadership challenges serves to enhance individual understanding, refine personal skill, and facilitate the process of learning the complex nature of leadership. Values clarification is advanced as an important reflective endeavor to guide readers in determining how to do the right thing in their own leadership journey.

Exploring leadership practices means that nurse faculty leaders reflect on their experiences, examining what is meaningful and significant. Reflection in this way uncovers the practical knowledge and innovation that is embedded in experience. Furthermore, it challenges leaders to consider the ways in which leading is a central part of who they are as teachers and nurses and how the practice of leading is interwoven with the practices of teaching and nursing (Stiles et al., 2011). Reflecting on experiences of leading—on the everyday practices of leading in which faculty engage—helps faculty to understand and claim leadership capacity and areas for growth and development as a leader (Stiles et al., 2011).

References

Corno, L. (2000). Looking at homework differently. *The Elementary School Journal,* *100*(5), 529–548.

Horowitz, S. (2006). Making the most of homework. *Children's Voice, 15,* 17–19.

Horton-Deutsch, S., Young, T., & Nelson, K. (2010). Becoming a nurse faculty leader: Facing challenges through reflecting, persevering, and learning to relate with others new ways. *Journal of Nursing Management, 18*(4), 487–493.

Horton-Deutsch, S., Pardue, K., Young, P. K., Morales, M. L., Halstead, J., & Pearsall, C. (2014). Becoming a nurse faculty leader: Taking risks by doing the right thing. *Nursing Outlook, 62*(2), 89–96.

Kouzes, J. M., & Posner, B. Z. (2003). *Academic administrator's guide to exemplary leadership.* San Francisco, CA: Jossey-Bass.

Kouzes, J. M., & Posner, B. Z. (2007). *The leadership challenge* (4th ed.). San Francisco, CA: Jossey-Bass.

Kouzes, J. M., & Posner, B. Z. (2012). *The leadership challenge* (5th ed.). San Francisco, CA: Jossey-Bass.

Pardue, K. T., Young, P., Horton-Deutsch, S., Pearsall, C., & Halstead, J. *Becoming a nurse faculty leader: Taking risks by being willing to fail.* Manuscript in preparation.

Patterson, K., Grenny, J., McMillan, R., & Switzler, A. (2012). *Crucial conversations: Tools for talking when stakes are high.* New York, NY: McGraw-Hill.

Pearsall, C., Pardue, K. T., Horton-Deustch, S., Young, P. K., Halstead, J., Nelson, K. A., … Zungolo, E. (2014). Becoming a nurse faculty leader: Doing your homework to minimize risk-taking. *Journal of Professional Nursing, 30*(1), 26–33.

Stiles, K., Pardue, K., Young, P., & Morales, M. L. (2011). Becoming a nurse faculty leader: Practices of leading illuminated through advancing reform in nursing education. *Nursing Forum, 46*(2), 94–101.

Stiles, K., Horton-Deutsch, S., & Andrews, C. (2014). The nurse's lived experience of becoming an interprofessional leader. *The Journal of Continuing Education in Nursing, 45*(11), 487–493.

Young, P. (2004). Trying something new: Reform as embracing the possible, the familiar, and the at-hand. *Nursing Education Perspectives, 25*(3), 124–130.

Young, P. (2011). Headlines from the NLN: Developing a portrait of a nursing education leader. *Nursing Education Perspectives, 32*(2), 136–137.

Young, P., Pearsall, C., Stiles, K., Nelson, K., & Horton-Deutsch, S. (2011). Becoming a nursing faculty leader. *Nursing Education Perspectives, 32*(4), 150–156.

Part II

Reflective Learning Environments in Academic Settings

Chapter 4
Developing Concept-Based Curricula

Jean Foret Giddens, PhD, RN, FAAN

A number of years ago, I taught health assessment in a baccalaureate prelicensure nursing program. I distinctly remember one particular student whom I observed during a skills check-off activity assessing the student's knowledge of the head and neck unit, which included examination of the eyes, ears, nose, throat, and mouth. I held the clinical skill checklist in one hand and a pen in the other, patiently watching the student proceed with the examination of the eye. After turning on the light, she held the ophthalmoscope against her eye, positioned herself in front of her lab partner, moved the diopter disc back and forth as she adjusted her focus, and told me what she was observing. She described seeing the red reflex and moved closer toward her lab partner. She noted that the optic disc was "round and creamy yellow"; she also described "light red arteries and darker veins running from the optic disc outward to the periphery." I smiled as I reviewed the instructor checklist, noting that she had perfectly described every single item on my list. Ordinarily, I would have considered this a stellar skills demonstration, but in this situation, I was dismayed. The student failed to notice that she was holding the ophthalmoscope backward—the light was shining into her own eye, not her lab partner's eye.

I clearly remember reflecting on this situation during my drive home from class. What went wrong? Did she not listen to me or watch my lab demonstration? Did she not watch the required videos? She attended laboratory practice sessions; did she not practice? The examination did not demonstrate what she had learned, but rather what she had memorized. It was also clear that the information she memorized lacked meaning.

On that particular day, I was thinking about eye exams, but these thoughts led to general concerns I had about health assessment for undergraduate students: How often do nurses use ophthalmoscopes? Why do we teach students to percuss a liver? Why do we teach measurement of diaphragmatic excursion? What is the value of teaching clinical skills that students might never perform in a clinical setting? What are we doing?

These thoughts did not stay contained in the area of health assessment, either. Over time, I questioned not only *what* we were teaching students, but also *how* we were going about it. Although I did not know it at the time, these thoughts were the seeds for future approaches to educating nurses. This chapter presents the initial development of a concept-based curriculum in an undergraduate program. Although the introduction of this curriculum was disruptive at the time, this approach led to curriculum transformation across the United States.

KNOWLEDGE STRUCTURES

Refers to the process of learning within the brain where connections are made between new information and existing knowledge to new information that results in new or deeper understandings.

Background

During the time of the skills demonstration I described earlier, I was in the midst of completing my doctoral education. Exposure to the education discipline literature helped me to see a need to rethink many of our educational approaches in nursing. One of the most profound influences for me at that time was the publication of *How People Learn* (Bransford, Brown, & Cocking, 2000), a synthesis of evidence on the science of learning, funded by the National Research Council. One important theme from this work is the formation of knowledge structures in the brain as a result of learning. This process occurs when the brain makes cognitive connections between previous understanding and new information; it is a key component needed for a learner to apply knowledge effectively to multiple situations. Since that time, further advances in educational neuroscience research have resulted in an enhanced understanding of human learning. These discoveries have fueled widespread interest across multiple disciplines to link human learning research with educational practice.

The conceptual approach is one of several educational trends that have emerged from the new understandings gained from the science of learning. Use of the term "conceptual approach" is purposeful in that it represents a spectrum of interrelated elements influenced by the science of human learning with implications for teaching, curriculum design, and learning (Giddens, Caputi, & Rodgers, 2015). Each of the five elements—concepts, exemplars, concept-based curriculum, concept-based instruction, and conceptual learning—is enhanced by the other elements. In other words, the greatest effect is achieved with the application of all five elements because of their interrelatedness. Here is a breakdown of these elements:

- **Concepts.** A *concept* is a mental construct or an organizing idea. Concepts are used to structure curriculum and guide instruction and learning. All disciplines have core concepts, and some concepts are shared by multiple disciplines. Although many nursing concepts are shared by other healthcare disciplines, the instructional and learning focus in a nursing curriculum is the application of those concepts to the practice of nursing.

- **Exemplars.** The word *exemplar*, derived from the word *example*, literally is just that—an example of the concept in the context of nursing practice. Typically, exemplars are health conditions and situations common to the practice of nursing. The use of exemplars is essential for learners to gain important content knowledge for deep understanding of the concept, which leads to the ability for recognition and application of other situations when encountered outside the formal classroom space. Carefully selected exemplars in the context of the conceptual approach free faculty and students from the burden of excessive curriculum content.

- **Concept-based curriculum.** As the term suggests, a *concept-based curriculum* uses concepts as foundational organizers for curriculum design, allowing faculty to shift from a teaching emphasis on content toward an environment that fosters conceptual learning. Concept categories (groups of like concepts) are often used as threads or structural elements. Featured concepts within a concept-based curriculum provide the necessary infrastructure for concept-based instruction and learning.

- **Concept-based instruction.** This element refers to the purposeful practice of teaching concepts and exemplars to promote conceptual learning. The approach requires a specific focus on the concept with linkages of exemplars back to the concept and interrelated concepts. Although there are really no specific instructional strategies unique for concept-based teaching, a variety of student-centered learning activities that require learners to apply information in a clinical context is used to facilitate students making the desired cognitive connections.

- **Conceptual learning.** This final element emphasizes *learning with understanding* as opposed to memorization of facts. Conceptual learning involves the cognitive organization of new information into logical mental structures (concepts) to draw meaning; thus, the learner becomes increasingly skilled at thinking. Specific information and facts are applied to situations to facilitate deeper understanding of concepts. Developing an understanding of the interrelationships of concepts and actively making cognitive connections leads to deep understanding and expert thinking. This explains why experts are able to see patterns and relationships of information that are not apparent to a novice learner, which is a key point that Patricia Benner makes in her description of expert nurses in her classic work, *From Novice to Expert* (Benner, 1984).

As I developed a greater understanding of human learning and developed a deep understanding of the conceptual approach, it became clear to me this was an important direction for nursing education. The generation of new knowledge within U.S. society has been exponential and will continue to accelerate. An understated skill set for nurses (and actually all healthcare providers) is information management: that is, the ability to locate, analyze, interpret, and apply information. Information management is a desired skill of lifelong learners and thus is critical for the delivery of healthcare based on current evidence. The conceptual approach offers a solution to educators with an over-burdened curriculum and to nursing graduates who achieve skills in information management though conceptual thinking.

INFORMATION MANAGEMENT

In this context, refers to the cognitive organization of new information and facts encountered by the learner.

Preparation

Following completion of my doctoral degree, and shortly after accepting a full-time faculty position, the dean made a formal request to the faculty for a revision to the undergraduate curriculum. She did not specify what it should look like but suggested that the curriculum should better prepare nurses for the rapidly changing healthcare environment—for example, increased complexity of care and integration of technology, and care coordination. Although most of my colleagues groaned at the thought of a curriculum revision, I saw this as an opportunity to apply some of my ideas about the conceptual approach to a new curriculum.

The continuum of opinion among the majority of faculty regarding a curriculum revision ranged from not doing a curriculum revision to making moderate modifications to the existing curriculum. As the outlier, I was thinking about starting with a clean slate and building something entirely new. My ideas were a radical departure from the traditional curricular approach, and I knew that convincing others would present a challenge. Using concepts as the cornerstone for the curriculum, as opposed to a medical model with an emphasis on body systems, was one example. Unfortunately, my ideas were not initially understood by others. At that time, my understanding of the conceptual approach was evolving, and thus I did not fully understand or consider the spectrum of the conceptual approach. I also lacked the ability to clearly describe to my colleagues what I was envisioning. Furthermore, examples of this work in the nursing discipline were not available.

Faculty members raised many concerns regarding a major curriculum revision such as the one I was proposing. One of the strongest arguments against a radical change was the fact that the first-time pass rate among our graduates on the National Council Licensure Examination for Registered Nurses (NCLEX-RN) was very strong—and for some, this fact alone provided sufficient evidence that revisions to the current curriculum were unnecessary. True, our first-time pass rates were high, but I wondered whether the NCLEX-RN pass rate was truly the best benchmark for success. Was it not also true that passing the NCLEX-RN was, in actuality, the minimum standard required needed to gain a nursing license?

My colleagues also argued that there was no evidence that what I was proposing would work. After all, the concept-based approach was not found in nursing education textbooks. My colleagues were justifiably skeptical because such an approach was inconsistent with the presentation of typical nursing curricula, and no evidence existed that it had been tested in nursing. This inconsistency represents a paradox for innovators: By definition, new ideas don't have evidence, yet the expectation is that standard practice is followed—particularly in academia. The only evidence I had came from the education discipline, and this was not acceptable to many of my colleagues. On the other hand, though, what evidence or proof did we have that the traditional curriculum platforms worked? How could we say we were adequately preparing nurses for the workforce? To what extent was the traditional curriculum responsible for excellent patient care by our nursing graduates?

A third argument against the conceptual approach verbalized by experienced faculty was that concept-based curricula had been used in nursing before, and it did not work. I had to do some thinking about this. Was the statement true?

Some grand nursing theories had been commonly used to guide nursing curricula in the 1970s. They were often referred to as "concept-based" because concepts used to guide the curriculum were drawn from the theory used. Concepts to support theories did not necessarily translate easily into curriculum, however, unless a great deal of work was done to either clarify the concepts or to use the theory concepts as broad concept categories with more specific concepts for learning within these. Furthermore, this approach happened decades before the science of human learning emerged. It is possible that students were exposed to abstract concepts; however, without concept-based instruction or the use of exemplars, it is unlikely that conceptual learning was routinely achieved.

I had to address these concerns before we could move forward. Had I not been persistent and persuasive, I likely would not have gotten the traction to move these ideas forward. A few faculty listened to my ideas, though, asking questions and beginning to understand—not all at once, but a little at a time. The more I discussed these ideas and explained what the conceptual approach meant, the better I was able to articulate my ideas. Over time (what might best be described as a *latency period*), I was able to gain a small group of faculty followers. And because we had the support of the dean and program directors, this was just enough support to begin the work.

The Project

The curriculum redesign was accomplished by a task force of the undergraduate curriculum committee. Because an inclusive process was desired, an initial general call invited all interested faculty to participate, regardless of the program in which they taught. An invitation for representation was also extended to our nurses from our partnering health systems and to nursing students so these important stakeholders could share in the process. Although many individuals attended off and on during the curriculum development process, approximately 10 core members regularly attended and shared the work. Values shared by the core task force members included a commitment for real change, openness to learn from other disciplines, and an overt awareness that the process would be difficult and also that we would not get it perfect the first time. These shared values ensured sustained progress toward acceptance of the curriculum.

REFLECTING ON ... HELP FROM OTHERS

- *Consider a project you are involved in. Who are the champions? Who are the challengers? What other stakeholders are available to provide input? Why is their input important?*

Innovative work involves trail blazing. We had no map or specific path to guide us, but we had a compass set to a general direction. We knew how to develop a traditional nursing curriculum, and we had a few references for concept-based curriculum from the education discipline. Thus, progression in the general direction intended depended on our ability to converge these two ideas.

Developing the Curriculum

The initial work of our task force group was dependent on gaining a greater understanding of concept-based curriculum. The work of Lynn Erikson (2002), a concept-based curriculum expert in the education discipline, and a book featuring pathophysiologic phenomena in nursing (Carrieri-Kohlman, Lindsey, & West, 2003) was especially helpful. Although details of how we developed the curriculum have previously been reported (Brady et al., 2008; Giddens et al., 2008), a general overview of the steps is presented here.

Setting a vision. Our curriculum work began by discussing, writing, and agreeing on the program description, program goals, and program outcomes. Because many members of the committee had completed these steps before with previous curriculum work, this familiar process felt safe. Setting the vision for our work in this way was helpful not only as a starting point, but also as a focal point for direction when the process became challenging.

Selecting concept categories. The first real steps to develop a concept-based curriculum were identifying and agreeing on concept categories and concepts. After much discussion, we agreed to two overarching concept categories: health and illness concepts, and professional nursing concepts. From there, we divided into two teams, each team charged with identifying concepts for each of the two categories. This proved to be very difficult work, primarily because we did not know how many concepts were the "right number," and we also lacked a clear and deep understanding of the level of concept needed; there was also a lack of clarity of the difference between exemplars and concepts. Our lack of expertise resulted in significant challenges and disagreements, which slowed the process. In some cases, we had to agree to disagree on the inclusion of some concepts just to move forward.

Developing the concepts. After concepts were selected, we began to develop the concepts using concept templates—writing a general outline of a concept presentation (definition, scope, attributes, and so on). The purpose of this work was to ensure some degree of consistency in how faculty and students would think about and use the concepts. Faculty members worked in teams to develop, review, and then approve the concepts as developed within the organizational templates.

Developing didactic and clinical courses. The next step in our process was to develop didactic and clinical courses. For the didactic courses, we agreed to an integration of populations to the concepts as opposed to an integration of concepts to population groups. This was a critical decision point because it represented a departure from our comfort zones (in our population-specific courses) and required future collaborations in teaching to ensure lifespan perspectives. Nonetheless, concern was raised that certain population groups (such as pediatric, child-bearing women, and older adults) would not be well represented in such an approach. These concerns were addressed through the careful selection of exemplars (that represented lifespan health conditions), plans for collaborative lifespan teaching, and plans for clinical education models. For example, instead of a lecture on heart failure, students would be introduced to the concept of perfusion and then would be engaged in various student-centered learning activities (such as pair and share, case study, or jigsaw) to learn about heart failure as an exemplar of perfusion. Clinical courses were envisioned as a mechanism for students to apply health and illness concepts and professional nursing concepts in the context of care with a shift in focus from a patient's specific medical condition to the response of the patient and family, resulting from health conditions and the appropriate nursing care indicated. This required designing specific learning activities for clinical education and changing the ritualistic approach in a decades-old clinical education model.

Managing Conflict and Opening the Lines of Communication

As our task force group worked, we gained greater understanding and commitment to what was being created; such commitment was essential to managing conflict. It was essential that we recognized and acknowledged when full agreement among task force members was unattainable but then found a way to move forward (sometimes by agreeing to disagree) as opposed to becoming immobilized by discontent. We also maintained awareness that some ideas might not work out as planned, and thus we challenged ourselves to remain open to reconsidering decisions. This mindset gave task force members permission to reevaluate processes when needed and not label such situations as mistakes or indecisiveness, but rather address unknown variables along the way.

REFLECTING ON ... HOW TO GET BUY-IN FOR YOUR IDEAS

- *Think of a time you wanted to try something new and your idea was not initially accepted. What would you do differently to gain acceptance?*

- *If you were to introduce a radically new idea in your organization, who are the key individuals that would need to be accepting of your idea? How would you gain their support?*

One of the greatest challenges, however, was addressing ongoing concerns verbalized by faculty not involved in the work. It was very difficult to understand what we were doing by looking in from the outside. Despite the fact that our task force meetings were open, it was rare when non–task force members attended. Knowing that a degree of faculty resistance existed and also that we needed to have the curriculum approved by the faculty, we began a very purposeful yearlong communication campaign to provide multiple avenues for faculty comment. We asked for time on the agenda at every faculty business meeting and held a series of special faculty forums to provide updates and opportunities for dialogue, with the specific intent to educate, answer questions, and address concerns. Furthermore, we regularly shared curriculum documents with all faculty via email with requests for comments, input, and feedback. Although it initially seemed that the issues and concerns raised by faculty were insurmountable, the strategy for open and regular communication provided an opportunity to address concerns and misunderstandings and also clarify perceptions. Regular communication and requests for input also defused the illusion that work was being done in secrecy and represented regular sensitizing doses to the innovative ideas found in the concept-based curriculum. *Critical mass* is a term used to describe the general level of acceptance needed for an innovation to be successful (Rogers, 2003). In this case, the communication campaign contributed to a critical mass of faculty acceptance and paved the way for curriculum approval.

REFLECTING ON ... CRITICAL MASS

- *Critical mass is a concept used to describe the amount of support needed to move forward with a decision. How do you know when critical mass has been achieved? How do you respond to those who remain against the idea after critical mass has been achieved?*

Outcomes

As one might expect, the implementation of a concept-based curriculum was associated with significant challenges due to an initial lack of understanding of the conceptual approach and the initial lack of expertise in conceptual teaching strategies among our faculty. However, the undergraduate committee and faculty who shared this work remained committed from the beginning. As the curriculum implementation progressed, the commitment, passion, and collaboration among faculty grew stronger. Student program outcomes were met, pass rates on the NCLEX-RN remained consistent with national standards, and student satisfaction remained high (Giddens & Morton, 2010).

Although the initial development of the concept-based curriculum at my university occurred several years ago, the impact has been substantial. Faculty from our nursing program disseminated this innovative work through presentations and publications leading to widespread interest. The release of the Institute of Medicine's *Future of Nursing* (IOM, 2011) and Benner's *Educating Nurses* (Benner, Sutphen, Leonard, & Day, 2010) further fueled interest in this approach, partly because of the close alignment in the call for educational change. Subsequently, there has been a significant proliferation of nursing schools adopting the conceptual approach, particularly for prelicensure nursing education; in fact, the conceptual approach has been adopted for many regional and statewide curriculum plans. Interest in the conceptual approach has gained momentum because it addresses several issues for nurse educators (particularly content saturation in the curriculum), but more importantly, nursing graduates are better equipped to enter the complex healthcare system because of their conceptual thinking skills. Long-term outcomes are yet to be determined, and so the story continues to be written!

Recommendations

One thing that has been gained from the initial and subsequent work is a deep appreciation for differences and recognizing the value of dissenting opinion. Dissension is often viewed from a negative perspective; it is annoying and can actually be quite painful when people don't agree with you. The gift of dissenting opinion emerges when you are forced to reflect on the alternative perspective and be open to the possibility that the dissenting view may hold value and can ultimately improve the outcome. This leads to a second major area of learning—seeking advice from stakeholders who are not the "usual suspects." All too often, we stay in a comfortable zone, asking advice and seeking from those who look like us and think like us. Diversity of thought—to include those outside your discipline, your projected area of impact, and your cultural group—can open your eyes to things you might have never considered.

The long-term future for concept curriculum is unknown. As more programs adopt this approach, possibly an authoritative board will recommend a standardized list of concepts. Also, possibly future interprofessional education (IPE) models will be built on a similar concept platform. Currently, many IPE courses or events focus on quality and safety, the only two concepts common to practice among all healthcare professionals. Could core IPE courses be developed with central and consistent understandings across all healthcare disciplines?

Final Reflections

Innovative work is extremely challenging. To be successful, you must have vision as well as the courage to try things even when not sure, trust in your instincts, and be willing to accept the possibility of failure. One of the greatest lessons learned from this work is that collaboration, commitment, reflection, and persistence are key behaviors for success. One of the most surprising and rewarding discoveries was the power of collective engagement. As faculty gained greater understanding, they became engaged; as engagement spread, a further commitment toward the project and toward others grew, leading to enhanced cooperation. Working together in this way produced a palpable energy and transformed the faculty to an innovative identity.

References

Benner, P. (1984). *From novice to expert*. Menlo Park, CA: Addison Wesley.

Benner, P., Sutphen, M., Leonard, V., & Day, L. (2010). *Educating nurses: A call for radical transformation*. San Francisco, CA: Jossey-Bass.

Brady, D., Brown, P., Smith, D., Giddens, J., Harris, J., Wright, M., & Nichols, R. (2008). Staying afloat: Surviving a curriculum change. *Nurse Educator, 33*(5), 198–201.

Bransford J. D., Brown, A. L., & Cocking, R. R. (2000). *How people learn: Brain, mind, experience, and school*. Washington, DC: National Academies Press.

Carrieri-Kohlman, V., Lindsey, A. M., & West, C. M. (2003). *Pathophysiological phenomena in nursing: Human response to illness* (3rd ed.). Philadelphia, PA: Saunders.

Erikson, L. (2002). *Concept-based curriculum and instruction*. Thousand Oaks, CA: Corwin Press.

Giddens, J., Brady, D., Brown, P., Wright, M., Smith, D., & Harris, J. (2008). A new curriculum for a new era of nursing education. *Nursing Education Perspectives*, *29*(4), 200–204.

Giddens, J., Caputi, L., & Rodgers, B. (2015). *Mastering concept-based teaching: A guide for nurse educators*. St. Louis, MO: Elsevier.

Giddens, J., & Morton, N. (2010). Report card: An evaluation of a concept-based curriculum. *Nursing Education Perspectives*, *31*(6), 372–377.

Institute of Medicine. (2011). *The future of nursing: Leading change, advancing health*. Washington, DC: National Academies Press.

Rogers, E. (2003). *Diffusion of innovations*. New York, NY: Free Press.

Chapter 5

Transformation of Teaching and Learning Through Debriefing for Meaningful Learning

Kristina Thomas Dreifuerst, PhD, RN, CNE, ANEF
Cynthia Sherraden Bradley, MSN, RN

Learning to think like a nurse is a challenging yet necessary process for students in prelicensure nursing education programs. Thinking like a nurse involves developing higher-order cognitive processes, including clinical judgment, clinical decision-making, and clinical reasoning. Curriculum is designed to assist students in the attainment of foundational knowledge, skills, and attitudes that novice nurses can use to launch their clinical practice and think like a nurse. Within the learning environments, faculty commonly use simulation as a pedagogy because they are able to easily manipulate the simulation to fit the curricular objectives and have it become whatever situation the student needs to experience, ultimately (and hopefully) resulting in meaningful learning.

DEBRIEFING

A teaching-learning process used by a facilitator with learners after a clinical or simulation learning experience where the student and teachers revisit the experience (Cantrell, 2008; Dreifuerst, 2009; Fanning & Gaba, 2007). Identified as the most significant component of simulation-based learning, debriefing is the time at the end of a simulation experience for learners to reexamine and think deeply on their simulation experience through guided reflection (Cantrell, 2004; Decker et al., 2013; Dreifuerst & Decker, 2012; Fanning & Gaba, 2007; Shinnick, Woo, Horwich, & Steadman, 2011). While the attributes of simulation debriefing include reflection, emotion, reception, integration, and assimilation (Dreifuerst, 2009), the hallmark of simulation debriefing is the reflective, bidirectional, interactive discussion between a facilitator and learners (Cheng et al., 2014).

Additionally, through debriefing, simulation becomes an opportunity to actively learn and develop a reflective practice (Shön, 1983). Reflection is an important developmental step in thinking, which potentiates metacognition, necessary for clinical reasoning, as the hallmark of the expert nurse (Benner, Sutphen, Leonard, & Day, 2010; Fowler, 1997; Pesut, 2004). Debriefing for Meaningful Learning (DML) is an active learning method that facilitates student development of clinical reasoning (Dreifuerst, 2012; Mariani, Cantrell, Meakim, Prieto, & Dreifuerst, 2012). This method, underpinned with concepts from experiential learning theory, reflective learning theory, and transformative learning theory, can make a difference in teaching and learning in nursing education. This chapter will describe how the use of DML in different settings can transform teaching and learning and foster thinking like a nurse.

Setting the Stage

Experiential learning, reflective learning, and transformative learning are constructs that underpin active teaching and learning. *Experiential learning* is not only knowledge created through the process of doing something, but also learning through reflecting on doing (Kolb, Boyatzis, & Mainemelis, 2001). In simulation, just as in clinical experiences, students have an opportunity to do both. Knowledge is created through the experience of being in the clinical simulation and through an opportunity for guided reflection through debriefing.

Reflection-in-Action

Similarly, learning to become a reflective nurse emphasizes reflection *in*, *on*, and *beyond* action, which are central tenets of reflective learning and the theory of reflection (Dreifuerst, 2009; Mann, Gordon, & MacLeod, 2009; Schön, 1983). Nurses often *reflect in-action* contextually while in their professional role. Teachers observing students describe this as "seeing the wheels turning" when the novices are putting together assessment findings, clinical judgments, and actioned decisions within the clinical situation (Dreifuerst, 2013). With experience, however, can come decreased awareness of reflection-in-action by individual nurses, yet more evidence of it is seen in their practice (Shön, 1983). Experienced nurses may not even be aware of engaging in reflection-in-action, yet in their practice, assimilation and accommodation are evident in each progressive patient situation that they encounter (Dreifuerst, 2009).

Assimilation theory (Ausubel, Novak, & Hanesian, 1986) describes the relationship between meaningful learning and the association of new meaning with existing frames, as the information in the new (clinical) situation is related to or adopted within what the nurse knows or has previously experienced. *Accommodation*, the complementary process to assimilation, occurs when the concepts from the existing frame do not fit and must be adapted to address the new (clinical) situation (Piaget, 1954). As nurses gain experience, each patient encounter is consciously or unconsciously put into

REFLECTION-IN-ACTION

The opportunity to focus on the thinking processes that were occurring in the moment during an experience (Schon, 1983). Guiding a learner to reflect-in-action requires Socratic questioning by the teacher to uncover the thinking processes and frames that influenced the decision-making process during the time of the action.

the existing frame during reflection-in-action and then adopted or adapted to meet the current context. This assimilation or accommodation process can be highly successful unless the existing frame has errors in the taken-for-granted assumptions because these errors are then carried into the new situation (Paget, 2001).

Although errors associated with taken-for-granted assumptions are more commonly seen in student and novice nurses, they are not limited to them: Seasoned nurses can also experience positive reinforcement errors in judgment. These types of errors lead to frames of reference with erroneous assumptions embedded within them. Unless someone challenges and corrects these errors, they will continue to incorrectly influence the thinking and clinical decisions nurses make. An emergency department (ED) nurse, Robert, describes this well:

> *During my orientation to the ED, I was precepted by the same nurse, Janice, most of the first month I worked there. She was an experienced nurse who had been working in this ED for more than 20 years. She moved through the shifts effortlessly, and I desperately wanted to be like that, so I followed and copied everything she did.*
>
> *We saw a lot of children and anxious adults in this facility, and using two identifiers could be challenging. Janice had a practice of putting one identification band on the patient and one on the bed or gurney. That way, we could scan two bands and satisfy the identifier clause even if the patient could not or would not communicate with us. It became such a standard practice that at some point, I stopped asking patients to confirm identity verbally after putting the band on their wrist or ankle because that was how Janice practiced. Every unit audit of patient identifiers lauded the excellent compliance of the ED, a leader in the organization for this important patient safety initiative.*

Further, each double-scan of the identification bands confirmed this practice for me, and I got so used to it that sometimes I would even scan the identification band on the bed twice if I had been caring for the patient all shift and visually recognized him or her rather than try to fish the person's wrist or ankle from under the sheets and blankets. I did this for years and honestly never gave it a second thought. That all changed, however, in a tragic way.

In the middle of the winter, I was working a double shift because my relief could not make it in due to hazardous road conditions. We got slammed that night as motor vehicle accident after motor vehicle accident occurred. A bus of high school girls basketball players went into the ditch, and 11 of the players were admitted with varying degrees of injury. I was assigned 4 of them and got them settled into four adjoining bays. They all had their team warm-up on, hair braided in similar ways, and 3 were blonde.

Everything was going fine, and I even got a quick break to have some coffee to keep me awake. When I returned, my co-worker advised me that a player in Bay 3 had nausea and vomiting while I was gone, but my co-worker had taken care of it and administered an antiemetic. Even though the patient was due for pain medication, my colleague said she held it to let the antiemetic take effect, so [the pain medication] was still due. Sure enough, the patient in Bay 3 was complaining of pain. I got the medication from the Pyxis and noted that it had been 15 minutes since the antiemetic was administered. The patient had no allergies according to the electronic MAR. I looked at the blonde girl in the bed and visually confirmed I knew her as Amanda, the patient in Bay 3. Then I scanned the identification band on the bed twice and administered the medication intravenously. Within

10 minutes, the patient had acute anaphylaxis, and a code was called. She was successfully treated.

As I was continuing to monitor her and trying to process what had just occurred, several of the teammates came to the door of Bay 3 and asked whether Allison was going to be okay. But wait, I thought … this wasn't Allison—she was in Bay 4. This was Amanda. I pulled the EMR closer and confirmed that we were documenting the resuscitation on patient Amanda. Then I looked up the census, and in horror, realized that Amanda was listed in Bay 5—there was no patient in Bay 4, and Allison was listed in Bay 3. How could that be true?

I looked at the identification bracelet on the bed, and it read Amanda. I grabbed for the bracelet on the patient, and it read Allison. My heart raced, and I tried to process it all. It made no sense! I knew that I personally had put the bracelets on the patients and also on the end of the beds and that I had carefully matched them. A second later, I realized that Allison had a known allergy to the pain medication I had given her, thinking that she was Amanda.

Later, after my error was reported, as a part of the root cause analysis (RCA) process, I learned that while I was on break, Amanda had vomited all over her bed. She also complained that it was so noisy she could not rest, and so my colleagues had moved her to quieter Bay 5 (without her bed), located at the end of the hallway. Bay 3 was quickly cleaned because they next realized they needed to move Allison to Bay 3 because a patient en route to the ED needed equipment available only in Bay 4. (That patient died before arriving.) As a result, the staff walked Allison next door into the freshly cleaned Bay 3, and she climbed into the bed that Amanda had previously occupied. In the haste of cleaning, the identification band listing Amanda's information was not removed from the bed in Bay 3, and the census switch in the computer was made by the Unit Secretary after I had given the wrong patient the medication. Both girls had similar build, coloring, clothes, and hairstyles. My visual identification did not discriminate between them, and by not scanning the band attached to the patient but only the one attached to the bed, I misidentified the patient to whom I was administering medications.

The RCA also determined that a majority of ED staff used this identification process, particularly the ones whom Janice had oriented. Although we were not aware of other errors that occurred from this procedure, clearly they were in the realm of possibility. Further, the RCA team recounted numerous stories from staff about how using this identification process was positively reinforced and therefore continued without any thought or reflection on what might be wrong with this assumption.

In this example, Robert speaks retrospectively about the situation but is able to articulate decision points and judgments during the scenario that were critical to what occurred. This is often the case with reflection-in-action. It is difficult to capture in the moment to teach novice nurses how to be aware of it. Often it is identified and shared retrospectively and is difficult for novices to discern from reflection-on-action.

REFLECTING ON ... REFLECTION-IN-ACTION

- *Knowing how difficult it is to demonstrate reflection-in-action to students, think of times where it is apparent that you can describe during preconference or preparation time to help students to be mindful or aware of this type of reflection during their clinical time.*

- *Recall a clinical experience that you as a teacher had which was important to you. Reflect-on-action about the particulars of that experience. Why is it one that you remember?*

REFLECTION-ON-ACTION

Retrospectively looking back at an experience to critically re-examine the thinking processes, interpretations, and responses during that experience (Schon, 1983; Tanner, 2007). Reflection-on-action includes reflection on the understanding that was implicit during the time of the action as well as the cues, frames, and prior experiences that influenced how the current situation was viewed.

Reflection-on-Action

Comparatively, however, *reflection-on-action* most definitely occurs after the fact. Nurses commonly describe reflecting on their day as they head home from work or when awakening during the night. This reflection is not only a recollection of events but also often an opportunity to revisit judgments, decisions, and actions that occurred. Reflection-on-action can also be thought of as the "coulda, woulda, shoulda" period of reflection as nurses describe alternatives to what they recollect occurred given that they are also engaged in sense-making and mindfulness which can transform thinking and learning from the episode of care (Dreifuerst, Horton-Deutsch, & Henao, 2014). Mary, a nurse who had been working in a busy oncology inpatient unit, describes one episode of reflection-on-action when she talks about caring for a patient named William, who experienced nausea and vomiting in addition to shaking chills several hours after receiving chemotherapy.

> *I was on the way home that evening. I was sitting in traffic and recalling how sick my patient William had become that day and how the last few patients who had received that therapeutic regime had very few symptoms. I was bothered by how quickly William was overcome with nausea and vomiting and also how his shaking chills concerned me despite his being afebrile. But then I got home from work, and my family needs absorbed my thoughts and attention, and I quickly put William out of my mind.*

That night as I was retiring to bed, I quietly wished for an easier day tomorrow at work and was relieved to fall asleep as my head hit the pillow. During the night, however, I woke suddenly and remembered that William and I had talked about the availability of PRN diphenhydramine and ondansetron, which he had agreed to take prior to the chemotherapy. However, before I could go and get those premedications, I got called away to another patient, and when I returned to William, I just gave him the chemotherapy agents. Shortly, he exhibited severe side effects.

I never gave those premedications, even though I know it is a good idea to do so, and William agreed to take them. In fact, I always give them; it is just what I do. It is my routine. I can't even believe that I did not give them to William and did not even realize it. That is why he got so sick! I just completely forgot, and it never crossed my mind again until right now. Clearly the fact that remembering woke me from a sound sleep is my brain telling me something important. All of that misery he went through was preventable, and it was my responsibility.

This revisiting of a clinical situation and sense-making demonstrates the power of reflection-on-action. Mary will remember the severity of William's response to her inaction and add it to the frame of her thinking, awareness, and understanding of giving chemotherapy drugs to patients. In fact, she later says, "I do this (give chemotherapy) so often that I was starting to do it by rote: you know, assuming and not thinking attentively. Just going through the motions really. Since William, however, I find that I am actively thinking and asking myself to go through almost a checklist with every patient. Like, 'Did I do this? Yep, check. Did I do that? Yep, check.' It has changed everything about how I attend to and pay attention in my practice despite the fact that it has become routine."

REFLECTING ON ... REFLECTION-ON-ACTION

- *Think about reflection-in-action and reflection-on-action. How would you describe these concepts to your students? Develop a sentence or two that you can use consistently in your teaching practice.*

- *The ability to reflect-on-action is dependent on prior experiences. As such, it is also a characteristic of a more experienced student. Think about ways to use reflection-on-action differently as students matriculate in your program.*

REFLECTION-BEYOND-ACTION

Involves anticipation in tandem with reflection, drawing the learner to think beyond the current situation in anticipation of a future encounter based on prior experience. Reflection-beyond-action is looking ahead while concurrently reflecting on the past (Dreifuerst, 2009).

Reflection-Beyond-Action

Transformative learning can also be evident in *reflection-beyond-action,* which represents the relationship between reflection and anticipation (Dreifuerst, 2009). Anticipation and reflection are complementary and dependent concepts of reference. Anticipation is based on reflection and reflection on anticipation. Reflection-beyond-action can be associated with the practice exemplified by expert nurses that has been referred to by other terms like intuition (Benner, 1984; Dreifuerst, 2009). For example, upon hearing details in report on a new patient, the expert nurse is already calling upon existing frames of reference and formulating a mental image of what to anticipate or expect during the assessment, planning, and implementation phases of care based on reflection of prior experiences and knowledge. Things that fit the mental frame are assimilated, and those that don't require thoughtful accommodation (Ausubel, Novak, & Hanesian, 1986; Piaget, 1954).

Time and an expansive cadre of experiences were once precursors to the development of the expert nurse, and this evolution often took 8 to 10 years or longer (Benner, 1984). This time frame, however, is not always possible today. It is not uncommon for the most senior nurses in the work environment to have fewer than 5 years of experience. This could be worrisome, yet in the clinical environment, nurses who have only a few years of experience can demonstrate expert practice. Likewise, highly experienced nurses can be known to practice at novice or competent levels for their entire career.

Because time on the job is not the only precursor to expert nursing practice, educators need to thoughtfully consider how to prepare students to potentiate this expertise. One option may be to develop the skill of anticipation. It is possible to teach student and novice nurses anticipation by making reflection-beyond-action explicit (Dreifuerst, 2012). Using debriefing methods like DML, the teacher moves from reflecting-on-action with the clinical or simulation experience that has just occurred to guiding the discussion into anticipation by creating a parallel scenario with unique details that is then processed as assimilation and accommodation transpire through Socratic discussion. In this way, reflection-beyond-action is modeled, imitated, and reinforced by relating the details of the new clinical situation to information that the novice knows and has experienced. Each experience then transforms the frame in a process of expansion and contraction of thought processes that build into experiential cognitive knowledge. A student nurse, Chris, and her clinical teacher, Renee, demonstrate reflection-beyond-action as they prepare to receive report at the start of their shift through Renee's recollection of the events.

Chris received her clinical assignment the night before and came to her third shift of clinical prepared to care for a 68-year-old female with pneumonia during her first clinical course on an inpatient medical floor in a community hospital. I caught Chris coming out of the locker room and pulled her aside to share that the patient she was assigned to care for that day had been transferred to the ICU during the night, so she (Chris) would need to care for a different patient. I had scanned the patient information on the census and saw that a 90-year-old male was admitted with complications from the flu and assigned him as an alternative patient for Chris to care for. Upon hearing this news,

Chris was flabbergasted and spit out, "But, Renee, I can't care for that patient. I prepared for a patient with viral pneumonia. I don't know how to care for a patient with the flu!"

I reassured Chris, and together we sat down for a few minutes to reflect-beyond-action. I remember walking Chris through the similarities and differences between viral pneumonia and the flu using her textbook and a Google search. We also talked about taking care of a 68-year-old female versus a 90-year-old male. Using Socratic questioning and guided reflection, I helped Chris to use the knowledge acquired in the classroom and from her clinical experiences the last 2 weeks to think about what would be the same about caring for the patient she anticipated and prepared for versus the one she would now have and what would be different. Chris took a few minutes to plan for what she needed to quickly review and look up before starting her shift and adjusted her plan of care for the experience. I observed Chris talking with several nurses throughout the shift about what happened and noted their conversation about what an important learning lesson this thinking on your feet and putting together what you know to face what you don't know was for novice nurses to have.

During post-conference, I had Chris share her experience with her peers and was pleasantly surprised at how well Chris talked about her fears at first and then, with my assistance, guided the class through how nurses anticipate and prepare for taking care of different types of patients as a part of their practice. It was a transformative experience for everyone and led to a discussion about when we as a clinical group would be transitioning away from preparing the night before clinical and how that would be done safely.

Renee's example is just one way transformative learning occurs within nursing education. This type of learning can be apparent in classroom, simulation, and clinical laboratory settings also. Orchestrating transformative learning experiences can be deliberate or serendipitous on the part of the instructor. When intentional, these experiences can have a significant impact on learning to think like a nurse.

REFLECTING ON ... REFLECTION-BEYOND-ACTION

- *Teaching reflection-beyond-action requires creating parallel situations for students to intentionally assimilate or accommodate while challenging their assumptions. Think of a recent clinical experience with a student and create a parallel case you could use to teach students the relationship between anticipation and reflection. Reflect on your own nursing practice. What are specific times you recall actively reflecting-beyond-action? How might you use those examples to further explicate this difficult concept to novices who are often concrete thinkers?*

Transformative Learning

Transformative learning is the process of challenging taken-for-granted assumptions or frames of reference in a manner that makes these frames more discriminate, inclusive, contextual, and reflective so that they warrant actioned decisions (Slavich & Zimbardo, 2012). Transformative learning theory includes the process of creating new habits of mind. This process can occur from repetition or practice, but it can also be prompted through reflection. For Mary, the experience with William transformed her approach to patient care from a passive thinking routine where she assumed that she always did something to an experience of active learning. For Robert, the experience with Amanda and Allison challenged his taken-for-granted assumptions on the practice of patient identification and transformed how he approached this process. For Renee, Chris, and the rest of the clinical students, learning that patient care transcends preparing to care for an individual to how patterns of care develop into thinking like a nurse was transformative in how they thought about clinical experiences going forward.

Traditionally, nursing educators often use passive teaching and learning environments in prelicensure programs. In *passive learning*, the students read and come to classes where predominantly they experience teacher lectures and dictated information and answers that lead to one thought process and second-hand knowledge. It is so familiar you can almost envision it. Learners sit, listen, take notes, memorize, and absorb all pertinent information and often silo it into individual and unrelated concepts much like Chris did with her thinking about the care of a patient with pneumonia. The results of such classes are often measured by multiple choice or true/false questions, and/or questions that require memorized answers. Little or no comparing, analyzing, hypothesizing, generalizing, or synthesizing occurs, yet these are both antecedents and referents of clinical reasoning.

Active Learning

Now, contrast passive learning with active teaching and learning environments where learners come prepared and are required to be engaged in the process. In *active learning*, reading must be done prior to class so that the student is prepared for the activities that ensue. Discussion is key, interaction is necessary, and reflection is encouraged and modeled. Moreover, activities in the class are designed to confront learners with their knowledge and skill levels, challenge their assumptions, and promote interaction with information in order to learn transformatively. In fact, in active teaching/learning environments, educators often model a way of thinking and interacting with information for a student through the process of information sharing.

Collins and O'Brien (2003) define active learning as

> *... the process of having students engage in some activity that forces them to reflect upon ideas and how they are using those ideas. It requires students to regularly assess their own degree of understanding and skill at handling concepts or problems in a particular discipline; attainment of knowledge by participating or contributing. The process of keeping students mentally, and often physically, active in their learning through activities that involves them in gathering information, thinking and problem solving. (p. 6)*

Turning traditional teaching and learning environments in nursing education into gateways of active learning can be facilitated by some of the lessons learned from clinical teaching in traditional environments, simulation, and debriefing. Positive outcomes from learning experiences using simulation in nursing are increasing (Hayden, Smiley, Alexander, Kardong-Edgren, & Jeffries, 2014), but the literature is limited in its generalizability because of the variation in the structure, objectives, and implementation of simulation. The same could be said for teaching and learning of nursing content within and between programs. Teachers struggle with how to create significant learning experiences in a way that is consistent so that incremental student learning can occur with each subsequent exposure, in simulated and traditional clinical learning environments. One way to embrace consistency is by adopting a consistent debriefing method throughout the simulation experiences in the curriculum.

DML is one method of debriefing that has demonstrated positive outcomes in the development of clinical reasoning (Dreifuerst, 2012; Mariani et al., 2012). DML is a faculty-facilitated debriefing method that uses Socratic questioning and a consistent process to teach and model comparing, analyzing, hypothesizing, generalizing, and synthesizing in a contextual frame. Worksheets guide the discussion and provide for *double-loop* teaching and learning processes to occur as teachers write and diagram the discussion on a whiteboard during debriefing while students do the same on copies of the worksheets. Reading, writing, thinking, and dialoguing occur concurrently as the teacher orchestrates the discussion into an active learning experience and helps students reflect in, on, and beyond action to unpeel the students' thinking related to the clinical experience they just engaged in.

Transforming Teaching

Teachers and students can use simulation and debriefing as an opportunity to develop clinical reasoning skills. Known best practices, evident in DML, include debriefing by a facilitator educated in the debriefing process and using discussion techniques that promote an open environment, confidentiality, self-reflection, assessment, and analysis (Decker et al. 2013). Debriefing should be conducted by someone who observed the simulation, be based on the objectives of the learning experience, use a structured framework, and encourage students to challenge taken-for-granted assumptions through active learning principles (Decker et al., 2013; Dreifuerst & Decker, 2012). Through DML, teachers and students can meet all these criteria. Many examples of DML are in the literature, and DML was most recently used by schools participating in the National Council of State Boards of Nursing (NCSBN) National Simulation Study (Hayden et al., 2014). Teachers involved in that study had an opportunity to reflect on the experience; many described the impact of using DML as transformational for teaching and learning in their programs. It is challenging to describe the powerful nature of transformational teaching and learning and attribute it to one particular intervention or method, but debriefing can transcend exigent explanations and provide a medium that depicts it. One story is shared here.

> As a new simulation director in a school of nursing, I was given the task of integrating simulation throughout the existing nursing curriculum. Because I was unfamiliar with the simulation pedagogy, I began to search for resources to support the development of a structured simulation program. Due to a shortage of clinical sites, the number of clinical hours using simulation was to be increased substantially within our program. In my strategy for developing a new simulation program, I was most concerned with maintaining the current standards of the present clinical education curriculum.

> I readily found resources for scenarios, moulage, props, and support for the technical aspects of teaching in the simulation setting. What I did not easily find was a method for what I likened to a post-clinical conference: a method for ensuring that students were leaving a simulation experience having achieved learning objectives similar to that of the clinical setting. Unlike the clinical setting, where a clinical group may encounter multiple diagnoses, in simulation, each student plans and provides care for a simulated patient with the same diagnosis. This difference prompted my search for a method or process to guide a process akin to post-clinical conference within this standardized environment.

While I knew that debriefing was an important component of a simulation learning experience, I was unsure of how to conduct an effective debriefing with students. As I began to inquire about existing debriefing models that local educators found valuable, I heard of two schools of nursing using DML in conjunction with the NCSBN national simulation study. After reaching out to Dr. Dreifuerst, I attended her DML workshop and began to implement the method with students while modeling DML to other simulation educators in my program. Because of my enthusiasm about the resulting changes that I witnessed in students' ability to deeply think and reflect in simulation, my program hosted a city-wide DML workshop with Dr. Dreifuerst to provide training for educators within my program and throughout the city.

As a collective learning organization, the impact of implementing DML was tangible. We first used DML in post-simulation debriefing for one semester; we then used DML in the clinical setting the following semester. Educators who previously had no structure to their debriefing in both settings were equipped with a framework that facilitated guided reflection for the students. Experienced educators expressed that they were seeing first-semester nursing students make connections between theory and practice with greater speed and increased depth, which further deepened and expanded thinking in the following semesters. New educators familiar with active learning and reflection now felt "all the pieces came together" in one teaching method and felt equipped to truly facilitate learning through an exhaustive and in-depth debriefing process. Many educators reported previously using elements present in DML in their "teaching style," yet following this method completely provided structure and "it made sense and seemed so obvious" in guiding a student through nurse thinking strategies.

As we began to visibly witness students making these profound connections between theory and practice, our perspective of the simulation pedagogy changed significantly. This perspective led to refining our simulation program; the ability of the student to reflect in-action, on-action, and beyond-action provided the impetus for designing more specific learning objectives, carefully constructing and revising scenarios, and thoughtfully facilitating scenarios based on our new perspective. Prior to using DML, simulation educators lacked consistency in debriefing methods, which was evident among students, particularly as they moved from course to course and semester to semester. Students became accustomed to the elements of structured, reflective thinking, promoting familiarity and knowing what to expect in debriefing; this greatly minimized anxiety and fear of the unknown while at the same time expanding their deep thinking.

Before the DML implementation, students were often assigned to write reflective journal entries post-simulation. After implementing DML, students' reflective journaling exhibited a richer nature, demonstrating a deeper connection and a more profound understanding of nursing content and supporting rationale. Previously, students may have been noted to perform correctly in a simulation scenario, but it was not discovered until students were debriefed that there was little or no understanding of why they implemented nursing interventions during a scenario. DML provided a framework for exposing students' lack of thought processes or erroneous thought processes; these thinking and reasoning processes would still be unknown without a method for making visible what was previously hidden.

What was most surprising was witnessing all manner of educators readily adapting to using DML in a variety of nursing programs: the highly organized and structured faculty as well as the spontaneous and eclectic-thinking faculty. Even the naysayers who began with trepidation and a lack of enthusiasm embraced reflective teaching quickly. Using DML in simulation debriefing also exposed a lack of structure to clinical post-conference. Much of this was driven by the expectations of students. Indeed, many educators within our organization and in surrounding programs have extended these principles beyond simulation into clinical and didactic teaching and learning environments because of the positive outcomes witnessed by both teacher and learner.

Whereas traditional lecture with sundry PowerPoint slides may have been the prominent and familiar teaching method in the past, the Socratic and reflective questioning style began to appear in multiple learning environments after DML was introduced in the school. Although guiding students through the processes of reflection-in-action and reflection-on-action may have been unfamiliar and intimidating initially, the results seen in the thinking processes of the students was undeniable. Lectures that may have occurred, inadvertently or not, during a simulation debriefing or a clinical post-conference were increasingly replaced with guiding reflective thought, facilitating a sense of wonderment, and thoughtful questioning. There were challenges to this, however. Teachers need to be prepared for this type of in-depth discussion and may have to refresh their understanding of the underlying pathophysiology and pharmacology driving nursing care. In many ways, then, because of DML, deep thinking was happening for both students and teachers.

Guiding students through reflection-beyond-action seemed to be particularly challenging for educators to learn. A solution for lessening this pain was to practice debriefing among educators. Trialing a variety of clinical situations that extended beyond a specific scenario provided experience in stretching our own reflection-beyond-action and equipped educators with possibilities to implement with students. Engaging students in reflection-beyond-action then became a rather competitive and fun art among faculty in challenging each other with alternative scenarios to propose to students.

What was most astonishing to me was the clarity that a structured reflective thinking process brought to my own thinking, both professionally and personally. As a nurse educator, engaging in DML exposed my misconceptions about learners and equipped me to ask more questions and give fewer answers. As a result, I began to see learners truly learn through increased self-regulation and a higher level of motivation. Rather than thinking I needed to impart knowledge and content, I became a facilitator of learners developing their own thinking and reasoning processes. On a personal level, I noticed that I began to ask more questions, assume less, and withhold judgment. This debriefing method promotes a type of childlike wonder and questioning that is possible to facilitate in any age group and in multiple settings.

In this example, the teacher identifies that the transformation of teaching is associated with embracing the role of facilitator of learning. This transformation not only changes the dynamic of the teaching/learning environment but also changes the relationships among teacher, learner, and learning. Students also articulate their perceptions of this transformation.

Transforming Learning

To gain insight into the students' experience with DML, we asked several of them to describe their experience using it and what aspects they found useful and challenging. We also asked them to describe how using DML influenced their thinking or facilitated their learning and how it influenced the way they interact with patients. And finally, we asked what they learned about themselves from using DML. Clearly, every student will have a unique experience with DML; however, we identified some common themes, including learning the power of anticipating and questioning as well as challenging assumptions. We start with Jamie, a junior nursing student in a traditional BSN program.

About 2 weeks before my clinical group's first simulation experience, Ms. Brown, our clinical teacher, introduced us to

DML. She described DML to us in a clinical post-conference, and then we walked through it together in the next post-conference using two students' patients for the day. It was really confusing, actually, and I was glad we were not using my patient because I felt like that student was on the hot seat and getting a lot of questions from Ms. Brown. Actually, we all were getting questioned a lot more than we were used to, and it made me nervous. The next week, the whole simulation experience was a range of emotions. I was nervous and excited. The simulator was really cool, and the equipment was very realistic during the orientation, so I was feeling confident.

But, when it was my turn to be the nurse, nothing went right. I could not hear the lungs, and I could not understand the patient speaking very much. I wasn't sure what I was supposed to pretend to do and what I was supposed to actually do. It felt very unrealistic and disappointing. The debriefing was rough. I was really nervous when Ms. Brown started asking me questions about what I was thinking and why I did things. I panicked because I thought if she is asking me, then it must have been wrong, so I doubted myself—only to find out in the discussion that I was right after all.

We had simulation every other week the rest of the semester, and we used DML to debrief. I got really comfortable with the worksheets and the way the conversation would go. The questioning did not bother me so much, and by the last simulation day, we were all asking the questions instead of just Ms. Brown.

I guess DML made me learn to ask questions of myself and others. She called it "thinking like a nurse," so I learned that nurses question as they think. I also learned to anticipate the questions that might be asked, and so I learned to insert questions into how I talked with patients and families to be sure I had their perspective in my train of thought. I have learned to be confident

*and that when I am questioned about what I do in patient
situations, it does not necessarily mean I did something wrong.
That is a big change.*

Because Jamie was a novice student to clinical and simulation, everything
was new, and so the learning curve was steep and anxiety high. This situation
is not uncommon for students who are early in their nursing program. As they
progress, however, students not only think differently, but also they may face less
anxiety when they approach new situations because they have experienced them
before. Lisa, a senior nursing student in a traditional BSN program, refers to this
in her responses.

*This was my third semester using DML. As a junior, we used it
first semester for simulation debriefing and second semester for
simulation and traditional clinical post-conference debriefing.
This year, I am a senior, and I have a preceptor clinical, not an
instructor from the school. I was so excited to start this clinical! It
is at [name of hospital] on [name of patient care unit], and I want
to get a job here after graduation, so I was thrilled to get my first
choice of clinical sites. I really like my preceptor and the other
nurses here, and I just feel like every day that I am on the unit, I
am learning things but also that I am contributing to the patient
care. I know that DML was hard to learn, but now it is so normal
and comes easy. We don't do post-conference because it is just
me and my preceptor, so we debrief as we go. I actually ask more
questions than he does, but he is starting to get it—that Socratic
thing. It's okay, though, because I am so used to the questioning
that now I actually ask myself why and what does that mean, and
how are these things related ... and then I answer myself, too.*

*So using DML taught me how to think deeper and ask questions.
I often ask myself—not out loud, but in my thoughts—"Does
this make sense?" or "Why does this make sense?" I have learned
that I can be really comfortable asking questions of myself
and others: that thinking in questions makes me think deeper*

and make relationships between things I have learned or know and experiences with patients. I also realized that through this questioning, I actually know more than I give myself credit for. I not only know the questions to ask, but also I know when I know the answers.

I am also at the point where I can do this in my head. I don't use the worksheets anymore, but sometimes I visualize the mapping or the relationship between what I did and what I expected to happen and what really happened. I see it in my brain. The other thing that I do is always think beyond with my preceptor. He always laughs when I start asking the what-if questions and says that I am picking his brain, but those are probably the most useful for me.

Lisa described using reflection-beyond-action to learn from the experiences of her preceptor in conversations that occur throughout their time together in the clinical setting and the confidence that comes from being comfortable with questioning and answering. Megan, a student in a second-degree accelerated BSN program, describes how the use of DML crept from clinical and simulation learning into the classroom setting.

[Laughing] I wonder if all of my teachers appreciate DML or if they dread the fact that we learned how to use it? I know it is supposed to be the way we debrief clinical and sim, but it keeps showing up in the classroom and Professor Taylor's lectures, and well, it has gotten a lot better. In the beginning, let's just say there were plenty of blank stares. I mean, we were learning to challenge ourselves and our thinking through all of these "why?" questions or "tell me more" statements. It was kinda funny: There was this point in post-conference when the tables just turned, and instead of the clinical instructor asking us everything, we started asking her and other students, like we just knew how to do that. Well, it wasn't long, and we were in Professor Taylor's lecture on ... gosh, I don't remember what, and Rachel (who is usually the teacher's

pet) raises her hand in the middle of a slide and asks Professor Taylor something like, "Why is that medication given and not this other one in this situation?" So the prof answers her, and then [Rachel] fires right back with, "But then why not do this instead?" So Professor Taylor explained what would happen in that situation and was about to go back to the slides when Rachel followed up with, "And if the patient situation was different and included these aspects instead, what would be the same and what would be different?"

Well, you could have heard a pin drop in that lecture hall because all of us knew she was doing DML with the prof, and Professor Taylor was clearly not comfortable. Let me just say, though, that the floodgates opened, and every lecture since there has been DML like questions and discussion, which never happened before. So I guess DML changed how we learn in lecture because we learned how to make sense of things by asking questions. Professor Taylor is getting used to it and even laughs now when she asks the class whether anyone has any questions because you know we are going to. The great thing is though that now we use less time in lecture slides and more time talking and asking questions in class. Professor Taylor even asked whether we would like some class time spent just in discussion instead of lecture. I know I do. I sometimes worry that when we discuss, we might miss important points that we need to know for the test, but actually I am doing fine with my test grades, and probably this way, I don't have to be as focused on memorizing because I actually understand why things are the way they are. [Laughs] "Why?, why?, why?" is our class motto!

Each of these examples demonstrates transformational teaching and learning using DML in different contexts, yet students are engaged in active learning: comparing, analyzing, hypothesizing, generalizing, synthesizing, and reflecting as they developed the skills needed for clinical reasoning. Teachers were also transformed in how they approached teaching with more emphasis on uncovering student thinking and correcting misunderstandings. Deep thinking, reflection, and anticipation occurred in teachers and learners, fostering the development of clinical reasoning. DML provides a method that transforms teaching and learning and prepares students for practice by learning to think like a nurse.

Final Reflections

Teaching and learning to think like a nurse is a complex yet necessary process to sustain the profession. One method is to intentionally teach and develop reflection-in-action, reflection-on-action, and reflection-beyond action in novices to foster higher-order thinking and expert practice. The use of debriefing methods like DML in clinical, simulation, and classroom settings provides a structure to foster and practice reflection and develop metacognition. Ultimately, the goal is to develop reflective nurses who can challenge taken-for-granted assumptions and begin to use Socratic questions of their own practice as they move from novice to expert nurse.

References

Ausubel, D. P., Novak, J. D., & Hanesian, H. (1986). *Educational psychology: A cognitive view* (2nd ed.). New York, NY: Werbel & Peck.

Benner, P. (1984). *From novice to expert: Excellence and power in clinical nursing practice.* Menlo Park, CA: Addison-Wesley.

Benner, P., Sutphen, M., Leonard, V., & Day, L. (2010). *Educating nurses: A call for radical transformation.* San Francisco, CA: Jossey-Bass.

Cheng, A., Eppich, W., Grant, V., Sherbino, J., Zendejas, B., & Cook, D. A. (2014). Debriefing for technology-enhanced simulation: A systematic review and meta-analysis. *Medical Education, 48*(7), 657–666. doi: 10.1111/medu.12432

Collins, J. W., & O'Brien, N. P. (2003). *The Greenwood dictionary of education.* Westport, CT: Greenwood Press.

Decker, S., Fey, M., Sideras, S., Caballero, S., Rockstraw, L., Boese, T., & Borum, J. C. (2013). Standards of best practice: Simulation standard VI: The debriefing process. *Clinical Simulation in Nursing*, *9*(6), S27–S29.

Dreifuerst, K. T. (2009). The essentials of debriefing in simulation learning: A concept analysis. *Nursing Education Perspectives*, *30*(2), 109–114.

Dreifuerst, K. T. (2012). Using debriefing for meaningful learning to foster development of clinical reasoning in simulation. *Journal of Nursing Education*, *51*(4), 1–8. doi:10.3928/01484834-20120409-02

Dreifuerst, K. T., & Decker, S. (2012). Debriefing: An essential component for learning in simulation pedagogy. In P. R. Jeffries (Ed.) *Simulation in nursing education: From conceptualization to evaluation* (2nd ed.). New York, NY: The National League for Nursing. Awarded a 2013 AJN Book of the Year in the Category of Nursing Education.

Dreifuerst, K. T., Horton-Deutsch, S., & Henao, H. (2014). Meaningful debriefing. In P. J. Jeffries (Ed.) *Clinical simulations in nursing education: Advanced concepts, trends, and opportunities* (pp. 44–57). Washington, DC: National League for Nursing.

Fanning, R. M., & Gaba, D. M. (2007). The role of debriefing in simulation-based learning. *Simulation in Healthcare*, *2*(2), 115–125. doi: 10.1097/SIH.0b013e3180315539

Fowler, L. P. (1997). Clinical reasoning strategies used during care planning. *Clinical Nursing Research*, *6*(4), 349–361.

Hayden, J., Smiley, R., Alexander, M. A., Kardong-Edgren, S., & Jeffries, P. (2014). The NCSBN National Simulation Study: A longitudinal, randomized, controlled study replacing clinical hours with simulation in prelicensure nursing education. *Journal of Nursing Regulation*, *5*(Suppl.2), S3–S40.

Kolb, D. A., Boyatzis, R. E., & Mainemelis, C. (2001). Experiential learning theory: Previous research and new directions. *Perspectives on Thinking, Learning, and Cognitive Styles*, *1*, 227–247.

Mann, K., Gordon, J., & MacLeod, A. (2009). Reflection and reflective practice in health professions education: A systematic review. *Advances in Health Sciences Education: Theory and Practice*, *14*(4), 595–621.

Mariani, B., Cantrell, M. A., Meakim, C., Prieto, P., & Dreifuerst, K. T. (2012). Structured debriefing and students' clinical judgment abilities in simulation. *Clinical Simulation in Nursing*. doi:10.1016/j.ecns.2011.11.009

Paget, T. (2001). Reflective practice and clinical outcomes: Practitioners' views on how reflective practice has influenced their clinical practice. *Journal of Clinical Nursing, 10*(2), 204–214.

Pesut, D. J. (2004). Reflective clinical reasoning. In L. Hayes, H. Butcher, & T. Boese (Eds.), *Nursing in contemporary society* (pp. 146–162). Upper Saddle River, NJ: Pearson Prentice Hall.

Piaget, J. (1954). *The construction of reality in the child.* Abingdon, UK: Routledge.

Schön, D. A. (1983). *The reflective practitioner: How professionals think in action.* London, UK: Temple Smith.

Slavich, G., & Zimbardo, P. (2012). Transformational teaching: Theoretical underpinnings, basic principles, and core methods. *Educational Psychology Review, 24*(4), 569–608. doi:10.1007/s10648-012-9199-6

Chapter 6
The Use of Visual Thinking Strategies in Healthcare Education

Meg Moorman, PhD, RN, WHNP-BC

As the pace and complexity of healthcare increases, nurse educators are challenged to create opportunities for students to develop observational and communication skills. The demand to do so is complicated by the desire to have classes that are more innovative and student-centered. And yet we teachers often teach in the same way that we were educated—with the "sage on stage" during class time. That tradition is changing, however. The use of arts and humanities is one way to infuse liberal arts into the nursing curriculum, as the National League for Nursing called for in its Bachelor of Science Essentials (NLN, 2011). Introducing art provides an opportunity to practice and improve observational skills, demanding fine attention to detail and nuance. Visual thinking strategies (VTS) is a teaching technique that holds potential to provide students with opportunities to improve observational and communication skills and also help infuse humanities into the nursing curriculum.

VISUAL THINKING STRATEGIES (VTS)

Abigail Housen and Philip Yenawine created VTS as a way to engage art viewers in more meaningful ways with museum art. VTS was eventually studied in primary education and found to increase observational skills, critical thinking, and communication. This teaching technique invites 8–10 participants to discuss three works of art in an art museum with a trained VTS facilitator over the course of a 1-hour session. (VTS is described in more detail in the section "Preparation" later in this chapter.)

VTS is a teaching technique that Abigail Housen and Philip Yenawine (2002) developed to engage museum visitors with artwork for a prolonged period of time. A former patient who was a docent at the local art museum introduced me to VTS early in my teaching career. I thought that taking students to the art museum sounded intriguing, although I was not clear what doing so would accomplish. Nonetheless, I offered the session to my students as an alternative to a written homework assignment. All 30 students chose to participate! They craved something new and innovative, and liked the idea of going as a group on a field trip.

As I watched the VTS facilitator hold discussions about three works of art over the course of an hour, the level of student participation and insight amazed me! Students who never spoke in class were revealing such a level of depth and insight that I knew something transformative was happening. The evaluations of this activity were all positive, and students told me that they craved more of this type of learning. So I decided to investigate for myself, and focused my doctoral dissertation on these questions:

- What meaning does VTS have for nursing students?

- How do students use VTS in caring for patients?

This chapter will discuss the need for expert communication and observational skills in healthcare and relate these needs specifically to nursing.

Background

As new nurse graduates enter the complex world of healthcare, they must work closely in large groups with each other and other healthcare members. Nurses spend more time with patients in a hospital setting than any other member of the healthcare team, so they must develop their communication skills and pay close attention to detail. Effective communication between patients and caregivers has been associated with improved patient satisfaction and safety, as well as improved patient outcomes (Paget et al., 2011). Because nurses' communication skills affect patient outcomes, nurse educators must provide students with opportunities to practice in creative ways and work with other disciplines to develop listening and communication.

Although teams provide most of the care delivered to patients, training remains focused on individual responsibilities. Consequently, care providers are often ill-prepared to work in complex settings from a team perspective (Geis, Pio, Pendergrass, Moyer, & Patterson, 2011). The Hospital Safety Goals (The Joint Commission, 2012) listed improving staff communications as a priority to improve healthcare safety and patient outcomes. In 2009, the Joint Commission for Hospitals revealed that 70% of inadvertent patient harm cases were due to lack of communication. Of those errors, 75% of patients died (Leonard, Graham, & Bonacum, 2004). Most of the time, communication skills are taught in didactic lectures with little opportunity for students to apply this knowledge. Krautcheid (2008) identified that although the theoretical base exists for nursing students to learn communication, students often lack both the opportunity to use communication skills and to be evaluated on them.

Application of group activities based on art, particularly in education, provides students an opportunity to practice communication with little stigmatization because art is accepted as a social activity. The NLN and the Institute of Medicine (IOM) specifically indicated the need for interdisciplinary education as a way to collaborate and communicate for better patient outcomes (NLN, 2011). These interdisciplinary educational endeavors can improve communication skills and provide students with practice working together.

Nurses must not only attend to their patients' needs, but also are required to constantly assess their patients' physical and emotional needs. To do this accurately, nurses must develop keen observational skills and learn to effectively communicate key issues back to the healthcare team. Observational skills are fundamental to physical examination and are the core technique that RNs use. These skills are not intuitive, thus necessitating the need for students to practice them in a variety of settings. Nurse educators are called on to teach students in creative, innovative ways (Benner, Sutphen, Leonard, & Day, 2010). Art can provide an opportunity to improve observational skills and demands "a high level of consciousness about what one sees ... a fine attention to detail and form: the perception of relations; the perception of nuance; and the perception of change" (Rogers, 2002, p. 230).

VTS has been studied in primary education and shown to improve critical thinking skills and aesthetic development, as well as communication skills (Housen, 2001; Housen & Yenawine, 2002; Yenawine, 1998). Klugman, Peel, and Beckmann-Mendez (2011) studied the use of VTS with medical and nursing students at a large medical center. Those students who were exposed to VTS were found to have higher tolerance for ambiguity and more of a willingness to communicate. Because of these studies, I wanted to explore what meaning VTS had for nursing students—and, specifically, how nursing students used VTS in caring for their patients.

REFLECTING ON ... CRITICAL THINKING

- *How do we model mutual respect for our students?*
- *How often do we give them an opportunity to explore other answers or consider alternative thinking in the classroom?*

Preparation

VTS is a teaching technique that typically occurs in an art museum with a trained VTS facilitator. With VTS, based on the educational philosophies of Lev Vygotsky (1993), students are more likely to synthesize learning when engaging and socializing together. To begin, the facilitator chooses three works of art for discussion. These works of art tend to be more abstract in context, which allows students to hear many interpretations about a particular work of art. As students gather around a work of art, the facilitator asks them a series of three questions (for the purpose of this exemplar, "she" refers to the facilitator and "he" refers to the student):

1. **What is going on in this picture?** This first question allows the participant to think aloud about what he is seeing, using a narrative to describe what he thinks he sees or interprets as meaning in the painting.

2. **Tell me what you see that makes you say that.** This directive invites the student to give visual evidence for what he saw and back it up with details. This directive also requires the students to look again at the painting and find factual evidence that contributes to understanding of what was meant. The facilitator gives no indication that she is judging or that the response was right or wrong. She listens intently and often points to the artwork while the student describes what made him come to that conclusion so that all participants are focusing on the painting. The facilitator paraphrases back to the student to seek understanding and may ask, "Did I understand you correctly? Is that right?" The student may agree, or may look again and clarify his meaning. The facilitator is very present as she paraphrases back to students, modeling for them what it feels like to be heard and acknowledged.

3. **What more can you find?** This final question invites other students to participate. After watching the initial interaction between the first student respondent and the facilitator, the students note that there was no judgment or correcting; rather, the facilitator respected and validated each student's answer. Other students are now more willing to give their interpretations in response to the question "What is going on in this painting?" After the student responds, again the facilitator listens and then paraphrases back with leading questions, such as, "What are you seeing that makes you say that?" Often students will build off each other's comments, and sometimes they have various interpretations about what is happening in the painting.

At the end of the discussion, the facilitator thanks the participants for their observations, and they move on to another work of art. The facilitator asks the same three questions about each work of art. Most of the discussions last about 20 minutes per piece of art, so in discussing three works of art, the total time for the VTS activity is approximately 1 hour.

REFLECTING ON ... THE ART OF LISTENING

- *How often do we really listen to what others are saying?*

- *Are we planning what we are going to say next, or are we attentive and present?*

- *How often do we validate and seek understanding while talking with others?*

The Project

This VTS experience was offered as a homework option during a sixth-semester obstetrics course in an eight-semester BSN program. Students who chose the VTS experience in their sixth semester were then recruited to participate in a study during their seventh semester to undergo another VTS experience while they were in a critical care course. These students voluntarily participated in another 1-hour VTS experience and agreed to individual interviews that focused on their experiences. The interviews were scheduled from 1 to 2 weeks after their second VTS experience and focused on the following guiding questions:

- What meaning does VTS have for you?

- How have you used VTS in caring for patients?

Using phenomenology based on the work of Martin Heidegger (1962), the students' responses were analyzed, and themes (discussed in the next section) were identified.

Outcomes

As data analysis was performed, I noticed that students often mentioned the work of the facilitator as important and significant in their enjoyment of this project. As I reflected on this, I then identified two themes from student responses that could be used in teaching and developed the term *facilitative teaching*. The two themes identified from student responses were feeling safe in learning, and seeing and thinking differently.

Feeling Safe in Learning

Students often spoke during their interviews of the fact that VTS made them feel safe to participate, and they often were encouraged by the manner in which the facilitator responded to their various answers. There was no negative feedback, which students often noted stifles their learning: All responses were treated with respect and validated. Students also noted that nursing school often had a level of scrutiny that was hard on them emotionally. For example, students who answer incorrectly in a large lecture often feel ashamed and embarrassed—and therefore less likely to participate again:

> We are mostly taught throughout school that if we make a mistake, our patient could die. That may be, so why would I want to volunteer to answer a question during a lecture when I may very well be humiliated by the instructor, knowing that a wrong answer would indicate I might have killed my patient? I'm not doing it. I won't answer during class, even if I am pretty sure I'm right. It's just too risky.

Students also sensed a similar feeling when participating in simulations:

> If you make a mistake during sims, everyone is watching, and you are completely humiliated. So sometimes, even if I see something wrong during a sim, I won't speak up. It's too embarrassing.

Other students spoke about the environment of learning in a place other than the hospital or classroom. Students found the art museum to be neutral territory, where there were no lab coats, no scrubs, and no name tags; everyone was treated with respect and attention. They found the art museum relaxing, comfortable, and welcoming. In the past, I have included medical students, physicians, nursing students, and nurses in VTS sessions. All participated without really knowing who was a nurse or a doctor. Even those with art history majors had no advantage over anyone else because everyone was treated equally, and all responses were treated with the same degree of attention.

REFLECTING ON ... JUDGING OTHERS

- *How do we give students the opportunity to communicate without fear of being wrong?*

- *How might we unintentionally shame students during class?*

- *What are strategies to encourage diverse thought in the classroom?*

Students also appreciated that this activity was not graded, and they felt much more open to go out on a limb or stretch their answers because there was no negative reaction from the instructor nor negative consequences for their answer.

This "high stakes learning" that students feel during class and clinical may stifle learning:

> *VTS felt open and free to me. I was able to express my thoughts and opinions about artwork in a way that felt much safer than the way we participate in class. The facilitator was really open and affirming.*

Most of the students appreciated the value in not being critiqued:

> *Just the fact that there are no demands on you. Like, you're allowed to just kind of perceive things as you do, especially the imperfect. I feel like with medicine, there's obviously, out of*

necessity, we have to be very precise and not make any mistakes. But I felt more open to explore here and go out on a limb, which really expanded my thinking.

Another student stated:

Everyone has an equal voice because ... no one has the expertise in the group unless they're trying to figure out the answer and compare the two comments. I think it puts everyone on an equal plane, to fully communicate your opinion, and that is validated by the facilitator.

Another student commented about the facilitator:

She was open to questions and interpretations. If you say something silly, she doesn't give you a weird look like, "That isn't the right answer." So she is very open and friendly. She didn't make me feel judged. There are sometimes when my opinion ... it wasn't probably right, but she was very open and listened to me.

Other students talked about how they could consider others' opinions, and at the same time, still hold onto their personal beliefs about what the painting meant.

At the end of a conversation, students often asked, "So, what's the right answer?" When the facilitator commented, "There really is no right answer. Your interpretation is your own," students replied with frustration, "There has to be a right answer! There always is in nursing school!" The facilitator then started a conversation with the students: "Do you ever have times in your clinical when patients have a complaint, and no one can find the cause of the problem?" When the students agreed that this situation happens often, the facilitator talked to them about tolerance of ambiguity and seeking more validation and fact finding.

Students find it frustrating that no one right answer exists and used exams as an example —usually, an exam question has only one right answer. As we discussed this, we talked about a diagnosis of headaches because often there is no explicit cause for why a patient might be suffering from headaches. Diagnostic tests can be performed, but after getting negative results, sometimes patients live with a symptom, not knowing what the cause is. Students really struggle with this concept that there is no one right answer, and this can be difficult as they transition from school to work as an RN. There is not always a right answer, and this ambiguity can be challenging. Learning to consider others' opinions and how others reached those conclusions can be insightful for nursing students. VTS can teach students how to tolerate this ambiguity—and thus consider that there may not be just one right answer.

Thinking and Seeing Differently

Because VTS is a systematic way for a group to look at art, it was not surprising that after experiencing VTS in two separate sessions, students noticed that they were able to more critically assess their patients and observe much more nuance and detail. They also found that they were much more precise in providing details to other nurses, doctors, and other members of the healthcare team. Consider the following student comment:

> In clinical, you get report about the big overview. Then you go in, and you start to see the patients and all of the other factors like their health history, their medicines, their diet, culture and their family, and these other components. All of those little things together kind of make up the big picture—like a work of art. You get a sense of the big picture, and then you go in for more details and data. You see it differently after getting the smaller pieces, and it validates the big picture.

Students noticed that their initial viewing of a work of art was broad and big, but as the conversations ensued, they discerned more detail, which helped inform them about the bigger picture of what was happening. They often saw details after another student pointed something out they had not initially seen. Students correlated this to working as a nurse by listening more intently to reports from respiratory therapists, dieticians, physicians, and social workers, who all gave details about the patient, but the student nurse was able to piece these together to form a "bigger picture" about what was going on with her patient.

Students also identified the value of hearing their fellow students' opinions during VTS. They found it fascinating to hear about how and what someone else saw, and they noted that it was easier for them to see the same thing after hearing someone else's rationale: "Oh! Okay. I see how you got to that!" This is based on Vygotsky's educational principle of hearing how others think: It can inform a learner's thinking and increase the ability to think critically (1993). One student noted, "Sometimes a fresh pair of eyes can really help you see what else is going on!"

Other students likened their experiences with VTS to walking into a critical care room for the first time:

> *You first walk in, and it's too much, and it's so overwhelming. But then you break it down into little pieces, and it's like that large work of art from Africa we looked at. It was way too busy when I first saw it. I didn't like it and wanted to walk away. But, after we started talking about it and everyone was looking at small details, we were able to find a common meaning for the large work of art and its meaning. We broke it down into little pieces, and it makes the big picture seem not so scary. That is what I ended up doing in the ICU the first day. I was overwhelmed, but then I just went to look at the medicines, then the vent, then the drains. ... I broke it down into small pieces, and it helped me to get a better understanding of the big picture! That was cool.*

Other students found that they gave more detail in their charting or reports to other nurses, stating facts to back up their observations:

> *I didn't just chart that she had swelling in her legs. ... I gave evidence to back it up. Her socks were tight, and she had imprints and pitting edema. She also had not had swelling the day before, so I compared and contrasted as I gave report to the resident. I was much more thorough about the swelling than before I did VTS.*

Even after graduation, students have commented how meaningful VTS is in their nursing practice. I recently received this email from a former nursing student:

> *I just wanted to send you a quick note to tell you how much I was impacted by the visual thinking strategies that you used as a class project in spring 2012. I have gone back to techniques I learned in that brief visit to the art museum again and again in my nursing practice. I feel like there are so many times that I just take things at face value, but when I pause for a moment to dig deeper into the clinical picture and reflect about what I'm seeing that makes me come to a certain conclusion, I find that my judgment is much better. I'm not sure if you are still incorporating this project into your teaching, but I just wanted to let you know that I value the experience, and I feel that it has made me a better nurse!*

Facilitative Teaching

While analyses of student responses were taking place, I kept hearing students talk about the role of the facilitator. Students who participated in VTS were particularly interested in how the facilitator guided the conversation and elicited participation, never making them feel criticized or judged.

Students felt that as they expressed an idea or thought, validation from the facilitator invited them to go deeper into their own thinking and explore other meanings that they would not have come to without that subtle prompt. Students felt respected and noticed that the facilitator's attempt to understand them by paraphrasing their thoughts really encouraged them in ways they had not experienced in the classroom. They found that this way of interaction made it much more likely that they would participate, and wondered out loud why nursing instructors couldn't be more open and encouraging. I went back and developed certain educational concepts from the perspective of a nurse educator and subsequently developed the term *facilitative teaching* (see Table 6.1).

Table 6.1: Facilitative Teaching

THEMES	RATIONALE	HOW TO IMPLEMENT INTO TEACHING
Validation	Promotes speaking out (Garon, 2012)	Paraphrase student response and ask, "Tell me how you got that answer" or "Did I understand you correctly?"
Reformation of VTS process into clinical practice	Encourages formulation/ reformulation (Vygotsky, 1993)	Display a complicated work of art in class and ask, "What is going on in this picture?" Ask, "What are you seeing to make you say that?" and paraphrase back to student for clarification. Provide a clinical picture of a complicated patient and provide scenario. Repeat the preceding VTS questioning, asking for evidential reasoning, paraphrasing, and inviting all participants to give input.
Mutual respect	Invites more	Invite participation (don't require it). Seek understanding and allow the student's point of view more insight and how he came to that conclusion without criticism; seek understanding of response without judgment through direct questioning.

The VTS experience revealed processes as expressed by students based on the role of the facilitator. Students identified with the facilitator and her role in facilitating a discussion. We call these processes and key components *facilitative teaching*, and they hold potential to enhance classroom learning for nurse educators.

Validation, formulation/reformulation, and mutual respect were all identified by participants as ways the facilitator was able to enhance learning. The facilitator listened attentively as students shared their individual interpretations of works of art. After each response, the facilitator listened, then paraphrased back to students what she understood them to say. She sought clarification and understanding, which, for students, displayed respect and validation that they very seldom felt in nursing education. Their answers were validated, giving them a sense of belonging. This process allowed students to actually experience presence and mutual respect, skills they were more likely to use in their own worlds. Students also commented that they were much more likely to participate after they witnessed the level of respect and attention the facilitator gave to the students who participated. When they witnessed that, others were much more likely to participate.

In the classroom, nurse educators often ask their students questions. Instead of simply validating whether a student's answer is right or wrong, I have found that asking students "Tell me how you came up with that answer" provides insight into student thinking and informs my teaching. By probing and trying to understand the process by which a student came to an answer, I am able to inform my own teaching and reflect on how I might be able to foster a better understanding in the future. Students also appreciate the respect and thoughtfulness of having my attention and my sincere quest to understand how they are drawing conclusions. My teaching is better because I take the time to listen and attempt to understand how they are thinking, and they feel respected. Student confidence in their observational skills related to the artwork also increases their confidence to respond in class. Facilitative teachers respect answers that may not be the answer expected and invite students to explain their thinking that arrived at that answer. This is consistent with developing creativity and encourages students to think deeply about difficult-to-solve problems.

VTS participants also were able to link their interactions with the artwork directly to patient care metaphorically. They even used the process of questioning as the facilitator did, as they inquired about patient care in the hospital. So, by literally looking at the "big picture" with VTS, then going closer, giving more detail, and then stepping back and looking at the whole, students had a process by which they could understand more clearly. They used this same analogy in patient care. One student spoke of a complex African work of art and said how overwhelmed he felt looking at it in the art museum during VTS. He related it to his first day in ICU as a student, looking at a complicated patient on a ventilator with multiple IVs, tubing, medications, and drains. He actually thought of the work of art, and, by a process he learned with VTS, he decided to look at individual components of the patient in the ICU. First he looked at the vent settings, then he looked at the IVs, then the medications. Then he literally stepped back and considered the whole person, with multiple smaller components making up the whole, similar to how he and the group had assessed the African work of art. When the respiratory therapist came in to change the ventilator settings, he asked her, "Tell me what you are seeing that makes you think you need to increase those settings." Vygotsky (1993) calls this process *formulation/reformulation* and identifies it as a key component of learning.

Facilitative teaching in the classroom is an opportunity for educators to model presence, active listening, and mutual respect. The act of validating student responses invites other participants to join in the conversation, giving the discussion a much richer dimension. Students are able to take this process of formulation/reformulation and use the same type of skill in clinical practice, drawing from their own experiences and discussions about art and applying them to the larger "picture" in caring for their patients.

Outcomes

Using VTS with students has been a wonderful, insightful experience. To provide a way of learning that is unconventional has been interesting and has really informed my teaching. VTS certainly provides a mode for students to learn to give more detail and evidence, which translates into a more thorough, accurate way to communicate, not only with patients but also among healthcare workers. After just one VTS experience, students start to provide evidence for their interpretations without prompting by the facilitator. Participants often start to look for rationale before even being asked, which lends itself to thoughtful, insightful discourse.

Learning to be more open and attentive to others' opinions can help inform students' thinking, which can enhance learning. VTS is a way to encourage interdisciplinary learning in a way that values all learners' opinions and invites them to listen attentively and respectfully to each other. This can expand participants' understanding of various healthcare team members and encourages them to listen to each other.

Students also spoke of the facilitator's ability to be present and listen to each person with attention and respect. The ability to be present was comforting to students, and they discussed how they might use it with patients. One student commented, "There are times when I can't fix a problem—say, after a patient gets a cancer diagnosis. The ability to really listen and be attentive is a gift I can give my patient. Nurses are good at that. The facilitator was really present as we all discussed our opinions, and she really listened. It felt good to be on the receiving end of that, and I want my patients to feel that."

Final Reflections

The role of the VTS facilitator can inform teaching. During a lecture, when a student volunteers an answer to a posed question, the facilitative teacher can query, "Tell me how you came up with that answer." As the student provides rationale for his answer, the teacher can validate and paraphrase back what the student says but may add an additional clarifying question to take the student into deeper thinking. By demonstrating an understanding of the student response, the teacher demonstrates mutual respect. This mutual respect is important to model for our students and might invite more participation and expansion of thought as conversations continue. If the teacher listens carefully to a student about the rationale, it can inform the teacher of incorrect thinking and help to inform her teaching. If a student provides rationale that is incorrect, the teacher must help the student to understand this, but can do it in a way that is gentle, respectful, and thoughtful. Preserving student dignity is important; shame and embarrassment stifle learning and stunt creative, insightful thinking to solve patient care problems.

References

Benner, P., Sutphen, M., Leonard, V., & Day, L. (2010). *Educating nurses: A call for radical transformation*. Stanford, CA: Jossey-Bass.

Garon, M. (2012). Speaking up, being heard: Registered nurses' perceptions of workplace communication. *Journal of Nursing Management*, 20(3), 361–371. doi:10.1111/j.1365-2834.2011.01296.x

Geis, G. L., Pio, B., Pendergrass, T., Moyer, M. R., & Patterson, M. D. (2011). Simulation to assess the safety of new healthcare teams and new facilities. *Journal of the Society for Simulation in Healthcare*, 6(3), 125–133. doi:10.1097/SIH.0b013e31820dff30

Heidegger, M. (1962). *Being and time*. Albany, NY: State University of New York Press.

Housen, A. (2001). Eye of the beholder: Research, theory and practice. *Visual Understanding in Education (VUE)*, 1–26. Retrieved from www.vtshome.org/system/resources/0000/0006/Eye_of_the_Beholder.pdf

Housen, A., & Yenawine, P. (2002). Aesthetic thought, critical thinking and transfer. *Arts and Learning Research Journal*, 18(1), 99–131. Retrieved from www.vtshome.org/system/resources/0000/0014/Aesthetic_thought.pdf

The Joint Commission (TJC). (2012). *Hospital national patient safety goals 2012*. Retrieved from www.jointcommission.org/assets/1/6/2012_NPSG_HAD.pdf

Klugman, C. M., Peel, J., & Beckmann-Mendez, D. (2011). Art rounds: Teaching interprofessional students visual thinking strategies at one school. *Academic Medicine*, 86(10), 1266–1271. doi:10.1097/ACM.0b013e31822c1427

Krautscheid, L. C. (2008). Improving communication among healthcare providers: Preparing student nurses for practice. *International Journal of Nursing Education Scholarship*, 5(1), 1–13. doi:10.2202/1548-923X.1647

Leonard, M., Graham, S., & Bonacum, D. (2004). The human factor: The critical importance of effective teamwork and communication in providing safe care. *Qualitative Safe Health Care*, 13, 85–90. doi:10.1136/qshc.2004.010033

National League for Nursing (NLN). (2011). *The future of nursing education: Ten trends to watch*. Retrieved from www.nln.org/nlnjournal/infotrends.htm#8

Paget, L., Han, P., Nedza, S., Kurtz, P., Racine, E., Russell, S., & Von Kohorn, I. (2011). Patient-clinician communication: Basic principles and expectations. *Institute of Medicine*. Retrieved from http://iom.edu/Activities/Quality/~/media/Files/Activity%20Files/Quality/VSRT/PCCwLogos.pdf

Rogers, C. R. (2002). Seeing student learning: Teacher change and the role of reflection. *Harvard Educational Review*, 72(2), 230–253. Eric: EJ648421

Vygotsky, L. S. (1993). *The collected works of L.S. Vygotsky* (vol. 2). New York, NY: Plenum Press.

Yenawine, P. (1998). Visual art and student-centered discussions. *Theory into Practice*, 37(4), 314–321. doi:10.1080/00405849809543821

Chapter 7

Interprofessional Education in Mental Health: Developing Practitioners Who Work Collaboratively and Provide Patient-Centered Care

Kathy Lay, PhD
Angela M. McNelis, PhD, RN, PMHCNS, ANEF, CNE
Sara Horton-Deutsch, PhD, RN, PMHCNS, FAAN, ANEF

The delivery of high-quality patient-centered care is a complex process that demands effective collaboration from healthcare professionals. Studies consistently demonstrate that collaborative healthcare improves quality, patient outcomes, patient satisfaction, efficiency, and job satisfaction through new knowledge and skills, communication, and interaction (Campion-Smith, Austin, Criswick, Dowling, & Francis, 2011; Curran, Sharpe, Flynn, & Button, 2010; Dacey, Murphy, Anderson, & McCloskey, 2010; Hammick, Freeth, Koppel,

Reeves, & Barr, 2007; Reeves et al., 2008). Collaborative healthcare delivery, however, requires further development (Reeves, Perrier, Goldman, Freeth, & Zwarenstein, 2013). Even though interprofessional education (IPE) is currently not the primary emphasis in most healthcare educational programs, it is slowly emerging as a pedagogically sound approach to advance interprofessional collaboration and patient care. Moreover, the need for interprofessional education expands beyond the United States as the world faces a shortage of healthcare workers. In 2010, the World Health Organization (WHO) called for innovative strategies to bolster the number of global health workers and develop a framework for action on interprofessional education and collaborative practice.

The WHO defined IPE as occurring when students from two or more professions learn about, from, and with each other to enable effective collaboration and improve health outcomes (2010). Building on this foundation, an Interprofessional Education Collaborative Practice Expert Panel developed core competencies for interprofessional collaborative practice: values/ethics for interprofessional practice, roles/responsibilities, interprofessional communication, and teams and teamwork (2011). These competencies overlap with those developed by the Quality and Safety Education for Nurses project (QSEN), which include patient-centered care, teamwork and collaboration, evidence-based practice (EBP), quality improvement, safety, and informatics (Sherwood & Barnsteiner, 2012). These expert groups all advocate for an independence-to-interdependence paradigm shift to optimize the quality care delivery.

Recognizing that interprofessional practice necessitates interactive, sustained interprofessional education, the three authors of this chapter—Kathy Lay, Angela McNelis, and Sara Horton-Deutsch—began the work that led ultimately to development of a graduate course co-taught and co-attended by faculty and students in social work and nursing. The goal was to develop mental health professionals who have the knowledge, skills, and attitudes to work collaboratively to provide quality patient-centered care. Our aim was to expose graduate social work and psychiatric nursing students to interprofessional collaborative practice and carry what they learned into their practice.

Background

The complexities of mental health provide clear demonstration of the need for collaboration. Worldwide, mental illness affects overall health, productivity, and longevity (Whiteford et al., 2013). Mental health is also a collaborative field requiring extensive interdisciplinary communication and cooperation among disciplines. Therefore, an interprofessional course combining graduate social work and psychiatric/mental health nursing students was a natural setting to practice interprofessional communication and relationship building.

The lack of access to mental health services is a global problem. Therefore, understanding and maximizing the strengths that each healthcare professional brings to the environment improves care delivery. Interprofessional teams, whose members' roles and accountabilities are clearly delineated, are able to reduce overlap, openly communicate, and make shared decisions. Building these teams, however, can come about only through intentional, directed, and sustained educational interactions among members.

REFLECTING ON ... SUPPORT FOR INTERPROFESSIONAL PRACTICE

- *How does the current healthcare system support or prohibit interprofessional practice: that is, a practice in which all members of the healthcare team have a voice?*

The Project

None of us three authors had experience developing an interprofessional course. Our initial plan was to schedule a few meetings to outline the course and divide the responsibilities. During these initial meetings, what became readily apparent was that in coming from different disciplines, we spoke different "languages." For example, as a social worker, Dr. Lay referred to recipients of care as "clients"; as nurses, Drs. McNelis and Horton-Deutsch often used the term "patients." We quickly recognized the need for a common dialogue regarding our theoretical orientations, as well as our professional roles and responsibilities, before we could proceed with a course outline. Therefore, we began by sharing resources and reading more about each other's disciplinary perspectives so that we could appreciate one another's contributions to mental healthcare.

Over the next few months, we engaged in an iterative process, moving back and forth from philosophical and theoretical perspectives to the practical considerations of what content we should include in the course and how we should present the course content. This process helped us to articulate, inform, and examine each other's viewpoints and assumptions. Because this process was both essential and integral for building the course, we recognized the value of having our students engage in a similar type of exercise and built this approach into our teaching/learning strategies.

Our pedagogical underpinnings were predominantly similar; we were all expert teachers who originally met through the university's Faculty Colloquium on Excellence in Teaching—and we readily agreed on the use of active learning strategies for our students. Because of our basic pedagogical synergy, our work primarily entailed philosophical conversations to deepen our understanding of one another's knowledge, skills, and attitudes prior to actual course development and delivery. Interestingly, through this process, we came to realize that the student growth we wanted the course to facilitate was similar to the growth that the three of us experienced during the development process.

REFLECTING ON ... UNDERLYING ISSUES

- *What underlying issues must be acknowledged and addressed for healthcare professionals to work within a true interprofessional framework that supports quality and safety?*

Laying the Foundation

The purpose of this project was to develop an interprofessional educational approach for graduate psychiatric mental health nursing and social work curricula. It was clear from the literature that the IPE course needed to address integrated treatment of *co-occurring disorders* (a mental illness and substance use disorder that occur together). Almost 9 million adults are struggling with a co-occurring disorder, and "only 7.4% receive treatment for both conditions with 55.8% receiving no treatment at all" (http://media.samhsa. gov/co-occuring/). Charles Curie, administrator for the Substance Abuse and Mental Health Services Administration (SAMHSA), states:

> All too often individuals are treated only for one of the two disorders—if they receive treatment at all. If one of the co-occurring disorders goes untreated, both usually get worse, and additional complications arise, including the risk for other serious medical problems, suicide, unemployment, homelessness, incarceration and separation from families and friends. People with co-occurring disorders cannot separate their addiction from their mental illness, so they should not have to negotiate separate service delivery systems. Our goal is to create a system that allows any door to be the right door for the services an individual needs. ("Co-Occurring Disorders," n.d.)

The silo approach to treatment rarely addresses the complex needs of individuals with co-occurring disorders, and it is for this reason that integrated treatment is considered a best practice (Maisto & Kiviahan, 2006). Treatment must be integrative, addressing all symptoms that individuals are struggling with, including mental illnesses, addictions, and

CO-OCCURRING DISORDERS

An individual having co-existing mental health and substance use disorders (www.samhsa.gov).

STRENGTHS PERSPECTIVE

Focuses on a client's abilities, talents, and resources.

FAMILY RESILIENCE THEORY

The ability to withstand and rebound from life struggles inclusive of a family adapting by tapping into their internal and external resources (Walsh, 2011).

environmental issues (www.samhsa.gov). Thus, it was imperative that the IPE course we developed demonstrate an integrative approach to treatment. As educators, we agreed that a primary focus would be for the course to carry forward to the students' practicum experiences.

Our first meeting focused on our approach to the treatment of individuals living with a co-occurring disorder. We were pleased that we shared similar philosophical approaches to treatment. Both nursing and social work curricula are grounded in the strengths perspective (Rapp & Goscha, 2011; Saleebey, 2012) and family resilience theory (Walsh, 2011). We discussed how diagnoses provide a generic language for care providers and that individuals are not defined by their diagnoses. We see individuals as bringing their own unique strengths and challenges to treatment; thus, positive outcomes require individualized recovery plans. Without this philosophical agreement, we most likely would have faced considerable challenges to the development of the IPE course.

We held several meetings over the course of an academic year to develop and refine the course. This process also included input from community stakeholders who were providers of community mental health and addictions treatment, as well as community partners who support student learning (nursing preceptors and social work field supervisors). Our collaborative approach manifested respect for one another's disciplines, practice experience, and pedagogies. Acknowledging common roles and differences was important to understanding our students' needs.

Developing and Implementing the Course

After establishing our intention to develop an IPE course that addressed co-occurring disorders and approaches to treatment, we developed the course description and objectives. We started with the description/objectives from a social work addictions practice course and revised them to incorporate IPE and co-occurring treatment (see the following boxed text). We made sure that the course built on other courses in the mental health and addictions curriculum in social work and psychiatric nursing. For example, most students in both disciplines have taken an assessment course as well as other practice courses.

COURSE DESCRIPTION AND OBJECTIVES

Course Rationale and Description

The purpose of this course is to provide learners with knowledge and skills relevant to interprofessional approaches to the treatment of substance use and co-occurring psychiatric disorders. The course includes prevention, intervention, and treatments of these disorders in diverse populations across the life span. Students draw upon previous and concurrent learning experiences and integrate values, knowledge, and skills relevant to their professional standards of practice. Consistent with strengths and ecosystems perspectives, students consider the impact of social environments, physical settings, community contexts, and political realities that influence the emergence of substance use and co-occurring disorders.

Objectives

Through active participation in the learning experiences and completion of the readings, assignments, and learning projects offered throughout this seminar, learners are expected to demonstrate the ability to:

1. *Critically analyze their own knowledge, skills, beliefs, and attitudes concerning substance use/psychiatric disorders within the context of professional practice.*

2. *Describe and apply the complex interplay of biological, genetic, psychological, social, ethnic, socioeconomic, and cultural factors relevant to holistic treatment of persons with substance use/psychiatric disorders.*

continues

3. *Describe the variety of professional practice roles within treatment settings and evaluate the application of values and ethics.*

4. *Discover, analyze, synthesize, and evaluate evidence of practice effectiveness and apply that knowledge in all aspects and processes of service delivery with persons affected by or at risk of substance use/psychiatric disorders.*

5. *Employ evidence-based treatment modalities and interventions in a variety of settings to meet the concerns and needs of diverse individuals, families, groups, and communities affected by or at risk for substance use/psychiatric disorders.*

6. *Collaborate with other community partners in tracking progress and evaluating the effectiveness of services with persons experiencing substance use/psychiatric disorders.*

TRANSTHEORETICAL MODEL OF CHANGE

A model that conceptualizes the process of intentional behavior change (Prochaska, DeClemente, & Norcross, 1992).

MOTIVATIONAL INTERVIEWING (MI)

A collaborative conversation helping people explore their own values and interests toward behavioral change (Miller & Rollick, 2012).

Next, we identified key course content. The neuroscience of addiction, the transtheoretical model of change, and motivational interviewing (MI) were seen as fundamental knowledge and skills necessary to practice with individuals living with co-occurring disorders. Additional content included IPE competencies; screening and assessment; ethics; and treatment approaches, such as MI, cognitive behavior therapy, dialectical behavior therapy, and mindfulness-based stress reduction. We designed the course as a hybrid format (face-to-face and asynchronous online), with face-to-face class meetings for skills practice and other experiential learning activities and content addressed in modules.

We designed assignments and learning strategies on best evidence for the adult learner (Knowles, Holton, & Swanson, 2011; Kolb, 1983). For example, the focal written assignment for the course was a structured, critical reflection using the Describe, Examine, and Articulate Learning (DEAL) model

(Ash & Clayton, 2004). DEAL is structured in a way that "generates, ... deepens and documents learning" (Ash & Clayton, 2009, p. 28). The DEAL assignment was adapted from a structured critical reflection assignment (Lay & McGuire, 2008) developed for a social work addictions practice course. Clayton had trained both Lay and McGuire in using the DEAL model of reflection in the context of service-learning assignments. Together, they subsequently adapted the model for other learning contexts. This DEAL model asks learners to describe either a personal or professional experience with addiction and provides them with specific reflection questions in the "Examine" section to facilitate the deconstruction of bias and prejudices individuals have toward those struggling with addictions. In addition, four articulated learning questions are included in all DEAL reflections. We modified those questions and added an additional one. We then designed these five articulated learning questions as prompts for further reflection and articulation of new understandings, enhanced communications and interactions, and setting future goals for practice (see Appendix A). Moreover, we encouraged students to demonstrate the universal intellectual standards for critical thinking (Paul & Elder, 2014) in their reflective writing. These standards include "clarity, accuracy, precision, relevance, depth, breadth, significance, and fairness" (Paul & Elder, 2014, p. 3).

Students completed an initial DEAL at the beginning of the semester and were then asked to revise it at the end of the course based on their learning. The second iteration provided students an opportunity to reflect on their thoughts and processes through time. This second iteration reinforced the importance of reflexivity, not only as related to scholarship, but also to clinical practice.

Because adult learners appreciate self-paced learning, we created and used online modules throughout the course. We also included forum discussions to serve as our dialogue with students and for students with each other. Forum discussions required students to participate with scholarly postings grounded in critical thinking. For these discussions and for face-to-face learning activities, we assigned students to a small interprofessional learning group (of approximately six members) for the duration of the course. This effort to assign social work and nursing students equally to each group facilitated learning from one another's discipline. For example, the ethics module assigned students to read each discipline's ethical codes/standards of practice and then discuss an assigned ethical dilemma. This assignment facilitated learning about others' disciplines and sparked interprofessional discussion.

We maximized face-to-face time with our students and incorporated as much active learning as was possible. The first face-to-face class focused on interprofessional collaborative practice. To begin, we presented and discussed interprofessional competencies. We then asked students, in their groups, to complete the "two-circle exercise." They drew two overlapping circles. Then, in one circle, they wrote roles and tasks that nurses perform; in the other circle, they wrote what social workers do. The overlap is what they have in common. The activity points out the many shared elements yet many unique elements that each discipline brings to an advanced practice healthcare team. During the class there was also a brief introduction to the neuroscience of addiction and its relationship to co-occurring disorders. The goal was to prepare students for the work they would do in the first module.

Finally, during the subsequent face-to-face class sessions, students practiced MI skills through role/real plays. Incorporating best practices of reciprocity and cooperation among students, time on task, and prompt feedback (Chickering & Gamson, 1987), these role and real plays were demonstrated and practiced in a variety of ways in order to increase students' comfort with MI and with receiving feedback. Following these class sessions, students completed an articulated learning assignment to reflect on their individual learning and their greatest challenge in the role/real plays.

ARTICULATED LEARNING ASSIGNMENT FOR ROLE/REAL PLAYS

Consider the following questions:

1. *What did I learn?*
2. *How specifically did I learn it?*
3. *Why does this learning matter, and why is it important?*

4. *In what ways will I use this learning?*

5. *What goals shall I set in accordance with what I have learned in order to improve myself and/or the quality of my learning and/or the quality of my future practice?*

Source: Ash & Clayton, 2009.

Outcomes

The IPE course on co-occurring disorders was taught for the fifth time (fall semester, 2014). Just as we encourage our students to engage in continuous and mindful reflection on their thinking, we continuously engaged in thinking about how to improve this course and responded accordingly. Each time the course was taught, we conducted mid-semester appreciative evaluations in which we asked students anonymously to share what was going well, what was not going well, what strategies or activities were facilitating or obstructing their learning, and what could be done to aid their learning in the second half of the semester. These evaluative data led to changes such as increased time for practicing MI skills, more activities and opportunities to "practice" as an interprofessional team (using case studies), and more balanced presentation of content from both nursing and social work. We also used end-semester evaluations to guide changes, such as increased clarity of written assignments and expectations for forum discussion postings. Because this was the first course developed and taught and attended by two different disciplines, we thought it necessary to conduct a deeper assessment beyond mid- and end-semester evaluations. To accomplish this, we conducted in-depth interviews with students who completed the course.

Three main ideas emerged from the interview data. First, students grew to have a broader perspective of approaches to patient care through understanding discipline-specific strengths and knowledge. Second, they described the need to "let go" of assumptions about the skills and scope of practice of the other professional group in order to fully engage in interprofessional education and practice. And finally, students expressed optimism that interprofessional practice would advance the health of the nation. Data revealed that overall perception of the course was positive. Students commented that they wanted more interprofessional courses and opportunities to learn with and from students in social work, and an expansion of this approach to include other disciplines, such as medicine and pharmacy. Students perceived that the face-to-face sessions facilitated their learning and suggested that more of the class be conducted that way. Students also generally observed that the course should be revised to have a greater emphasis on the theoretical underpinnings of IPE and more opportunities to work in interprofessional teams on patient-centered care and treatment case studies.

> ### REFLECTING ON ... IPE COURSE DEVELOPMENT
>
> - *How does reading this chapter influence your ideas/plans to develop or facilitate an IPE course?*

Recommendations

As with any new initiative, reflection is essential for improvement. Our process for the ongoing development of course content continues to be a critical reflexive (Timmins, 2006) and collaborative process—one that involves student, faculty, field supervisor, and preceptor feedback. "Reflexivity is finding strategies to question our own attitudes, theories-in-use, values, assumptions, prejudices and habitual action; to understand our complex roles in relation to others" (Bolton, 2014, p. 7). This is an important part of clinical practice, and, if our curriculum development team aims to prepare students for interprofessional practice, we must model reflection and reflexivity, which includes building therapeutic relationships with colleagues. We are transparent in soliciting and making available frequent feedback; we share information about upcoming data-driven course changes with our key stakeholders: students, faculty, and practice partners. We find it equally important to share these ideas with colleagues across the United States so that we can expand the IPE initiative. The collaborative model that we used to develop and implement this course can be used by other disciplines and universities in a concerted effort to move forward the state of IPE science and improve patient care.

REFLECTING ON ... INCLUSION OF OTHER HEALTHCARE PROFESSIONS

- *What are other ways interprofessional education can honor the different lenses that different professions bring to healthcare?*

Final Reflections

The process of developing this interprofessional course not only provided our students with new ways of being in their practice settings, but also jump-started a variety of collaborative research projects in which we brought together faculty from social work, nursing, and medicine, and established a broader team for partnership. This team of faculty has morphed into multiple groups that are now working together in the university as practice settings, launching projects to benefit patients as well as interprofessional research, and expanding now to other universities outside our community. Stepping back and looking at our small start, the work of three colleagues with a desire to provide an IPE experience that positively impacts patient care has led to a multitude of IPE projects.

References

Ash, S. L., & Clayton, P. H. (2004). The articulated learning: An approach to guided reflection and assessment. *Innovative Higher Education, 29*(2), 137–154.

Ash, S. L., & Clayton, P. H. (2009). Generating, deepening, and documenting learning: The power of critical reflection in applied learning. *Journal of Applied Learning in Higher Education, 1*(Fall), 25–48.

Bolton, G. (2014). *Reflective practice: Writing and professional development.* Los Angeles, CA: Sage.

Campion-Smith, C., Austin, H., Criswick, S., Dowling, B., & Francis, G. (2011). Can sharing stories change practice? A qualitative study of an interprofessional narrative-based palliative care course. *Journal of Interprofessional Care, 25*(2), 105–111.

Chickering, A. W., & Gamson, Z. F. (1987). Seven principles for good practice in undergraduate education. *American Association for Higher Education Bulletin, 39*(7), 3–7.

Co-Occurring disorders. (n.d.). Retrieved from http://www.nattc.org/respubs/cooccurring/

Curran, V. R., Sharpe, D., Flynn, K., & Button, P. (2010). A longitudinal study of the effect of an interprofessional education curriculum on student satisfaction and attitudes toward interprofessional teamwork and education. *Journal of Interprofessional Care, 24*(1), 41–52.

Dacey, M., Murphy, J. I., Anderson, D. C., & McCloskey, W. W. (2010). An interprofessional service-learning course: Uniting students across educational levels and promoting patient-centered care. *Journal of Nursing Education, 49*(12), 696–699.

Hammick, M., Freeth, D., Koppel, I., Reeves, S., & Barr, H. (2007). A best evidence systematic review of interprofessional education: BEME guide no. 9. *Medical Teacher, 29*(8), 735–751.

Interprofessional Education Collaborative Practice Expert Panel. (2011). *Core competencies for interprofessional collaborative practice: Report of an expert panel.* Washington, DC: Interprofessional Education Collaborative.

Knowles, M., Holton, E. F., & Swanson, R. A. (2011). *The adult learner* (7th ed.). New York, NY: Taylor Francis Publishers.

Kolb, D. A. (1983). *Experiential learning: Experience as the source of learning and development.* New York, NY: Prentice Hall.

Lay, K., & McGuire, L. (2008). Teaching students to deconstruct life experience with addictions: A structured reflection exercise. *Journal of Teaching in the Addictions, 7*(2), 145–163.

Maisto, S., & Kiviahan, D. (2006). Screening for psychiatric disorders among adults presenting for substance use disorder treatment: Current practices in the United States. *International Journal of Mental Health & Addiction, 6*(1), 32–36.

Miller, W. R., & Rollnick, S. (2012). *Motivational interviewing: Helping people change* (3rd ed.). New York, NY: Guilford Press.

Paul, R., & Elder, L. (2014). *The miniature guide to critical thinking concepts and tools* (7th ed.). Santa Rosa, CA: The Foundation for Critical Thinking.

Prochaska, J., Diclemente, C., & Norcross, J. (1992). In search of how people change: Applications to addictive behaviors. *American Psychologist, 47*(9), 1102–1114.

Rapp, C. A., & Goscha, R. J. (2011). *The strengths model: A recovery-oriented approach to mental health services.* New York, NY: Oxford University Press.

Reeves, S., Perrier, L., Goldman, J., Freeth, D., & Zwarenstein, M. (2013). *Interprofessional education: Effects on professional practice and healthcare outcomes* (update). The Cochrane Collaboration. Hoboken, NJ: Johns Wiley & Sons. doi:1002/14651858.CD002213.pub3

Reeves, S., Zwarenstein, M., Goldman, J., Barr, H., Freeth, D., Hammick, M., & Koppel, I. (2008). Interprofessional education: Effects on professional practice and health care outcomes. *Cochrane Database of Systematic reviews*, 2008, Issue. Art. No. CD002213. doi:10. 1002/14651858

Saleebey, D. (2012). *The strengths perspective in social work practice* (6th ed.). Advancing core competencies. Upper Saddle River, NJ: Pearson.

Sherwood, G. & Barnsteiner, J. (2012). *Quality and safety in nursing: A competency approach to improving outcomes.* Oxford, UK: Wiley-Blackwell.

Timmins, F. (2006). Clinical practice in nursing care: Analysis, action and reflexivity. *Nursing Standard, 20*(39), 49–54.

Walsh, F. (2011). *Strengthening family resilience* (2nd ed.). New York, NY: Guilford.

Whiteford, H., Degenhardt, L., Rehm, J., Baxter, A., Ferrari, A., Erskine, H., ... Vos, T. (2013). Global burden of disease attributable to mental and substance use disorders: Findings from the Global Burden of Disease Study 2010. *Lancet, 382*(9904), 1575–1586.

World Health Organization (2010). Framework for action on interprofessional education and collaborative practice. Retrieved from http://www.who.int/hrh/resources/framework_action/en/

Chapter 8

An Online Teaching Framework: Using Quality Norms and Caring Science to Build Presence and Engagement in Online Learning Environments

Sara Horton-Deutsch, PhD, RN, PMHCNS, FAAN, ANEF
Jason Drysdale, MA in ILT

Creating authentic presence and engaging students in transformative caring–healing learning is a challenge, even with face-to-face contact in a brick-and-mortar setting; accomplishing those objectives in an *online* setting requires effective evidence-based pedagogies and online-specific teaching strategies. Toward that end, the authors of this chapter—Sara Horton-Deutsch (nursing faculty) and Jason Drysdale (instructional designer)—partnered to create and begin to test an online teaching framework that incorporates Caring Science, Caritas Processes™, action-oriented student/teacher relations, reflective pedagogical practices, creativity, and thoughtful consideration of power/relation dynamics (Hills & Watson, 2011). The goal is a more "tactile," consciousness-heightening online learning environment: a place where students learn omnivorously, reflect critically on critical assumptions and beliefs, become aware of their levels of awareness, and decipher the compositions of their composite identities.

To meet the needs of current online learners, educators must appreciate the significant changes in students' ways of learning over the past 30 years. The Internet gives students ready access to staggering amounts of factual information: As of this writing, Google (2014) reported that there are more than 60 trillion individual pages online. The result is paradigmatic change in how students learn and what educators value. This change does not preclude the need for facts—it simply means that students need data access more than data storage. As educators, then, we need to adjust our online-education focus to *ways of thinking* and *ways of applying* knowledge in service of *building* meaningful skills and *developing* core professional and personal values. The students thereby obtain a dynamic mental skill set rather than a static data folder.

Educators must see online learning not as an adapted version of a brick-and-mortar-based pedagogy but rather as a completely native platform with its own set of challenges, benefits, methodologies, and pedagogies. Building an online curriculum indigenous to the operational online learning culture creates genuine online presence and builds genuine online engagement.

Background

Even though many have demanded a transformation of nursing education (Benner, Sutphen, Leonard, & Day, 2010; Institute of Medicine [IOM], 2011), few research-based pedagogical strategies exist to address this demand. The project described in this chapter contributes to meeting this demand. In this chapter, we evaluate the ability of different online course construction frameworks to create presence and engage students in reflecting on experiences, thinking from multiple perspectives, challenging assumptions, and exploring new possibilities.

Overcoming the Obstacles to Quality Online Education

Distance educators and learners face the same problem today as they faced when correspondence courses, educational radio, and educational television were the tools of choice: That is, physical distance between teacher and learner engenders cognitive distance that can inhibit student learning. This transactional distance contributes to online students' feelings of isolation, and maintenance of heavily text-based curricula yields an awkward "disconnect" between medium and message. The combination of these factors limits the utility of online education (Moore, 1993). If the pedagogy and instructional design of online courses fail to shorten the transactional distance between teacher and learner, there is significant risk of minimal student engagement—a disservice to both students and faculty.

With advances in modern technology—such as persistent broadband Internet, learning management systems (LMS), and mobile devices—instructional designers and faculty have new tools to shrink the cognitive distance between learners and instructors. Our project used tools, methodologies, and pedagogies that fit with online learning environments to build an online course that has unique *value* as a learning medium rather than being just a convenient alternative to the traditional classroom. We added Caring Science to the online course to reduce transactional distance, create presence, foster deep engagement, and give students a transformational learning experience.

TRANSACTIONAL DISTANCE

Theory from Roger Moore (1993) that says when there is physical distance between learner and teacher, there is cognitive, emotional, and psychological distance as well that can act as a barrier to learning.

CARING SCIENCE AND THE CARITAS PROCESSES

According to Watson (2008), Caring Science is defined as follows:

> *Caring Science is an evolving philosophical-ethical-epistemic field of study, grounded in the discipline of nursing and informed by related fields. Caring is considered as one central feature within the metaparadigm of nursing knowledge and practice. Caring Science is informed by an ethical-moral-spiritual stance that encompasses a humanitarian, human science orientation to human caring processes, phenomena, and experiences. It is located within a worldview that is non-dualistic, rational, and unified, wherein there is connectedness to ALL; the universal field of Infinity: Cosmic LOVE. Caring Science within this worldview intersects with the arts and humanities and related fields of study and practice (pp.18–19).*

Caritas Processes bring love and caring together to form a deep transpersonal caring focusing on how to Be while doing the work of nursing. The 10 Caritas Processes include (Watson, 2007):

1. *Embrace altruistic values and practice loving kindness with self and others.*

2. *Instill faith and hope and honor others.*

3. *Be sensitive to self and others by nurturing individual beliefs and practices.*

4. *Develop helping-trusting-caring relationships.*

5. *Promote and accept positive and negative feelings as you authentically listen to another's story.*

6. *Use creative scientific problem-solving methods for caring decision-making.*

7. *Share teaching and learning that addresses the individual needs and comprehension styles.*

8. *Create a healing environment for the physical and spiritual self which respects human dignity.*

9. *Assist with basic physical, emotional, and spiritual human needs.*

10. *Be open to mystery and allow miracles to enter.*

The rocketing pervasiveness of online education has made online educators scramble to establish quality norms and best practices. The following quality norms guided our pedagogical design: consistent navigation, visible competency alignment, clear accessibility of instructional materials, clearly stated expectations for the use of media and technology, and a welcoming, intuitive home page. This set of norms, informed by both the Quality Matters Rubric and the Online Learning Consortium Quality Scorecard, tailors learning structures to learners' needs (Quality Matters, 2011). Both of these resources have been widely adopted in higher education for formalized design evaluation. We aimed to build on this foundation, using the rubric and scorecard to inform our design but not determine it.

REFLECTING ON ... TRANSFORMATIONAL LEARNING

- *What intentionally threaded framework(s) can you use to bridge distance and provide students space and structure for transformational learning?*

Humanizing Online Education Through Caring Science

To humanize an online course, Caring Science, the Caritas Processes and Noddings' four ingredients of a caring curriculum underpinned online learning: modeling, practice, authentic dialogue, and confirmation/affirmation (Noddings, 1984). Through modeling, faculty members assist others in being their best selves and create a caring environment between and among students and faculty and also inside and outside virtual, clinical, and classroom settings. Through practice, faculty members create a caring environment through being in day-to-day relationships with students. This includes supporting relationships between and among students and faculty, between and among students, and in and out of classroom and virtual settings (Hills & Watson, 2011). Through authentic dialogue, faculty members create dialectic space for students to reciprocate authentic dialogue. Finally, through confirmation and affirmation, faculty members hold students in the highest ethical regard, prompting the students to assume their respective ideal forms, even if the students cannot track this idealization process *in medias res* (Benner et al., 2010; Johns, 2009; Ironside, 2001, 2005; Sherwood & Horton-Deutsch, 2012).

Infusing an online curriculum with Noddings' four components (1984)—amplifying student connection and student engagement beyond the levels that they normally experience in an online learning environment—requires "authentic presence." Lombard and Horton-Deutsch (2012) define *authentic presence* as a practice of genuineness, self-knowledge, and ability to self-reflect; of caring communication; of being in the moment; and of being honest with oneself and others. Authentic presence in any interpersonal moment captures the human-to-human spirit (Watson, 2015), encourages full inhabitation of all aspects of ourselves and use of all our senses (Paterson & Zderad, 2007), and forces one to endure the pull of turbulence and risks staying open/connected to what is emerging (Parse, 1999).

Combining Online Education, Caring Science, Presence, and Engagement

Remaining "open to what is emerging" creates vulnerability and humanity. This persistent, practiced, intentional openness—the quintessence of authentic presence, which is the quintessence of humanity—is also the quintessence of quality nursing. Facilitating the development of authentic presence in nursing requires creating safe spaces for students to explore where they have been, where they are, and where they want to go in their nursing practice. Providing opportunities for students to replace negative experiences with positive experiences of connection, emotion, and authenticity can rewire neural pathways (Selhub, 2010). The question for this project was, then, how to model authentic presence in our Doctor of Nursing Practice (DNP) nursing students' online environment so that the students could capture that presence and re-create it in their respective internal environments.

Creating learning experiences that support *authentic presence* entails incorporation of self-care practices where students are encouraged to cultivate and reflect on individualized health-promoting behaviors and activities (Dossey & Keagan, 2013; Orem, 2001). Breathing exercises, guided imagery, and loving/

kindness meditations pave the way for learning by opening the students to their own fears or vulnerabilities and stimulating compassion. These practices aim to develop authentic presence and create an environment where deep learning can occur.

Authentic presence space prepares students to *engage* in learning within self and with others. Research demonstrates that students who are more engaged in learning have more desirable learning outcomes, such as better critical thinking, more profound satisfaction, and higher grade performance (Carini, Kuh, & Klein, 2006; Kuh, 2009; Salamonson, Andrew, & Everett, 2009). Nursing students' engagement, interaction, and participation in their educational experiences improves learning outcomes (Kuh, 2003) and occurs across traditional and online learning environments (Giddens, Fogg, & Carlson-Sabelli, 2010). In addition, student engagement is a basic tenet of reflective practice (Horton-Deutsch, Sherwood, & Armstrong, 2012).

Learning experiences that support engagement also include the use of quality norms that intentionally facilitate students' navigation through the learning process. When designing engaging courses, leaving space for reflection is as important as curating resources for students. This balance between space and structure does not happen without an intentional design process that foregrounds context: building learning experiences that caringly guide students into discovery via contact with content, classmates, instructors, and themselves.

REFLECTING ON … STUDENT ENGAGEMENT

- *In what ways can you balance structure and freedom in your online courses?*

- *How can you capture the spirit of the content to challenge and engage students authentically?*

The Project

The purpose of our project was to explore teaching strategies *designed* to create authentic presence and engage students in online learning and those strategies' *actual effect* on DNP students.

MIND MAP

A diagram used to visually organize information.

Course Mapping

The authors created a mind map (we used the bubbl.us online tool available at www.bubbl.us) to visually present the course description, technology requirements, weekly topics, theoretical orientation/readings/viewings, and learning activities. The map allowed the team to visually align those elements with course competencies (see Figure 8.1).

Using a course-mapping process—with a map designed from the student perspective—is a helpful way to keep a course student centered, giving instructors the tools to evaluate flow, pedagogy, methodology, workload, space, and structure in an objective format. The map acts as both a visually organized planning document and an evaluative tool. It allows the instructor and designer to target meaningful change, structuring the course intentionally and incorporating time and activities for reflective practice.

For example, in this specific project, beginning each assignment with a "presencing" exercise served to focus thoughts and attention. Having students then engage in reading assignments and complete learning activities (reflections and discussions, videos, and written assignments) required them to reflect on their experiences, reflect on their readings, and respond to questions that helped them begin to think in new ways and through multiple perspectives. In addition, incorporating aesthetic expression into reflection and discussion assignments further prompted students' interest and emotions. Mapping the course facilitated this balance between structure and space, creating an intentional online learning environment where students had both the freedom and the support to meaningfully reflect and grow.

Learning Activities

After a course map was completed, learning activities were developed to support meaningful learning. The course emphasized components of learning in two segments, based on Shulman's (2002) longitudinal study of knowledge growth (see Figure 8.2). The first segment focused on engagement, understanding, and action; the second segment focused on reflection, judgment, and commitment. In segment 1, students received presencing activities, received an overview of a particular topic, completed introductory readings, and completed a learning assignment focused on engagement, understanding, and action. Students were then asked to connect the topic to what they already knew, consider how the readings contribute to a fuller understanding, and consider how they would apply this understanding to their nursing practice in an ethical manner (action). Subsequently, in segment 2, students received a presencing exercise; received an overview of how they might take further their learning on the topic; completed theoretical readings centered on Caring Science and multiple ways of knowing; and completed a learning assignment focusing on reflection (reflecting on experiences, thinking from multiple perspectives, challenging assumptions, and exploring new possibilities), judgment, and commitment.

Shulman's reflective-learning approach to knowledge growth was incorporated into the following learning activities: online dialogue and discussion assignments; two 5-minute video assignments, completed at the beginning and end of each course; a written Describe, Examine, and Articulate Learning (DEAL) (Ash & Clayton, 2004; Ash, Clayton, & Atkinson, 2005) assignment that built on learning throughout the course; and a written commitment-to-change assignment.

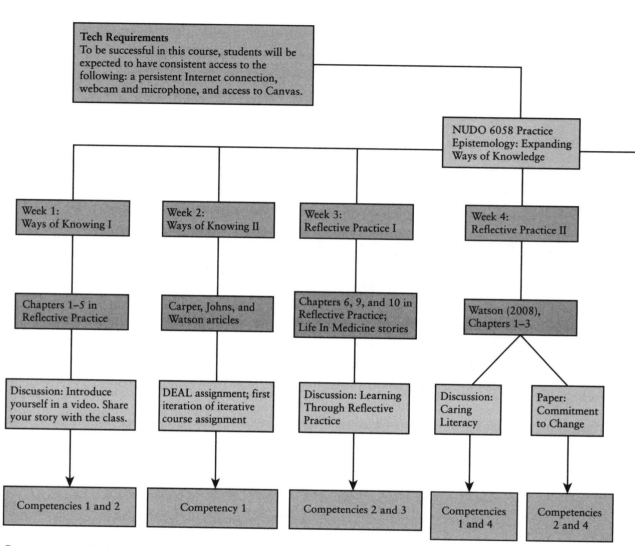

Competency 1: Understand (analyze) the complexities of the client's lived experience.

Competency 2: Obtain (create and evaluate) a detailed life story or client narrative.

FIGURE 8.1

Mind Map of DNP
Epistemology Course

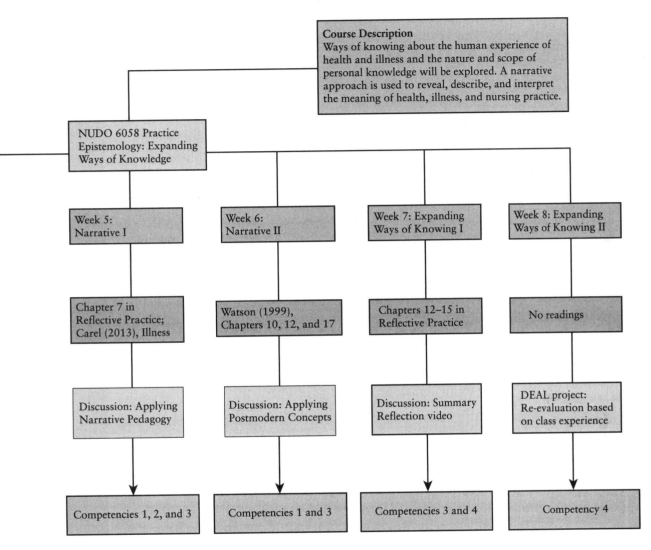

Competency 3: Identify (synthesize) common themes in life stories.

Competency 4: Increase awareness of (interpret) the empathic and caring nature of nursing practice (in light of transformational experience).

FIGURE 8.2

Shulman's Table of Learning

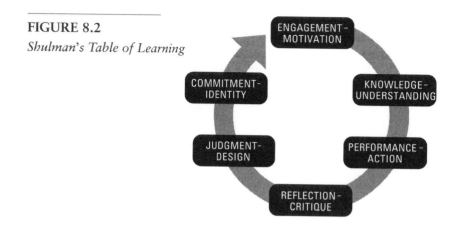

For the first video assignment, we asked students to begin by sharing what they value most about their life and work. Next, we asked them to share their current understanding of the course topic, practice epistemology. Then, we asked them the following two questions:

- What does authentic presence mean to you?

- What does engagement mean to you?

At the end of the course, we asked students to reconsider the preceding questions as well as the following:

- How has the course influenced your understanding of authentic presence?

- In what ways did this course influence your understanding of engagement in learning?

A written DEAL assignment (Ash & Clayton, 2004; Ash, Clayton, & Atkinson, 2005; Ash, Clayton, & Moses, 2008), described in detail in Chapter 7, focused on a personal or professional experience with illness. The first iteration focused on students' current understanding of the illness by writing a thick description; completing an examination to externalize, deconstruct, and critique the dominant understanding; and articulating their learning. The second iteration was used to support reflexivity and inform learning experiences in the course.

We used the commitment-to-change assignment to assess student learning at midpoint in the course. For this assignment, we asked students to reflect on what they had learned so far in light of their current professional context. The goal of the paper was for students to see how their experiences in the course were transforming their practice. We then asked students to write a two-to-three–page single-spaced paper, identifying two or three possible changes that they planned to make in their nursing practice and identifying the level of commitment to making these changes as well as their resistance to change.

In addition, employing learning activities founded in the arts and humanities strengthened this approach. These activities included presencing exercises (e.g., breathing, guided imagery, meditations) and artistic expression (e.g., photos, music, poems) to further capture/elucidate the topic of discussion (caring/healing). They support aesthetic ways of knowing/being to enhance the understanding of caring and support intentional conscious practice.

Evaluation

Using a Caring Science curriculum also required evaluation strategies congruent with Noddings' four components (modeling, practice, authentic dialogue, and confirmation/affirmation). The previous assignments modeled equitable, respectful, caring relations and cultivated a disciplined scholarship necessary for developing expertise. They promoted dialogue through online discussions that gained depth through time and required students to link theoretical concepts to ethical practice. We were interested in students' ability to "acquire insights, see patterns, find meanings and significance, see balance and wholeness, make compassionate and wise judgments, while acquiring foresight, generating creative flexible strategies, developing informed skilled intentionality, identifying ethical and cultural traditions of the field, grasping the deeper structures of the knowledge base, enlarging the ability to think critically and creatively and find pathways to new knowledge" (Bevis, 2000, p. 265). Facilitating instruction in this manner held to the ideals of practice (affirmation/confirmation), aimed to access students' thinking, and captured the essence of a Caring Science curriculum.

Integration of Quality Norms

After a course map is completed and the course is developed, quality norms come into play. Norms help instructors influence the way students experience the course online. The goal is to make navigating the course as intuitive as possible, with technology acting as an invisible enabler to learning rather than a barrier. As such, a set of quality norms can guide a course into an LMS. Most LMSs act as toolboxes for instructors: They provide the necessary means to develop a course but give no instructions on how or what to build. As with web design, the inclination is to look at the layout of a course like a puzzle: "[E]ach content element is a puzzle piece, and you put all the pieces in the middle and rearrange until they fit together" (Drysdale, 2011, p. 27). This seemingly logical approach tends to result in "a cluttered layout with elements jammed into every available space" (Drysdale, 2011). For instructors, quality norms provide the framework that gives intentional shape to the course, enabling students to effortlessly navigate their learning online (Quality Matters, 2011).

Outcomes

We taught this course for the first time in summer 2014 with 11 DNP students. Nearly three-quarters (72%) of the students completed the course evaluation. On a 5-point scale, with 5 denoting "exceeded expectations," the mean score for the course evaluation was 4.4, and the instructor evaluation was 4.7. Over the course of the semester, we received only three questions regarding navigation of the course, suggesting that both the course structure and directions for navigation were clear and effective.

On the second iteration of the DEAL project, students spoke of the value of reflection and developing a deeper appreciation of multiple ways of knowing. For example, one student wrote, "I learned that reflection takes time and is a process. However, simply thinking is not enough. … The structure of the iterative reflective questions was important in my ability to look at this experience in different ways and ask myself questions I might not have considered."

Another student wrote about how strong emotions such as anger and fear clouded her perception through the first writing of the DEAL project but how the repetitive nature of the assignment helped her to work through her emotions. As a result, during the second writing, she remarked, "I was able to ask questions I hadn't thought of and take time to consider the situation within a broader context."

Similarly, another student wrote that she had an expanded appreciation of the body/mind/spirit connection and how her feelings and emotions influenced communication and treatment plans. "I learned the importance of emotional intelligence and that taking care of myself is an important part of being more present for others."

Finally, one student remarked that the assignment taught her to be more conscious and curious in her daily activities, helping her appreciate their beauty and significance.

In response to the commitment-to-change project, students identified changes that they were planning for their nursing practice. Broadly, papers focused on obstacles to making these changes, the value of making changes, and how remaining connected to their values would support their efforts toward achieving their goals. More specifically, nearly all the students identified the need to create time for themselves each day to care for themselves so they could be more present for others, whether patients or their own students. Students identified these practices as essential for modeling caring relations with others. Interestingly, these papers were filled with examples of Noddings' four components of evaluation.

We received the least direct feedback on the learning activities that incorporated the arts and humanities. Most likely, this was due to these assignments not being formally evaluated but used as a way to set the tone for the learning environment and create a safe space for authentic dialogue. Within assignments, such as the commitment-to-change project, students did identify the value of finding particular arts and humanities activities, such as breathing exercises or artistic expressions, that would fit with their particular patient or student populations. This suggested that the students found value in activities that support intentional practices and caring.

To gauge the growth of students from the beginning of the course to the end of the course, students recorded a second 5-minute video readdressing the following questions:

- What does authentic presence mean to you?

- What does engagement mean to you?

- How has the course influenced your understanding of authentic presence?

- In what ways did this course influence your understanding of engagement in learning?

The majority of students exhibited substantial growth in their understanding and experience of engagement and authentic presence. One student began by defining authentic presence as "sincere and genuine care" that was worth the extra time it takes with patients. Upon reflection, that understanding grew:

> *Authentic presence is more than just being sincere and preventing cell phone interruptions during your patient encounters. It's a constellation of things that comes together to provide an experience for our patients. It's a constantly growing and developing skill set that will become more refined with time. It's the environment in which your encounter takes place, and it's a mindfulness of not only your own emotions and feelings, but also that of the patients. From the things you say down to the way you breathe, these all play a part in your authentic presence you provide. It is taking yourself off autopilot and recognizing the uniqueness of every moment and encounter.*

Another student began with no prior knowledge of epistemology, coming to the course with excitement about the potential for impact on her teaching but without a tangible sense of meaning to authentic presence. A third student reflected, "What we're really teaching through reflective learning is clinical judgment, and clinical judgment is a way to take that static learning, those stats, and those bits of information and really apply them to the person that's in front of us."

A fourth student—embarrassed, but open—shared at the beginning that she knew little about epistemology and had to look up the definition. Her understanding of authentic presence was much more sophisticated at the end of the course: Intuition and experience led to seeing authentic presence as active listening, providing for patients with body, soul, and knowledge.

A fifth student's reflection breathed life into her experiences, giving them shape and purpose:

> *Authentic presence is more than just being there physically, but it's when you are able to be honest with yourself, and self-reflect on your values, and cultural meanings, and intentions that you have and how those things come into play when you're interacting with others—and accepting that others might come with their own intentions and own goals—and come to middle ground when you are interacting with people in general.*

Although some students started out with a clearer understanding of epistemology, engagement, and authentic presence, others began with little or no knowledge. Most students exhibited significant growth, assimilating this knowledge into new ways of knowing that will significantly affect the care they provide for patients. All students—even those with worldviews and experiences that made the content of the course difficult to internalize—questioned, reflected, engaged with classmates and themselves, and came away changed by their experiences.

Final Reflections

Designing an online course can be taxing—much like transcribing a piece of music that, although beautiful, can be difficult to put into notes. Instructors and designers working together can create online courses that balance structure and freedom, capturing quality norms for online learning, critical reflection, and the spirit of the content. Online courses created in this way can challenge and authentically engage students in learning. Through this project, it became clear that both students and instructors benefit when courses are developed with intention—where maps and frameworks guide course development, quality norms guide instructional design, and reflective pedagogies and learning activities support presence and engagement. This approach—when used to design online courses that bridge transactional distance, employ the use of media intentionally, and provide students both the space and structure needed for transformational learning—is an effective and practical methodology for designing meaningful learning experiences.

References

Ash, S. L., & Clayton, P. H. (2004). The articulated learning: An approach to reflection and assessment. *Innovative Higher Education, 29*(2), 137–154.

Ash, S. L., Clayton, P. H., & Atkinson, M. P. (2005). Integrating reflection and assessment to improve and capture student learning. *Michigan Journal of Community Service-Learning, 11*(2), 49–59.

Ash, S. L., Clayton, P. H., & Moses, M. G. (2008). *Learning through critical reflection: A tutorial for service-learning students.* Accompanying *Instructor's Version.* Raleigh, NC: Center for Excellence in Curricular Engagement, North Carolina State University.

Benner, P., Sutphen, M., Leonard, V., & Day, L. (2010). *Educating nurses: A call for radical transformation.* San Francisco, CA: Jossey-Bass.

Bevis, E. (2000). Accessing learning: Determining worth or developing or excellence—from a behaviorist toward an interpretative criticism model. In E. Bevis, & J. Watson (Eds.), *Toward a caring curriculum: A new pedagogy for nursing* (pp. 67–107). Boston, MA: Jones & Bartlett Learning.

Carini, R. M., Kuh, G. D., & Klein, S. P. (2006). Student engagement and student learning: Testing the linkages. *Research in Higher Education, 47*(1), 1–32.

Dossey, B., & Keegan, L. (2013). *Holistic nursing: A handbook for practice* (6th ed.). Burlington, MA: Jones & Bartlett Learning.

Drysdale, J. (2011). *Bootstrapping design.* Publisher: Author.

Giddens, J., Fogg, L., & Carlson-Sabelli, L. (2010). Learning and engagement with a virtual community by undergraduate nursing students. *Nursing Outlook, 58*(5), 261–267. doi:10.1016/j.outlook.2010.08.001

Google (2014). *How search works.* Retrieved from https://www.google.com/insidesearch/howsearchworks/thestory/index.html

Hills, M., & Watson, J. (2011). *Creating a caring science curriculum: An emancipatory pedagogy of nursing.* New York, NY: Springer.

Horton-Deutsch, S., Sherwood, G., & Armstrong, G. (2012). Reflection in classroom and clinical contexts: Assessment and evaluation. In G. Sherwood, & S. Horton-Deutsch (Eds.), *Reflective practice: Transforming education and improving outcomes.* Indianapolis, IN: Sigma Theta Tau International.

Institute of Medicine (IOM). (2011). *The future of nursing: Leading change, advancing health.* Washington, DC: National Academies Press.

Ironside, P. M. (2001). Creating a research base for nursing education: An interpretative review of conventional, critical, feminist and postmodern, and phenomenological pedagogies. *Advances in Nursing Science, 23*(3), 72–87.

Ironside, P. M. (2005). Teaching, thinking, and reaching the limits of memorization: Enacting new pedagogies. *Journal of Nursing Education, 44*(10), 441–449.

Johns, C. (2009). *Becoming a reflective practitioner.* (3rd ed.). Oxford, UK: Wiley-Blackwell.

Kuh, G. D. (2003). *The national survey of student engagement: Conceptual framework and overview of psychometric properties.* Indiana University Center for Postsecondary Research. Retrieved from http://nsse.iub.edu/pdf/conceptual_framework_2003.pdf

Kuh, G. D. (2009). The national survey of student engagement: Conceptual framework empirical foundations. *New Directions for Institutional Research, 141,* 5–20. doi:10.1002/ir.283

Lombard, K., & Horton-Deutsch, S. (2012). Creating space for reflection: The importance of presence in the teaching-learning process. In G. Sherwood & S. Horton-Deutsch (Eds.). *Reflective practice: Transforming education and improving outcomes* (pp. 22–38). Indianapolis, IN: Sigma Theta Tau International.

Moore, M. G. (1993). Theory of transactional distance. In D. Keegan (Ed.), *Theoretical principles of distance education.* New York, NY: Routledge.

Noddings, N. (1984). *Caring: A feminine approach to ethics and moral education.* Berkeley, CA: University of California Press.

Orem, D. (2001). *Nursing: Concepts of practice.* (6th ed.). St. Louis, MO: Mosby.

Parse, R. (1999). *Illuminations: The human becoming theory in practice and research.* Sudbury, MA: Jones & Bartlett Learning.

Paterson, J., & Zderad, L. (2007). *Humanistic nursing.* Retrieved from http://www.gutenberr.org/files/25020/25020-8.txt

Quality Matters. (2011). *2011–2013 Quality Matters Rubric with Points.* Retrieved from https://www.qualitymatters.org/rubric

Salamonson, Y., Andrew, S., & Everett, B. (2009). Academic engagement and disengagement as predictors of performance in pathophysiology among nursing students. *Contemporary Nurse, 32*(1), 123–132.

Selhub, D. (2010). *The love response. Your prescription to turn off fear, anger, and anxiety to achieve vibrant health and transform your life.* New York, NY: Ballantine.

Sherwood, G., & Horton-Deutsch, S. (2012). *Reflective practice: Transforming education and improving outcomes.* Indianapolis, IN: Sigma Theta Tau International.

Shulman, L. (2002). Making a difference. A table of learning. *Change, 34*(6), 36–44.

Watson, J. (2007). Global Translations—10 Caritas Processes. Retrieved from http://watsoncaringscience.org/about-us/caring-science-definitions-processes-theory/global-translations-10-caritas-processes/

Watson, J. (2008). *Nursing: The philosophy and science of caring* (Rev. ed.). Boulder, CO: University Press of Colorado.

Watson, J. (2015). *Presence: An elusive and spirit-filled concept and practice.* Manuscript submitted for publication.

Part III

Reflective Learning Environments Within Healthcare Systems

Chapter 9

Transformational Reflective Organizations: Front-Line Challenges and Changes Guided by Caring Science

Jean Watson, PhD, RN, AHN-BC, FAAN

No organization can be reflective. No organization can be ethical.

It is the people, the human consciousness of those within the organization—they are the ones who live out the ethics and reflective stance for true organizational transformation.

The worldview, the philosophy, and consciousness of the leader— that makes all the difference. ...

–Jean Watson

Knowing that no organization truly can be reflective or ethical—only that the humans within it can internalize such a skill or value—how can nursing leaders create reflective, values-guided organizations? How can nursing organizational leaders and administrators transcend this outdated era that we continue to experience and give their own vocational reflective voice, values, and forms of authentic leadership to guide the human/organizational change now so needed for humankind and society alike?

This chapter offers a background for conscious, intentional change guided by a new era in science and an evolving unitary worldview. It explores two reflective leadership experiences that sought transformative change from within one university's college of nursing. These changes emerged from Caring Science consciousness, providing the core values and the ethical/philosophical context, as well as the intellectual scholarly foundation for nursing's scholarly advancement.

Background

In the 1990s and 2000s, nursing education and clinical nursing care models made remarkable strides with regard to influencing system-wide healthcare practices. These remarkable educational/clinical and system changes represent deep cultural consciousness shifts. One of the greatest influences of these shifts is nursing, maturing within its evolution of knowledge, research, caring practices, and philosophies and theories underpinning nursing as a distinct discipline and profession. Another influence of these changes includes wise leaders willing to transcend the dominant worldview systems and open new space for creative, imaginative, and inspired visions of possibilities—those beyond the usual mindsets and status quo.

We witness today some dramatic new openings representing nursing's mature, disciplinary theoretical stance. The national Magnet Recognition Program, which introduced the quality national hospital nursing practice standards, is one example. These new criteria include hospital nursing practices, guided by nursing theories and defined professional practice models. Indeed, there is a steady and consistent trail of magnet hospital research evidence, demonstrating patient outcomes and affecting, for example, mortality, length of stay, and better work environments (Kelly, McHugh, & Aiken, 2011; McHugh et al., 2013; Needleman, 2013). Nursing magnet research captures the significant relationship between nursing care and patient/system outcomes; embedded in the magnet outcome research is an identified professional practice model, indicating that nursing practice success is influenced by use of a professional nursing theory/model.

This maturing of nursing professional practice models, in spite of the dominant medical disease–founded hospital system, is revolutionary and indeed has had a major impact on hospital staff, patients, and society. However, even with these best practice hospital successes—and even with the maturing of nursing as a distinct discipline and profession—the professional practices of nursing are still surrounded by an outdated scientific worldview of medical disease and sick care practices, as well as latent and overt norms established by the historic, institutional, industrial, modern era hospital culture.

In light of the driving norms, forces, and the powerful hospital culture, which has led to noncaring and nonhuman practices against nursing's phenomenon of focus (human caring/healing, health, and human experiences), it remains remarkable that hospital nursing has made such major leaps toward improving nursing practice and outcomes.

And as great as these accomplishments have been and continue to be, what is missing within the hospital sick-care culture is the worldview shifts surrounding and engulfing our daily existence and reality about healthy living and life itself. For example, a global quantum, scientific, spirit-filled, evolved consciousness is emerging throughout all of humankind today. These global shifts are moving toward inner healing, human caring, mental health, self-caring, self-knowledge, self-control, and self-healing approaches, addressing individual and collective human suffering.

EVOLVED CONSCIOUSNESS

Both Western medicine and nursing have evolved from Era I thinking, focusing on body physical parts; to Era II mindsets, focusing on mind-body interaction; to Era III, focusing on evolved view of oneness, connectedness—referred to a transformative unitary consciousness (Watson, 2008, 2010).

CARING ECONOMICS

A focus on economics that includes human caring as an economic variable and critical resource regarding the real wealth of a nation (Eisler, 2010).

What is happening in this era in human history demands an expanded and dramatically different worldview—a cosmic, unitary view of our world and planet Earth. This new cosmic demand points us seemingly in the opposite directions of the dominant physical treatment–cure model. The quantum move is away from hospital and sick-care, away from what has been defined as *Era I* (body physical thinking), and away from material medicine and external interventions and cure of body at all cost—physically, mentality, economically, spiritually. Now the move is into quantum field views; nonlocal consciousness; energetic view of all of life; and views related to inner health, inner healing, healthy communities, and human and environment planetary health.

Developments are even occurring in the field of caring economics. For example, Eisler (2008) calls for a partnership economics of caring—in contrast to a domination control-over economics—acknowledging that human caring becomes a foundational necessity for survival of our world, not only economically but in actuality. Richard Layard, professor at the London School of Economics, poses that the big breakthrough in economics was finding that "[Y]ou can ask people how they feel about their lives" as an economic indicator of well-being rather than wealth (2014, p. 2). He advises governments around the world to focus their economic policies on happiness and well-being; his work is related to thriving, addressing widespread depression, anxiety, and mental health as forms of evidence for economic decisions for nations. The small kingdom of Bhutan, on the borders of China and Nepal, prefers a Global National Happiness Index

(GNHI) over the gross national product (GNP) mentality. Layard has consulted with, for example, the German and British governments to explore the option to substitute GNHI for GNP.

This new thinking is emerging from an evolved consciousness of humanity and survival beyond material wealth. We are at a point in human history, now surrendering to the universal, shared humanity reality—that is, everything is connected, reflecting the view we all "belong to the infinite field of universal Love" (Levinas, 1969), one of the foundations of Caring Science.

REFLECTING ON ... YOURSELF

- *What is your inner guide asking of you?*
- *How can you break set with conventional norms expecting conformity?*

Reflective Leadership in an Age of Caring Science

This infinite field of life spirit, from which we all come and to which we all return, can be the source of economics and other new thought systems on which Caring Science is built.

We can now draw upon this reality in guiding forms of reflective leadership, attending to health, healing, and our spiritual harmony with All (Levinas, 1969; Watson, 2008, 2011, 2014). This view is not only consistent with new science trends for medical science and technology, but also with indigenous teachings and wisdom traditions across all time—to which we now have to return and honor for our individual/collective survival, as well as our daily health. Rhetorical, existential, and spiritual questions remain as touchstones for our time if we take reflective leadership seriously:

- How do we as a society and global village learn to give new meaning to living, dying, suffering, and human existence?

- What is nursing in this new world?

- What will it be when the systems behind us, in the medical physical science world, are no longer there, defining and dominating the health-healing culture of our evolved practice world?

- What will nursing and healthcare become when nursing has a universal worldview of health, healing for all?

These are the big quantum calls, challenges, and questions for each of us and for nursing and the world today. Consistent with Al Gore's views on the human–environment relation, these are not just scientific questions but spiritual questions as well:

- Are we here for a purpose?

- Does nursing have a covenant with humanity?

- Is there a reason for nursing's existence?

- Are we alone?

- Is there a greater intelligence we can draw upon for life's living?

- Is body physical the only plane to consider for treatment of disease, organizing structures, policies, and practices for individual/societal global health/healing and graceful living?

- Or are we here to focus solely on the physical science objective plane of humanity, and basic medical treatment of disease, after the fact?

- Are we participating in wielding power and control over our hearts and souls and other human beings and our planet Earth?

- Is nursing poised and confident to develop and mature nursing *qua* nursing or succumb to advancing nursing *qua* medicine?

These are the dominant existential/spiritual survival questions facing nursing and all of humankind today. These global existential/spiritual awakenings in humanity affect nursing and how it defines and redefines itself for a new era in human evolution. This evolution brings dramatically different worldviews and approaches to caring and healing.

The good news is that as we face this turning point for our world, new values begin to emerge, and we can look for new symbols for change—signs of rebirth—as old things must die. Perhaps at the cosmic level, this is a timeless era, where the world is undergoing ancient cycles of human/life/environment existence.

Ancient global symbols and archetypes exist to remind humanity of the normal life/death cycles. For example, the Indian divinity, *Vishnu*, stands as a universal symbol for creation and destruction, ruling all cycles of birth/rebirth by nature's universal principles and not the full control of mankind. Other universal symbols are the circle and mandala, shamanic visions that see humans as luminous beings connected to all of humanity in a universal cosmic field.

Native and ancient world traditions have called up a universal spirit world. For example, Brazilian healers (*cueranderos*) and other shamanic indigenous practices, such as distant healing, chanting, drumming, and soul retrieval, all are in communication with the broader field of connections with universe spirit, our Source—all energetic connections that transcend time, space, and physicality.

These ancient symbols, codes, and archetypal reminders reflect the contemporary Era III, scientific emergence in quantum physics and global unitary views of science and human beings, à *la* Martha Rogers in nursing, deep philosophical starting points for science from Levinas, positing the "ethic of belonging" as first principle of science. These all lead to global unitary views for survival, and require—if not demand—new reflective approaches to humanity and organizations.

These reflective, ancient, and converging contemporary mindsets are located within new discourses identified as *Era III thinking* (Dossey, 1991; Newman, 1994; Watson, 1999, 2008, 2012). This discourse is consistent with notions of "unitary science unitary field" (Rogers, 1970, 1992; Watson & Smith, 2002). Concepts such as *transpersonal, trans-disciplinary, integrative medicine, mind/body medicine, mind/body/spirit medicine, unitary caring field, caritas field* (Watson, 2014), and other similar terms reflect a new reality and worldview shift. These words and concepts are all attempts to capture creative imaginative images, a new emerging consciousness toward body as energy, life as energy-spirit–filled existence. This shift in worldview invites inner approaches to health, well-being, and post-hospital community-based, home-based human environment "survival of humanity and our world"–based realities.

REFLECTING ON ... TRANSFORMATION

- *With such quantum shifts in front of and before us then, how are we to consider new liberating structures, evolved systems, reflective learning communities, and environments for transformational, front-line leadership?*

- *How do we move contemporary successes, such as exemplary magnet hospitals, toward futuristic visions, embracing authentic creative spirit-filled changes—changes that can take us into a brave new worldview of actualizing human caring/healing/healthy educational and moral value-guided practice communities, organizations, and our broader world?*

Unitary Caring Science as One Way Forward

While from the bounded level of our mind
Short views we take not see the lengths behind;
But more advanced, behold with strange surprise
New distant scenes of endless science arise!

–Alexander Pope (in Watson, 2002, p. 453)

In the past two decades or more, Caring Science has evolved toward a higher, deeper level of maturity to underpin and guide nursing and healthcare, while ushering in new transformative models of science with hope for an evolved civilization for humanity. As this work has evolved and transformed itself, it now finds itself intersecting and converging with quantum thinking, with some of the latest thinking in integrative medicine, and specifically, integrative nursing

(Kreitzer & Koithan, 2014). Further, the evolution of Caring Science scholarship with science of unitary human beings (Rogers, 1970, 1992, 1994) likewise offers another foundation for a transtheoretical and transdisciplinary discourse for nursing and organizations. New explanatory models are needed, and unitary Caring Science and integrative thinking offer a new worldview explanatory model for reflective change.

Background of Caring Science and Unitary Worldview

A framework of Caring Science and *caritas* (a Latin word conveying universal love, charity, and caring) intersecting with Rogerian science of unitary human relocates our existing medical system thinking into a quantum field of possibilities, drawing upon the evolution of humans and One World—awakening to the unitary view, that everything in the universe is connected, even if we cannot physically "see" this oneness. Nevertheless, we currently are experiencing our unitary connections, physically and virtually, via the Internet, social media, television, space travels internally and externally, and other dimensions waiting to happen that we cannot imagine at this time. This era is and can be called a *revolution of human consciousness*—a profound worldview shift, from separation to connections, from distance-separating to distance-connecting.

Thus, moving from the current system of thinking toward reflective front-line changes takes us into a path of consciousness, attending to the patterns of unity, diversity, and a global universal field of Oneness. This path has been referred to as a *quantum world*, or even a *quantum cosmology* (Watson, 2014).

Unitary Caring Science and integrative principles serve as an emerging area of nursing and trans-disciplinary focus and ground the quantum Era III worldview—acknowledging a deeper *Ethic of Belonging* (Levinas, 1969; Watson, 2006, 2008), making it explicit that we all "belong" to the infinity and universal cosmic energetic quantum field of whole (Watson, 2014). This basic starting point as the first principle of unitary science helps us to understand that a nurse's consciousness as a leader has an individual and a global effect at the same time.

From Limited Consciousness to Liberated Consciousness: A Personal/Professional Story

My background in developing and implementing Caring Science and Watson's theory of human caring in education and practice, combined with my views of a global unitary quantum consciousness field, contribute to my story. My story embraces and builds upon the reality that humanity and educational and healthcare organizations have to move beyond the status quo, toward the future, with renewed focus on human/environmental, caring, healing, and health; these are inner models of unitary caring and well-being, beyond medical disease and physical care. From this line of thinking, I offer two personal/professional examples of being on the front line of change, transforming organizations from inside out representing whole-system Caring Science projects. Two experiences serve as personal exemplars from education and clinical care:

- Creation of the Colorado Center for Human Caring as Dean of Nursing

- Implementing the Denver Nursing Project in Human Caring

REFLECTING ON ... SERVICE

- *How are you willing to translate your passion into coherent, informed, moral social action?*

- *How can you give your authentic voice and leadership in human caring to systems embedded in limited thinking?*

- *How can you offer yourself in reflective service to humanity to fulfill your destiny?*

- *How can you language and message nursing and human caring as ancient and noble service to humanity?*

- *How can you find your purpose and calling from within?*

Colorado Center for Human Caring

The 1980s were an interesting time, especially for the University of Colorado (CU) School of Nursing on the Health Sciences Campus in Denver. The school has a long history of leadership and national standing, being one of the early schools offering master's degrees in nursing before systems knew exactly what a master's-prepared nurse was, or even how to use or benefit from a master's-level nurse. The history and origins of the now-international nurse practitioner (NP) model began in 1965 at the University of Colorado under the vision and leadership of Dr. Loretta Ford and Dr. Henry Silver, a pediatrician in the medical school. This program led to what is now considered mainstream NP programs, offered at both the master's and doctoral levels, changing the nature of professional nursing.

The CU School of Nursing in the 1980s and early 1990s developed the first publicly funded nursing clinical doctorate as the career professional practice degree ("ND" in those days; later it became the foundation at CU, allowing for the transition of the ND into the now-standard doctor of nursing practice degree [DNP]). However, in Colorado, the clinical doctorate was focused on caring–healing and health and was designed for nursing beyond hospital disease/medical-focused care. Other historic programs and changes have put CU College of Nursing on the national map once again. The school and entire CU Health Science Center campus moved to a new campus, uniting hospitals, research, and education for all health/medical care professionals on one campus. This is the now prominently recognized University of Colorado Anschutz Medical Center Campus (interesting fact that the name change, paradoxically, went retro—from "Health Sciences" to "Medical Sciences"—in naming the Anschutz campus).

> **NOTE**
>
> *This very phenomenon of language continues to reflect the consciousness of medical systems and offers another message for this chapter.*

In spite of the history of innovative leadership and visionary programs before their time, and while we witness the dominant thinking of medicine's presence, the School of Nursing on the Health Science Campus during the late 1970s and early 1980s was in the throes of chaos and decline. The chancellor later confided in me that he was considering closing the school. Probably the public does not realize this history, but I did, as I experienced it as a new faculty, having just completed my PhD in 1978, and immediately joining the university faculty.

This era of national nursing chaos included Boston University abruptly closing its school of nursing after a long history, and Duke University closing its undergraduate program, threatening undergraduate nursing programs in other parts of the United States. Abrupt national activities were affecting nursing education, combined with a large national nursing hospital shortage.

During this era, the CU School of Nursing went through a series of successive deans, all with brief tenures for a variety of reasons. After national searches and the school navigating inner and outer turmoil, I was appointed Dean of Nursing at CU in 1983. The hope and expectation was to bring new vision, new life, and new directions to nursing in the university—to set the course for actualizing the profession, as the School of Nursing soon would be celebrating its 100-year history.

The big question before the school in the mid-'80s was that if it were to survive, two essential questions needed to be asked and addressed:

- Where should the School of Nursing be in the 21st century?

- Where should nursing be in the year 2000 when the School of Nursing will be 100 years old?

These were my inspired dean challenges in the mid-'80s that came to me both from our university-wide, multicampus system President, Arnold Weber, and Health Science Center Chancellor, John Cowee. These rhetorical and futuristic questions influenced my decision to become dean (as it was not a career goal of mine to be a dean, especially at that early point in my own career).

Nevertheless, accepting the challenge and serving as dean set a path for new philosophical organizational standards for the faculty, students, colleagues, clinical agencies, and the broader health and public community. I was intent on helping the faculty and school succeed in meeting these exciting challenges and invitations to create our preferred future.

Two major initiatives during my tenure as dean may offer some insight about a reflective organization and how a leader's worldview, value system, and creative innovation can open new possibilities of what might be, rather than conforming to the status quo. The two projects and programs can be seen as living examples of reflective change and a glimpse into reflective organizational leadership, guided by a higher/deeper vision of nursing and Caring Science; focusing on redefining nursing scholarship and practices as human caring, healing, and health, beyond conventional science models and beyond medical/sick hospital-care approaches. The two initiatives conveying reflective organization examples are:

- The Center for Human Caring
- The Denver Nursing Project in Human Caring

The Center for Human Caring (CHC) in the School of Nursing became an international center for practice, research, education, and scholarship in Caring Science. The CHC established new relationships with clinical partners and other departments and faculty within the broader university—for example, philosophy, arts, humanities, classics, music, drama, existential studies, and religious studies—and the broader public. These broader relationships and programs brought new life and new connections, inspired programs for nontraditional scholarship and methods of research, and explored underdeveloped connections between and among disciplines.

The CHC sponsored monthly open seminars to the university community as well as the public. These seminars included series such as Caring and Art, Caring and Music, Caring in Dance/Movement, Caring in Film, and Caring in Literature. The CHC and School of Nursing held concert series, inviting faculty at the Boulder Campus College of Music to be on the Health Science Campus. Faculty scholars' presentations in philosophy, literature, English studies, and religious studies, as well as experts in phenomenology, physics, and great literature and so on, were offered monthly.

Each series was framed around Caring Science, identifying and acknowledging how each area program contributed to understanding human caring as a serious ethical, philosophical, ontological, epistemological, methodological, pedagogical, praxis, policy endeavor, integrating arts and humanities within nursing and healthcare, beyond conventional thinking. The scholarly notes and opening remarks helped to introduce our faculty, students, clinical colleagues, other disciplines, and the larger public to see the connection among Caring Science and arts, literature, philosophy, music, sound, and movement, and all ways of knowing, being, doing, becoming, as part of deep dimensions of human caring/healing, health.

Another specific example included co-teaching with Hazel Barnes, the internationally acclaimed Distinguished University Professor of Classics (the first woman in our university to be named a Distinguished Professor, the highest honor for scholarly work) known for her translation from French to English of Jean-Paul Sartre's existential writings and books. She was a visiting professor, coming in once per week to offer open noon seminars in the School of Nursing on the existential meaning of selected human conditions. Faculty and graduate students, as well as professors of medicine and psychiatry, attended her seminars. In addition, to expand the pedagogies of our curriculum, some of the faculty and I applied for and were funded by the university's humanities fund to integrate humanities and use of literary works into the existing curriculum. We shared nursing arts seminars with a professor of fine arts from the Boulder Campus, helping students integrate art and artistry of their being and knowing and learning as part of their journey into nursing and exploration of subjective human experiences.

All these combined efforts and many, many more occurred under a new vision for nursing and human caring scholarship, education, and practice. The nursing curriculum was redefined and reframed with faculty and clinical colleagues' involvement and commitments. The curriculum was organized within lines of Caring Science; thus, faculty and students could see how everything they were doing was contributing to the larger field of Caring Science. This consistent framework guided nursing, giving voice to its maturing as a distinct discipline and profession with its own unique standing.

Within this same era, the Center for Nursing Research was also created, helping the school to generate substantial research support through federal grants. This focus on Caring Science research and expanded methodologies led to the School of Nursing, during my deanship, being ranked fifth in the United States for its nursing federal research funding.

UNDERSTANDING CARING SCIENCE AS A BROADER VIEW OF SCIENCE

In my conversations and meetings with the University Board of Regents, with our University President and members of a newly created School of Nursing National Advisory Visiting Board, I helped others to understand Caring Science as a broader view of science, encompassing the values of sustaining humanity, which is beyond medical science. I worked to assist others in understanding nursing as the science, art, and practice of human caring, healing, and health—helping us and our publics to see nursing beyond medical hospital floor-duty nursing.

As one of the members of the Board of Regents asked me, "So, you are not preparing floor nurses anymore?"

My reply, with a touch of light humor, was, "No. Didn't you know? Nurses do not 'do floors' anymore. Now they are going to be 'doing windows.'"

I am not sure that the board member got it, but I loved that moment.

Of course, it is impossible to go into all the happenings, but they included many faculty meetings and retreats. These sessions always included our clinical colleagues and nursing leaders of healthcare systems as partners in transforming and merging values and cultures for advancing nursing as the science and art of caring/healing and health. We together developed new clinical teaching associate models and new clinical-educational practitioners, and established formal clinical teaching hospital partnerships. The Chief Nursing Officer (CNO) was designated Clinical Associate Dean of Nursing, leading to piloting of new professional models of caring/healing within their settings.

These new patterns of curriculum reform—of redefining nursing with a Caring Science framework—were transformative for staff, faculty, and our university and larger public. The school's renewed internal faculty relationships, combined with clinical agencies and clinical leaders, led to an evolved and exciting era in the School of Nursing. The creation of the CHC serves as a symbol of innovative cultural change from within, guided by a core philosophy to expand nursing to serve humanity. This reflective approach opened new horizons of advancements of seemingly miraculous changes by inviting the human spirit to emerge from the people within, celebrating diversity, and opening new partnership and new connections where before there were none.

Overall, the School of Nursing during the mid-'80s into the 1990s, during my era as dean, represented an era of excitement, an exemplar of creating structure to support a reflective organization, offering new hope and concrete liberating programs that emerged from authentic leadership and authentic presence, giving voice and action to an expanded consciousness of Caring Science. It still opens my heart to hear that faculty who experienced that era in the School of Nursing affectionately referred to it as the "Camelot Years."

Denver Nursing Project in Human Caring

In addition to the CHC academic programs, offered to an international community, which included speakers and programs from around the world and from diverse departments in the university, the CHC housed the Denver Nursing Project in Human Caring, which was the site of a nurse-run, interdisciplinary clinical practice center that served the healthcare of persons with AIDS or who were HIV–infected. This "Caring Center," as it became known, was guided by the theory of human caring (Watson, 1979), and it served as the cultural norm for the caring/healing relationship between and among practitioners, the patients, their partners, and the larger public. This center generated new models of professional practice, allowing for and offering new caring/healing modalities, such as therapeutic touch, intentional touch, music, massage, exercise physiology, counseling, group sessions, psychiatric help, and care partnerships with other patients and staff. Nursing staff did education in local bars with patients from the center and attended patient funerals as part of their loving, continuous-care commitments.

New forms of documentation of patient care records were developed and systematically used in the records (documenting, at that time, the original 10 carative factors from Watson theory [1979 publication]) while adding "administrating medical treatments" (to allow for the respiratory and blood work that was done in the center). Every week, King Soopers donated food for an open lunch time for all staff as well as patients and their partners; local Denver florists donated flowers; and patients and community members donated a piano, artwork, furniture, and other furnishings to make the Caring Center non-institutional. It generated research on outcomes and economics, and up to $1 million annually was saved by keeping persons out of the hospital (Leenerts, Koehler, & Neil, 1996).

The Caring Center was federally funded for the maximum years possible, and became a destination site for students and practitioners from around the world. It was adopted as a national model at its time for community support and caring community. As one young man said to me, "Why do you have to get AIDS to get this kind of care? It should be available for everyone."

In summary, perhaps my story as a new dean, intentionally breaking set and holding deep reflective values and a higher vision and image for all, can be a hopeful example. By recognizing and participating in the life cycle of the organization, and understanding the contraction/expansion phenomenon and need for organizational maturity, I invited space for creative emergence through an engaged caring process and structure for reflective change. It may be viewed as one exemplar of human/organizational transformation from within.

When organizations are in crisis and experiencing chaos, it is precisely the time to go back to core values and core mission as the ground of purpose and direction. From this core value foundation, a reflective leader lifts up the vision and purpose for all. It is from this solid core foundation that participants are more able to navigate their way through the chaos and find order emerging from the foundation. As the participants navigate from this foundation, they are simultaneously repatterning themselves and their organization into a reflective, transformed system. What they gain is self-knowledge and self-control over chaos and crises, co-creating their preferred future.

I hope my personal story will invite others to consider new patterns, visions, and versions for how they may trust their inner self as a leader, and how they too can create reflective transformative structures and systems for a still evolving world and evolving unitary worldview.

Final Reflections

A reflective organization requires a reflective leader. A reflective leader invites reflection from all his or her constituents, as no organization can be reflective given that it comes from within the people. Reflective leadership is guided by a goal of human/organizational transformation, grounded in timeless values and a higher vision. Timeless values sustain and inspire humanity and invite evolution of the individuals and the organization. Vision goes beyond change of status quo, and instead invites transformation. Transformation implies an inner and outer journey, going back to core foundation.

A reflective leader assesses and participates in the patterns and cycles of life of the people and the organization. Reflective leadership requires knowledge of the organization's pattern and history, always understanding that organizations have a high and low cycle, just like the rhythm of the universe. Organizational patterns are expanding and contracting, just like the breath of life, the seasons of time.

This understanding of humans and organizations is ancient knowledge; this is not based upon leadership theory 101. To grasp the co-creation of reflective leadership—to create a reflective organization—requires understanding basic change, but invites transformation from within and moves with the rhythmic cycles of the organization.

We do this by adhering to dynamics of consciousness evolution—by knowing when to expand and when to contract.

Reflective leaders are successful when they inspire and invite the participants to engage in a shared purpose greater than self, co-creating a larger vision for themselves and the organization.

If leaders of this time are able to hold and act upon a consciousness of honoring the whole and moving beyond physical material reality as the dominant worldview—if they/you are open to change from within and are able to draw upon the creativity and human spirit of the whole—then there is hope for a new era of nursing and healthcare for all.

We no longer are bound by an outdated worldview of separation science; rather, nursing leaders creating reflective organizational patterns become global Caring Science–consciousness leaders in service to humanity and our world. Leadership from a Caring Science worldview, paired with belief in the human spirit and creative emergence and transformation from within, will usher in new yet-to-be imagined structures and processes for reflective organizations.

References

Dossey, L. (1991). *Meaning and medicine.* New York, NY: Bantam.

Eisler, R. (2007). *The real wealth of nations: Creating a caring economics.* San Francisco, CA: Berrett-Koehler.

Kelly, L. A., McHugh, M. D., & Aiken, L. H. (2011). Nurse outcomes in magnet and non-magnet hospitals. *Journal of Nursing Administration, 41*(101), 428–433.

Kreitzer, M., & Koithan, M. (2014). *Integrative nursing.* New York, NY: Oxford Press.

Layard, R. (2014). Happy in his work. *Financial Times.* September 13, 2014, p. 2.

Leenerts, M. H., Koehler, J. A., & Neil, R. M. (1996). Nursing care model increases care quality while reducing costs. *Journal of Association of Nurses in AIDS Care, 7*(4), 37-49.

Levinas, E. (1969). *Totality and infinity.* Pittsburgh, PA: Duquesne University.

McHugh, M. D., Kelly, L. A., Smith, H. L., Wu, E. S., Vanak, J. M., & Aiken, L. H. (2013). Lower mortality in magnet hospitals. *Medical Care, 51*(5), 382–388.

Needleman, J. (2013). Assessing low mortality in magnet hospitals. *Medical Care, 51*(5), 379–381.

Newman, M. A. (1994). *Health as expanding consciousness.* Philadelphia, PA: FA Davis.

Rogers, M. (1970). *An introduction to the theoretical basis of nursing.* Philadelphia, PA: FA Davis.

Roger, M. (1992). Nursing science and the space age. *Nursing Science Quarterly, 5*(1), 27–34.

Roger, M. (1994). The science of unitary human beings: Current perspectives. *Nursing Science Quarterly, 7*(1), 33–35.

Watson, J. (1979). *Nursing: The philosophy and science of caring.* Boston, MA: Little Brown.

Watson, J. (1999). *Postmodern nursing and beyond.* Edinburgh, UK: Churchill-Livingston.

Watson, J. (2006). *Caring science as sacred science.* Philadelphia, PA: FA Davis.

Watson, J. (2008). *Nursing: The philosophy and science of caring* (rev. ed.). Boulder, CO: University Press of Colorado.

Watson, J. (2012). *Human caring science.* Sudbury, MA: Jones & Bartlett.

Watson, J. (2014). Integrative nursing – human caring and peace. In M. Kreitzer, & M. Koithan, *Integrative Nursing* (pp. 101–108). New York, NY: Oxford University Press.

Watson J., & Smith, M. C. (2002). Caring science and the science of unitary human beings: A trans-theoretical discourse for nursing knowledge development. *Journal of Advanced Nursing, 37*(5), 452–461.

Chapter 10
Building Interprofessional Teams

Kelly L. Scolaro, PharmD
Donald J. Woodyard, BS
Benny L. Joyner, Jr., MD, MPH
Carol Fowler Durham, EdD, RN, ANEF, FAAN

The Joint Commission (TJC, formerly the Joint Commission on Accreditation of Healthcare Organizations) and other regulatory agencies have identified interprofessional teamwork and communication as being essential for patient quality and safety (TJC, 2013). Administrators, faculty, and students acknowledge the importance of interprofessional education (IPE) yet struggle to create meaningful and longitudinal learning experiences with potential to impact patient outcomes.

The quote "be the change that you wish to see in the world," derived from Mahatma Gandhi's work, describes the spirit of a small group of University of North Carolina–Chapel Hill Nursing, Medicine, and Pharmacy faculty who collaborated in 2010 to deliver an interprofessional elective course titled "Interprofessional Teamwork (IPT) and Communication – Keys to Patient Safety." Our group understood that effectively training the next generation of nurses and other healthcare providers called for a new paradigm of education. Through teaching the value of interprofessional teamwork and communication, our ultimate goal has been to inspire and equip each of our students with the tools to be a champion for patient safety. This chapter will describe the importance of building interprofessional teams within healthcare education and how to use these teams to model educational and healthcare practices that save lives.

Background

The groundbreaking and revolutionary report that the Institute of Medicine (IOM) released in 2000 created a climate of change in healthcare (Kohn, Corrigan, & Donaldson, 2000). That report brought patient safety to the forefront by highlighting the number of deadly adverse events and medical errors that occur within the United States healthcare system. According to the report, as many as 98,000 Americans die each year as a result of medical error—more deaths than are attributable to motor vehicle accidents, breast cancer, or AIDS (Kohn, et al., 2000; Martin, Smith, Mathews, & Ventura, 1999). Costs of these preventable adverse events are estimated to be between $17 billion and $29 billion (Thomas et al., 1999; Van Den Bos et al., 2011). These IOM findings, coupled with a federal government call to action, made addressing the problem of preventable adverse events and medical error a high priority. However, 2013 data—the latest available data—show that number has not decreased and may even have been underrepresented (James, 2013). Premature deaths associated with preventable harm to patients are now estimated at more than 400,000 per year, and serious harm seems to be 10- to 20-fold more common than lethal harm (James, 2013).

Root-cause analyses of these errors identify poor communication, ineffective leadership, and human factors as the leading causes (TJC, 2013). Leaders in nursing—and more broadly, the healthcare industry—recognize and acknowledge these errors as significant problems, yet they continue to address them within intraprofessional silos, wherein each profession independently addresses the perceived challenges. The fact that the last two decades have seen no significant reductions in the rates of error occurrence demonstrates the fallacy of this silo approach (TJC, 2013). Indeed, there are increased opportunities for errors with the advent of new regulations restricting work hours for healthcare professionals, increasing patient complexity as well as system complexity, increasing turnover within all healthcare professions, and more frequent handoffs between care providers.

To address the real root of the problems and break down silos, focus is needed on teamwork, collaboration, and communication. To this end, some agencies have turned toward Team Strategies and Tools to Enhance Performance and Patient Safety (TeamSTEPPS), a tool developed by the Department of Defense (DoD) and the Agency for Healthcare Research and Quality (AHRQ). TeamSTEPPS has been useful for improving and standardizing communication among healthcare providers (Haynes, 2014; King, Toomey, Salisbury, Webster, & Almeida, 2006; King et al., 2008). Numerous healthcare institutions have adopted the TeamSTEPPS framework for communication in their everyday processes (AHRQ, 2014). The body of evidence demonstrating the impact of TeamSTEPPS training in the improvement of patient safety outcomes continues to grow (Guimond, Sole, & Salas, 2009; Haynes, 2014; Keebler et al., 2014; Spiva et al., 2014; Weaver et al., 2010).

REFLECTING ON ... PREVENTABLE ERRORS

- *What role might you have you played in the current estimate of 400,000 preventable deaths per year? If you are an educator: Are you preparing learners to change this outcome? If you are in practice: What are you doing to mitigate the changes of preventable errors to improve from last year?*

- *What will you say to the next patient/family who has a preventable error? Can you assure them this will not happen again to someone else?*

The Need for Interprofessional Education

For sustained change to occur in healthcare, health professional education must change. Traditionally, health professions training begins intraprofessionally (i.e., education "siloed" within one's own profession) until students progress to the clinical phase of their education, at which time they are immersed in a multiprofessional setting (i.e., students learning about how to care for patients alongside each other but still within their own profession), continuing to contribute to fragmented care (Aase, Aase, & Dieckmann, 2013). Since 2010, the emphasis shifted to creating and delivering education to students interprofessionally. True *interprofessional education* (IPE) is defined as "when two or more professionals learn about, from, and with each other to enable effective collaboration and improve health outcomes" (WHO, 2010, p. 7).

In 2011, the release of the Core Competencies for Interprofessional Collaborative Practice further validated the call to action (IPEC, 2011). This groundbreaking report created by national associations of nursing, medicine, pharmacy, and other health professions educators was truly an interprofessional effort. The report emphasized four domains of IPE: values and ethics of interprofessional practice; roles and responsibilities; interprofessional communication; and teams and teamwork (IPEC, 2011). Following this report, the accreditation standards for medicine, nursing, and pharmacy were updated to include requirements for IPE (see Table 10.1). This change in accreditation standards provides the structure and organization necessary to develop and deliver an interprofessional curriculum. However, after decades of teaching in an intraprofessional manner, changing to a truly interprofessional curriculum remains a daunting and mostly unfulfilled task.

Table 10.1: Summary Comparisons of Interprofessional Education Accreditation Standards Across Medicine, Nursing, and Pharmacy

PROFESSION	ACCREDITATION STANDARDS
Medicine	**ED-19-A.** The core curriculum of a medical education program must prepare medical students to function collaboratively on healthcare teams that include health professionals from other disciplines as they provide coordinated services to patients. These curricular experiences include practitioners and/or students from the other health professions.
	ED-29. The faculty of each discipline should set standards of achievement in that discipline and contribute to the setting of such standards in interdisciplinary and interprofessional learning experiences, as appropriate.
	Sources: Accreditation Council for Continuing Medical Education, 2012; Liaison Committee on Medical Education, 2013a; and Liaison Committee on Medical Education, 2013b.

PROFESSION	ACCREDITATION STANDARDS
Nursing	**Essential VI:** Interprofessional Communication and Collaboration for Improving Patient Health Outcomes

The baccalaureate program prepares the graduate to:

1. Compare/contrast the roles and perspectives of the nursing profession with other care professionals on the healthcare team (i.e., scope of discipline, education, and licensure requirements).

2. Use inter- and intraprofessional communication and collaborative skills to deliver evidence-based, patient-centered care.

3. Incorporate effective communication techniques, including negotiation and conflict resolution to produce positive professional working relationships.

4. Contribute the unique nursing perspective to interprofessional teams to optimize patient outcomes.

5. Demonstrate appropriate team-building and collaborative strategies when working with interprofessional teams.

6. Advocate for high-quality and safe patient care as a member of the interprofessional team.

Essential VII: Interprofessional Collaboration for Improving Patient and Population Health Outcomes

The master's degree program prepares the graduate to:

1. Advocate for the value and role of the professional nurse as member and leader of interprofessional healthcare teams.

2. Understand other health professions' scopes of practice to maximize contributions within the healthcare team.

3. Employ collaborative strategies in the design, coordination, and evaluation of patient-centered care.

4. Use effective communication strategies to develop, participate, and lead interprofessional teams and partnerships.

5. Mentor and coach new and experienced nurses and other members of the healthcare team.

6. Functions as an effective group leader or member based on an in-depth understanding of team dynamics and group processes.

Sources: American Association of Colleges of Nursing, 2008; American Association of Colleges of Nursing, 2011.

continues

Table 10.1: *Continued*

PROFESSION	ACCREDITATION STANDARDS
Pharmacy	**Guideline 1.6** The college or school's values should include a stated commitment to a culture that, in general, respects and promotes development of interprofessional learning and collaborative practice in didactic and experiential education. **Standard No. 3: Evaluation of Achievement of Mission and Goals** The college or school must establish and implement an evaluation plan that assesses achievement of the mission and goals. **Guideline 3.2** In general, the evaluation plan should describe the desired outcomes of the college or school's mission and goals, including the educational program(s), research and other scholarly activities, professional and community service, interprofessional education, and pharmacy practice programs. **Standard No. 6: College or School and other Administrative Relationships** The college or school, with the full support of the university, must develop suitable academic, research, and other scholarly activity; and practice and service relationships, collaborations, and partnerships, within and outside the university, to support and advance its mission and goals. **Guideline 6.1** The relationships, collaborations, and partnerships should advance the desired outcomes of the college or school's mission and goals, including student learning, research and other scholarly activities, professional and community service, interprofessional education, and pharmacy practice programs. **Guideline 6.2** In general, the relationships, collaborations, and partnerships collectively should: • Promote integrated and synergistic interprofessional and interdisciplinary activities.

Source: Accreditation Council for Pharmacy Education (2011).

Health professions educators face many obstacles when attempting to incorporate IPE into curricula. Some of the obstacles include:

- Determining the optimal time to introduce IPE into the curriculum while matching the current level of the learner (e.g., first year vs. fourth year)

- Managing enrollment around markedly varied schedules and differentials in course credit requirements across professional schools

- Working in the absence of standardized and validated assessments

- Space (specifically classroom) availability

- Faculty trained in IPE methodology

- Administrative support

- Funding

    Sources: Aase et al., 2013; Brock et al., 2013; Headrick et al., 2012; Smith et al., 2009; Sullivan & Godfrey, 2012.

Two institutions that have successfully overcome these obstacles are the University of Washington and the University of Minnesota. Both institutions acknowledge that while their faculty and commitment to IPE are no different from many other institutions, the distinguishing characteristic of their successes is their investment in IPE, largely through grant funding, that allowed them to create interprofessional centers (Brandt, 2014; Headrick et al., 2012). These successful examples highlight the critical role of overall resources, but particularly the availability of grant support to initiate transforming IPE, clinical practice, and patient care.

REFLECTING ON ... IPE EXPERIENCES

- *If I had to give an "elevator speech" (a concise passionate statement) on why we need IPE experiences to the dean of my school, what would it be?*

- *If the accrediting body for my profession were to visit tomorrow, would we demonstrate sufficient IPE experiences? If not, what do we need to implement now to meet those standards?*

The Delivery of Interprofessional Education

Just as the practical aspects of delivering IPE have vexed IPE efforts, the way in which IPE is delivered has also been a challenge. Currently, many different methods are used to deliver IPE. Some of the most popular efforts consist of single-day intense workshops (Brock et al., 2013; Hobgood et al., 2010; Van Winkle et al., 2012). Single-day workshops offer ease of scheduling; however, single "doses" of IPE have not been shown to have a large impact on practice because students need more opportunities to practice newly learned teamwork and communication skills than can happen in a single day (Kurosawa et al., 2014). More sustained trainings are designed to expose students to IPE over the course of several weeks (Buring et al., 2009; Odegard et al., 2009; Owen & Schmitt, 2013; Smith et al., 2009). Semester-long courses are rarer but offer classmates across professional schools the advantage of opportunities to learn with, from, and about each other (Vyas, McCulloh, Dyer, Gregory, & Higbee, 2012). Executive course models, course offerings that occur regularly during off-duty or nonstandard times (i.e., nights and weekends), have grown in popularity and offer an alternative to the traditional academic calendar. Albeit well-documented in the business literature as successful, the executive model has not been studied for delivering IPE in healthcare professions.

Even though methods of delivery have varied, the use of TeamSTEPPS as a basis for IPE is a common underpinning. Brock and colleagues used TeamSTEPPS training among a group of interprofessional students and demonstrated significant gains in team attitudes and motivation. The authors also found significant gains in all areas of teamwork, especially in situation monitoring and communication (Brock et al., 2013). Additional studies have demonstrated similar gains in teamwork skills when TeamSTEPPS curriculum is used in interprofessional courses (Aase et al., 2013; Baker & Durham, 2013; Headrick et al., 2012).

Using the IPEC competencies as an organizing framework and TeamSTEPPS as a foundational tenet of interaction, we needed a meaningful way to immerse learners into clinical settings. Simulation is a popular and effective method for teaching students about interprofessional teamwork and communication (Brock et al., 2013; Headrick et al., 2012; Reese, Jeffries, & Engum, 2010; Sullivan & Godfrey, 2012). Simulation, in the purest sense, is simply the opportunity to practice in a scenario that is very near to real life. As such, it comes in several forms, including low-fidelity and high-fidelity, using patient simulators, standardized patients, and computer-based simulators/simulation.

Engum and Jeffries (2012) suggest that simulation is one of the best ways to dismantle the "culture" of each profession that is usually based on power and hierarchy. By offering near real-life scenarios for patient care, simulations help provide a context for students to apply what they know as well as learn how they can rely on each other during patient care encounters (Reese et al., 2010). Simulated competitions at local, regional, and national conferences (e.g., SimWars developed by Godwin, Okuda, and Wingart) allow students to practice interprofessional teamwork and communication and also become more familiar with how differences in professional training manifest in similar patient-care scenarios. However, these experiences traditionally exclude professions outside medicine and nursing. Despite these and other innovative ideas and projects being done nationally, to actualize a true shift in the educational paradigm and see improved patient outcomes, we suggest that faculty work in interprofessional teams and that IPE must be taught early and reinforced throughout a learner's training both in the classroom and during clinical rotations, and we have sought to create this at our institution.

FIDELITY

Fidelity is also referred to as realism or authenticity. Fidelity or realism is determined by many factors including the equipment, tools, environment, and believability of the scenario (Meakim et al., 2013). Dieckmann and colleagues (2007) describe five dimensions that contribute to fidelity: physical, psychological, social, cultural, and trust.

Preparation

Building our interprofessional team and development of the interprofessional elective occurred over several years, and we based the course on several interprofessional projects spanning 2001–2008. Beginning in 2001, the Provost's Office at UNC–Chapel Hill sponsored the Health Affairs Interdisciplinary Case Conference (HAICC), a one-evening effort to expose students to interprofessional learning that included students from the 10 health affairs schools on campus. Students were assigned to interprofessional small groups with one faculty facilitator, and, using the World Health Organization (WHO) International Classification of Functioning and Disability (ICFD), the students interviewed a standardized patient before developing a patient-centered management plan (Harward, Tresolini, & Davis, 2006). To demonstrate the effectiveness of shared decision-making, students developed a plan individually before working with the group on a comprehensive care plan. A pre-/post-survey about their knowledge of and attitudes toward working with other professions administered to all participants showed a significant improvement. More than 5,600 students participated in the HAICC over an 8-year period.

Another one-day event, the Interprofessional Patient Safety and Education Collaborative (IPSEC) project, funded by GlaxoSmithKline, was developed in 2006. This project included more than 900 medical and nursing students from UNC–Chapel Hill and Duke University over 2 years. The goals of the project were to expose students to team training using TeamSTEPPS and reinforce the didactics through team-based simulations. Pre-/post-surveys showed improved knowledge and attitudes similar to HAICC (Hobgood et al, 2010). Faced with budget reductions and the logistical difficulties of administering to such large numbers of students in 1-day events, these two projects were terminated, but they served as important precursors to our elective course. Even though the logistics and budget issues were immense, these two projects created pathways and relationships that helped our interprofessional team and course.

Using the lessons learned from HAICC and IPSEC, a small group of nursing, medicine, and pharmacy faculty came together to create a pilot project called Simulation for Interdisciplinary Education (SIDE) in 2008. This project brought together a group of IPE champions and fostered good will, respect, and sharing of resources and ideas. Like the IPSEC project, the SIDE project incorporated TeamSTEPPS and asked students to apply the TeamSTEPPS knowledge in a simulation. Additionally, the SIDE project added the inclusion of pharmacy students and was structured to test retention over time as students were recruited to participate in the simulation one time and then again 6 months later. We assessed TeamSTEPPS knowledge and teamwork skills at the initial simulation and again after the time lapse. The SIDE project was voluntary, and we struggled to recruit students because we could not offer course credit or a certificate of completion. However, reaction from those students who did participate was overwhelmingly positive. These students suggested that we needed more than just a volunteer experience: something with more investment and value to the learner. Students wanted a course, and from this, our interprofessional course was designed and launched.

The Project

Since January 2010, we have offered an interprofessional elective for prelicensure students from the schools of nursing, medicine, and pharmacy. The ultimate goal of the course is to create a collaborative, practice-ready, health professions workforce. By allowing students from these professional schools to engage with and also learn about and from each other in an immersive simulation-based environment, we advance learners from siloed and fragmented professionalization to collaboration-based transprofessionalization, and ultimately to communicate and coordinate care more effectively as a team to improve patient health outcomes.

REFLECTING ON ... THE KNOWLEDGE OF OTHERS

- *Critically reflect on what you know about other professionals: their education, roles, and responsibilities. How confident are you that you know what that professional does?*

- *Consider how you feel when people say they know exactly what you do in your profession. Do you find you are uncomfortable? Have you ever done the same regarding another profession?*

The foundation of this semester-long course is TeamSTEPPS curriculum, which focuses on understanding different healthcare professional roles, promoting teamwork, and developing communication skills and strategies to improve collaboration among health professionals. In 2011, when IPEC was published, the course faculty appreciated that the domains were widely present throughout the course and aligned the course terminology to link directly with the four IPEC competencies: values/ethics for interprofessional practice, roles/responsibilities, interprofessional communication, and teams and teamwork (IPEC, 2011).

When designing and implementing our course, we faced many of the obstacles outlined previously in this chapter. Our schools have vastly different requirements and deadlines for creating new courses. We were not allowed to create one course with one course number due to concerns about which school receives the tuition dollars. Our schools have different grading requirements—for example, pass/fail versus plus/minus letter grades—which made creating assessments and calculating final grades difficult. We also had difficulty recruiting and retaining nursing and medical students because our school of nursing does not require, nor provide time for, electives; and our school of medicine requires electives, but only in the fourth year and only in 2-week blocks. Our school of pharmacy both encourages and requires students to pursue elective opportunities; thus, it is not surprising that pharmacy students outnumber nursing and medicine students in our elective course every year. This leads to unbalanced teams when we run simulations. Despite all these obstacles, the course has been a success, and enrollment has grown every year. Overcoming these obstacles emphasizes the need for healthcare educators—and, specifically, administrators—to reprioritize their curriculums and create space to allow for interprofessional learning.

Our course has an emphasis on patient-centeredness and assists learners with quality improvement to improve patient safety as outlined in the Quality and Safety Education for Nurses (QSEN) competencies (Cronenwett et al., 2007). The course requires the participants to apply what is learned about teamwork and communication into immersive, simulation-based scenarios with immediate feedback focusing on anchored teamwork skills and continual improvement. They participate in multiple team configurations, experiencing simulation with high-fidelity simulator scenarios and standardized patients scenarios; and in teams as they disclose errors to family members (standardized patients); complete patient handoffs; conduct root-cause analysis; complete a medical malpractice mock trial; and learn not only to understand differences in interprofessional roles and responsibilities, but also to rely on the complementary skills of their interprofessional team members to assist them in providing optimal care (Woodyard et al., 2009, 2010, 2013).

REFLECTING ON ... THE VALUE OF PERSONAL EXPERIENCES

- *What intraprofessional, multiprofessional, and interprofessional experiences have I experienced? How has each of these experiences differed?*

- *What experiences, both personal and professional, could I use to highlight the value of IPE and teamwork training to my students?*

Outcomes

Although efforts to educate students and practitioners of interprofessional teamwork and communication have been studied and are reported in the literature, the impact of interprofessional education on patient care is not fully known or understood beyond some positive impact on patient safety and quality care (Baker & Durham, 2013; Malec et al., 2007; Remington, Foulk, & Williams, 2006). Through assessments in our course, our students have demonstrated measurable improvement in teamwork skills, TeamSTEPPS knowledge, error-disclosure skills, and attitudes toward other professions over the duration of the course.

The course has continued to grow every year that it has been offered. For example, the first time we offered the course, not a single medical student enrolled. Now, we have almost equal numbers of medical, nursing, and pharmacy students. We feel that the growth is a result of our increased recruiting efforts and, most importantly, positive word of mouth from our former students. The course has also been noticed by our school administrators, and the faculty are now a regular part of the Health Affairs Collaborative Group, which is a committee comprising associate deans working to bring more interprofessional opportunities to all the health affairs schools.

Course Impact

Personal experiences of the faculty with medical error were an important factor in developing this course. Also bringing to light concerns about health professionals excluding the patient and family in care is central to what we do in the course. We are continuously thankful to our students who learn about these issues and become champions for patient-centered care. We believe that we are impacting healthcare one student at a time. Students are transformed through this opportunity to work together. They realize the impact that collaborating with other professionals can have on improving patient care. To illustrate this impact, take a moment to review the following quotes our former students provided with regard to the impact of our course.

> As a seasoned registered nurse, I learned my communication skills by trial and error. I wish I had had the opportunity to take this course. It would have been such a great asset if somewhere I learned how to effectively communicate and collaborate with physicians and pharmacists before I started working in the hospital.
>
> —Maureen Baker, RN, MS

> This course truly gets at the heart of why developing interprofessional relationships is important. It's not just about communication and teamwork—it's about the patients and their safety. It may take a little time to get comfortable assessing patients (some of whom act belligerent), making recommendations, and adjusting your treatment to the patient's response, but you will become more confident in your role as part of an interprofessional team. I would definitely recommend this course to all students in the healthcare profession!
>
> —Jennifer Kim, PharmD

The opportunity to run simulations with colleagues from pharmacy, nursing, and medicine introduced me to the broad range of skills that are necessary to deliver safe and effective care. Time and again, I found that when I came to a hole in my clinical knowledge or skills, another member of the team would have more familiarity with resources or more developed skills than I. Having this experience as a preclinical student helped me to understand how to reach out to and utilize members of my team in a way that lectures do not. I gained a deeper understanding and therefore a deeper respect for other members of my team.

–Jewel Sheehan, MD

Faculty Learnings

We learned so much through developing and executing this course. For example, we learned how to deal with barriers among our three schools and the university as a whole. We learned to deal with adversity and keep moving on. We learned how to market our course to students and administrators. The first year we offered the course, our ratio was 3 faculty to 7 students. Through our collective marketing efforts, we are now up to 24 students. Looking back, we could have tried to engage students and school leadership sooner. We could have brought the two groups together to allow the students to express what they learned to leadership. This advocacy, which has occurred only recently, is what has really captured the attention of the leadership of the schools of medicine, nursing, and pharmacy and has allowed further growth and development of our course.

We also learned to capitalize on our resources and our strengths, clinical and educational. We learned the power of being role models for our students. All three course directors engage and demonstrate collaboration by being present at every class, and by doing this, model teamwork and communication for our students. Each profession is represented throughout the IPE experience from design, implementation, and evaluation through to refinement.

Another lesson we learned is to level the playing field and set aside traditional hierarchal authoritative roles. The course does not just belong to one school: It is a joint effort with alternating leads. The concept of shared leadership and responsibility has allowed for all three schools to feel a shared sense of pride and accomplishment. Given this, each school remains committed to the success of this program.

Developing this course had its share of surprises as well. We came to realize that despite all our practice experience (more than 60 years combined) working in environments with physicians, nurses, and pharmacists, how little we really knew about the other professions. We realized that we never fully appreciated the differences in how we organize our work, problem-solve clinical issues, and approach patient care. Teaching this course and working alongside each of these professions exposed us to the way in which the training differs among the schools of medicine, nursing, and pharmacy—from when each profession is introduced to clinical experiences to how each profession approaches patient care. This realization made us better clinicians and educators. What surprised us the most, however, was how much interest there was to incorporate IPE into our collective curricula. As we began to explore ways to grow this effort, we were stunned by the reception that we received. At every turn, there was interest in our course. Our students were our biggest champions. Indeed, their advocacy of IPE led this growth of our IPE efforts.

Final Reflections

We enjoyed many successes in this course. Students who elected to take this course self-selected into a topic in which they were already curious. However, the content they were exposed to and the experiences they received as part of the course helped to equip them with fundamental skills to both practice collaboratively and advocate for more efficient teamwork in the healthcare setting. Watching our students progress across the semester—for some, feeling empowered to take a situational leadership role, while others learned mutual respect and began to "listen" to their colleagues—is hugely rewarding for us as faculty. At the end of every semester, we receive hugs from students, words of thanks, and praise for the course, as well as requests for more IPE educational opportunities. They advocate for this experience to be offered to all health affairs students. They are inspired to be the change that we hope to see in healthcare. The course also opened doors for the course directors to share their work with others who are interested in IPE at state and national conferences.

Moving forward, we would like to bring IPE to practitioners, especially new graduates. Just as trying to incorporate IPE into the health professional schools brings many challenges, we know that bringing IPE to practitioners is fraught with obstacles. However, it is essential that practitioners receive training, especially new graduates not previously trained interprofessionally. Currently, no standardized, scalable approach for delivering and reinforcing IPE to students and practitioners exists (Reeves, Perrier, Goldman, Freeth, & Zwarenstein, 2013).

We are examining several methods to educate practitioners on interprofessional teamwork and communication that have been recommended in the literature. Patrician and associates (2012) describe a successful fellowship model used within the Veteran's Administration (VA). The VA Quality Scholars Fellowship Program is for predoctoral and postdoctoral nurses and physicians. Fellows are tasked with developing quality-improvement projects, and several successful projects have centered on interprofessional training (Patrician et al., 2012). Continuing education is a way to reach clinicians, and many of the national accreditation bodies have developed processes for accrediting providers of IPE (Owen & Schmitt, 2013). Owen and Schmitt (2013) describe four examples of how to provide IPE to practitioners: a 1-day program offered by the VA; integration of the LEAN quality-improvement process into University of Minnesota outpatient clinics in a limited longitudinal approach; and two longitudinal, integrated programs at the University of Virginia (UVA) and the University of Rochester. At the University of Rochester, TeamSTEPPS is used in a longitudinal continuing education program within the workplace; UVA uses continuing education and interprofessional education for practitioners and students (Owen & Schmitt, 2013). We know that additional research is needed to continue the momentum created by our course and these other examples.

Our course has overcome many challenges and seen much success over the five semesters it has been offered. Widespread national recognition of the need for IPE experiences and new accreditation requirements for IPE curricula are establishing an environment favorable for change. We are optimistic that the content of our course is well developed and will prove an invaluable resource for UNC–Chapel Hill and other institutions as they seek to answer the call and incorporate IPE into their training requirements. We know that our course makes our students better providers and will improve the quality and safety of the care for our patients. As for us, as faculty, we have certainly learned how to build and be a part of an interprofessional team, grown professionally, and enjoyed being instrumental in beginning this paradigm shift at our institutions.

References

Aase, I., Aase, K., & Dieckmann, P. (2013). Teaching interprofessional teamwork in medical and nursing education in Norway: A content analysis. *Journal of Interprofessional Care*, 27(3), 238–245. doi:10.3109/13561820.2012.745489

Accreditation Council for Pharmacy Education. (2011). *Accreditation standards and guidelines for the professional program in pharmacy leading to the doctor of pharmacy degree.* (Adopted: January 15, 2006). Guidelines 2.0 Retrieved from www.acpe-accredit.org/standards/

Accreditation Council for Continuing Medical Education. (June 2012). *The accreditation requirements of the Accreditation Council for Continuing Medical Education (ACCME).* Retrieved from www.accme.org/sites/default/files/626_20131016_Accreditation_Requirements_Document_0.pdf

Agency for Healthcare Research and Quality (AHRQ). (2014). TeamSTEPPS: National Implementation. Retrieved from http://teamstepps.ahrq.gov/about-2cl_3.htm

American Association of Colleges of Nursing. (Oct. 20, 2008). The essentials of baccalaureate education for professional nursing practice. Retrieved from www.aacn.nche.edu//education-resources/baccessentials08.pdf

American Association of Colleges of Nursing. (March 21, 2011). The essentials of master's education in nursing. Retrieved from www.aacn.nche.edu/education-resources/MastersEssentials11.pdf

Baker, M. J., & Durham, C. F. (2013). Interprofessional education: a survey of students' collaborative competency outcomes. *Journal of Nursing Education*, *52*(12), 713–718. doi:10.3928/01484834-20131118-04

Brandt, B. F. (2014). Update on the US National Center for Interprofessional Practice and Education. *Journal of Interprofessional Care*, *28*(1), 5–7. doi:10.3109/13561820.20 13.852365

Brock, D., Abu-Rish, E., Chiu, C. R., Hammer, D., Wilson, S., Vorvick, L., ... Zierler, B. (2013). Interprofessional education in team communication: Working together to improve patient safety. *BMJ Quality & Safety*, *22*(5), 414–423. doi:10.1136/bmjqs-2012-000952

Buring, S. M., Bhushan, A., Brazeau, G., Conway, S., Hansen, L., & Westberg, S. (2009). Keys to successful implementation of interprofessional education: Learning, location, faculty development, and curricular themes. *American Journal of Pharmaceutical Education*, *73*(4), 1–11. doi:10.5688/aj730460

Cronenwett, L., Sherwood, G., Barnsteiner, J., Disch, J., Johnson, J., Mitchell, P., ... Warren, J. (2007). Quality and safety education for nurses. *Nursing Outlook*, *55*(3), 122–131. doi:10.1016/j.outlook.2007.02.006

Dieckman, P., Gaba, D., & Rall, M. (2007). Deepening the theoretical foundations of patient simulation as social practice. *Simulation in Healthcare*, *2*(3), 183–193.

Engum, S. A., & Jeffries, P. R. (2012). Interdisciplinary collisions: Bringing healthcare professionals together. *Collegian*, *19*(3), 145–151. Retrieved from http://dx.doi.org/10.1016/j.colegn.2012.05.005

Guimond, M. E., Sole, M. L., & Salas, E. (2009). TeamSTEPPS: An educational program seeks to improve teamwork and ultimately patient safety. *American Journal of Nursing*, *109*(11), 66–68. doi:10.1097/01.naj.0000363359.84377.27

Harward, D. H., Tresolini, C. P., & Davis, W. A. (2006). Can participation in a health affairs interdisciplinary case conference improve medical students' knowledge and attitudes? *Academic Medicine*, *81*(3), 257–261.

Haynes, J. (2014). TeamSTEPPS makes strides for better communication. *Nursing*, *44*(1), 62–63. doi.10-1097/01.NURSE.0000438725.66087.89

Headrick, L. A., Barton, A. J., Ogrinc, G., Strang, C., Aboumatar, H. J., Aud, M. A., ... Patterson, J. E. (2012). Results of an effort to integrate quality and safety into medical and nursing school curricula and foster joint learning. *Health Affairs* (Millwood), *31*(12), 2669–2680. doi:10.1377/hlthaff.2011.0121

Hobgood, C., Sherwood, G., Frush, K., Hollar, D., Maynard, L., Foster, B., ... Taekman, J. (2010). Teamwork training with nursing and medical students: Does the method matter? Results of an interinstitutional, interdisciplinary collaboration. *Quality Safety in Health Care, 19*(6), e25. doi:10.1136/qshc.2008.031732

Interprofessional Education Collaborative Expert Panel (IPEC). (2011). Core competencies for interprofessional collaborative practice: Report of an expert panel. Washington, DC: Interprofessional Education Collaborative. Retrieved from http://www.aacn.nche.edu/education-resources/ipecreport.pdf

James, J. T. (2013). A new, evidence-based estimate of patient harms associated with hospital care. *Journal of Patient Safety, 9*(3), 122–128.

Keebler, J. R., Dietz, A. S., Lazzara, E. H., Benishek, L. E., Almeida, S. A., Toor, P. A., ... Salas, E. (2014). Validation of a teamwork perceptions measure to increase patient safety. *BMJ Quality & Safety.* doi:10.1136/bmjqs-2013-001942

King, H. B., Battles, J., Baker, D. P., Alonso, A., Salas, E., Webster, J., ... Salisbury, M. (2008). *TeamSTEPPS: Team strategies and tools to enhance performance and patient safety advances in patient safety: New directions and alternative approaches* (vol. 3: Performance and Tools). Rockville, MD: Agency for Healthcare Research and Quality.

King, H. B., Toomey, L., Salisbury, M., Webster, J., & Almeida, S. (2006). *TeamSTEPPS: Team strategies and tools to enhance performance and patient safety.* Developed by the Department of Defense (DoD) in collaboration with the Agency for Healthcare Research and Quality (AHRQ). Retrieved from http://teamstepps.ahrq.gov/aboutnationalIP.htm

Kohn, L. T., Corrigan, J. M., & Donaldson, M. S. (2000). *To err is human: Building a safer health system. Committee on Quality of Health Care in America, Institute of Medicine.* Washington, DC: National Academies Press.

Kurosawa, H., Ikeyama, T., Achuff, P., Perkel, M., Watson, C., Monachino, A., ... Nishisaki, A. (2014). A randomized, controlled trial of in situ pediatric advanced life support recertification ("pediatric advanced life support reconstructed") compared with standard pediatric advanced life support recertification for ICU frontline providers. *Critical Care Medicine, 42*(3), 610–618. doi:10.1097/ccm.0000000000000024

Liaison Committee on Medical Education. (2013a). Functions and structure of a medical school. Standards for accreditation of medical education programs leading to the M.D. degree. Retrieved from www.lcme.org/publications/functions2013june.pdf

Liaison Committee on Medical Education. (2013b). Summary of new and revised LCME accreditation standards and annotations. Retrieved from www.lcme.org/2013-new-and_revised-standards-summary.pdf

Malec, J. F., Torsher, L. C., Dunn, W. F., Wiegmann, D. A., Arnold, J. J., Brown, D. A., & Phatak, V. (2007). The Mayo High Performance Teamwork Scale: Reliability and validity for evaluating key crew resource management skills. *Simulation in Healthcare*, 2(1), 4–10. doi:10.1097/SIH.0b013e31802b68ee

Martin, J. A. , Smith, B. L., Mathews, T. J., & Ventura, S. J. (1999). *Births and deaths: Preliminary data for 1998*. (Department of Vital Statistics, Trans.) National Vital Statistics Reports (vol. 47). Atlanta, GA: Centers for Disease Control and Prevention, National Center for Health Statistics.

Meakim, C., Boese, T., Decker, S., Franklin, S. E., Gloe, D., Lioce, L., ... Borum, J. C. (2013, June). Standards of Best Practice: Simulation Standard I: Terminology. *Clinical Simulation in Nursing*, 9(6S), s3–s11. Retrieved from http://dx.doi.org//10.1016/j.ecns.2013.04.001

Odegard, P. S., Robins, L., Murphy, N., Belza, B., Brock, D., Gallagher, T. H., ... Mitchell, P. (2009). Interprofessional initiatives at the University of Washington. *American Journal of Pharmaceutical Education*, 73(4), 1–7. doi:10.5688/aj730463

Owen, J. A., & Schmitt, M. H. (2013). Integrating interprofessional education into continuing education: A planning process for continuing interprofessional education programs. *Journal of Continuing Education in the Health Professions*, 33(2), 109–117. doi:10.1002/chp.21173

Patrician, P. A., Dolansky, M., Estrada, C., Brennan, C., Miltner, R., Newsom, J., ... Moore, S. (2012). Interprofessional education in action: The VA Quality Scholars fellowship program. *Nuring Clinics of North America*, 47(3), 347–354. doi:10.1016/j.cnur.2012.05.006

Reese, C. E., Jeffries, P. R., & Engum, S. A. (2010). Learning together: Using simulations to develop nursing and medical student collaboration. *Nursing Education Perspectives*, 31(1), 33–37.

Reeves, S., Perrier, L., Goldman, J., Freeth, D., & Zwarenstein, M. (2013). Interprofessional education: Effects on professional practice and healthcare outcomes (update). Cochrane Database Systematic Reviews, 3, CD002213. doi:10.1002/14651858.CD002213.pub3

Remington, T. L., Foulk, M. A., & Williams, B. C. (2006). Evaluation of evidence for interprofessional education. *American Journal of Pharmaceutical Education*, 70(3), 1–7. doi:10.5688/aj700366

Smith, K. M., Scott, D. R., Barner, J. C., DeHart, R. M., Scott, J. D., & Martin, S. J. (2009). Interprofessional education in six US colleges of pharmacy. *American Journal of Pharmaceutical Education, 73*(4), 1–7. doi:10.5688/aj730461

Spiva, L., Robertson, B., Delk, M. L., Patrick, S., Kimrey, M. M., Green, B., & Gallagher, E. (2014). Effectiveness of team training on fall prevention. *Journal of Nursing Care Quality, 29*(2), 164–173. doi:10.1097/NCQ.0b013e3182a98247

Sullivan, D. T., & Godfrey, N. S. (2012). Preparing nursing students to be effective health team partners through interprofessional education. *Creative Nurse, 18*(2), 57–63.

Thomas, E. J., Studdert, D. M., Newhouse, J. P., Zbar, B. I., Howard, K. M., Williams, E. J., & Brennan, T. A. (1999). Costs of medical injuries in Utah and Colorado. *Inquiry, 36*(3), 255–264.

TJC. (2013). Sentinel event data-root causes by event type. In The Joint Commission (Ed.), (vol. 2014, Sentinel Event Statistics Data - Root Causes by Event Type (2004 – Q2002 2013)).

Van Den Bos, J., Rustagi, K., Gray, T., Halford, M., Ziemkiewicz, E., & Shreve, J. (2011). The $17.1 billion problem: The annual cost of measurable medical errors. *Health Affairs, 30*(4), 596–603. doi:10.1377/hlthaff.2011.0084

Van Winkle, L. J., Bjork, B. C., Chandar, N., Cornell, S., Fjortoft, N., Green, J. M., ... Burdick, P. (2012). Interprofessional workshop to improve mutual understanding between pharmacy and medical students. *American Journal of Pharmaceutical Education, 76*(8), 1–6. doi:10.5688/ajpe768150

Vyas, D., McCulloh, R., Dyer, C., Gregory, G., & Higbee, D. (2012). An interprofessional course using human patient simulation to teach patient safety and teamwork skills. *American Journal of Pharmaceutical Education, 76*(4), 1–9. doi:10.5688/ajpe76471

Weaver, S. J., Rosen, M. A., DiazGranados, D., Lazzara, E. H., Lyons, R., Salas, E., ... King, H. B. (2010). Does teamwork improve performance in the operating room? A multilevel evaluation. *Joint Commission Journal on Quality and Patient Safety, 36*(3), 133–142.

Woodyard, D., Durham, C., Scolaro, K., Barrick, J., Stegall-Zanation, J., Biese, K., ... Hobgood, C. (2009). Simulations for Inter-Disciplinary Education (SIDE) Project: Teaching the communication aspect of patient care. *Simulation in Healthcare, 4*(4), 294.

Woodyard, C., Woodyard, D., Scolaro, K., & Durham, C. (2010). The mock medical malpractice trial: Introducing health professional students to the legal field using simulation. *Simulation in Healthcare, 5*(6), 420.

Woodyard, D., Chatterji, D., Cowherd, S., Durham, C., Scolaro, K., & Barrick, J. (2013). Teaching interprofessional root cause analysis using simulation. *Simulation in Healthcare, 8*(6), 506.

Woodyard, D., Scolaro, K., Durham, C., Shelly, J., & Hobgood, C. (2013). b-SAFER: A systematic approach to delivering effective interprofessional handoffs. *Simulation in Healthcare, 8*(6), 506.

Woodyard, D., & Woodyard, C. (2013). The standardized (patient) jury: An insight into deliberations for law students during a mock medical malpractice trial. *Simulation in Healthcare, 8*(6), 505.

World Health Organization (WHO). (2010). Framework for action on interprofessional education & collaborative practice. Geneva, Switzerland: World Health Organization. Retrieved from http://whqlibdoc.who.int/hq/2010/WHO_HRH_HPN_10.3_eng.pdf

Resources
General Interprofessional Education Resources

Accreditation Council for Pharmacy Education
www.acpe-accredit.org

Interprofessional Education Collaborative Expert Panel
www.aacn.nche.edu/education-resources/IPECReport.pdf

IPEC Interprofessional Education Collaborative – Connecting Health Professions for Better Care
https://ipecollaborative.org/Recommended_Links.html

Liaison Committee on Medical Education
www.lcme.org

National Center for Interprofessional Practice and Education
https://nexusipe.org/

Nursing-Specific Interprofessional Education Resources

American Association of Colleges of Nursing (AACN) Teamwork and Collaboration – Joanne Disch, PhD, RN, FAAN

- AACN Member Collaboration Community State of the Science for Teamwork and Collaboration
www.aacn.nche.edu/qsen/Teamwork-Resource-Paper.pdf

- Learning Module Teamwork and Collaboration
www.icpre.com/Presentations/AACN/TC/player.html

World Health Organization – Framework for Action on Interprofessional Education & Collaborative Practice
http://whqlibdoc.who.int/hq/2010/WHO_HRH_HPN_10.3_eng.pdf

A Nursing Perspective on Simulation and Interprofessional Education (IPE)
www.nln.org/facultyprograms/facultyresources/pdf/nursing_perspective_sim_education.pdf

The Simulation Innovation Resource Center (SIRC) National League for Nursing
http://sirc.nln.org/

Simulation-Based Interprofessional Education
http://sirc.nln.org/mod/resource/view.php?id=789

Quality and Safety Resources

Agency for Healthcare Research and Quality (AHRQ)
www.ahrq.gov

Agency for Healthcare Research and Quality (AHRQ) – Mortality and Morbidity Cases
www.webmm.ahrq.gov

Agency for Healthcare Research and Quality (AHRQ) – High Reliability Organizations (HRO)
www.ahrq.gov/professionals/quality-patient-safety/quality-resources/hroadvice/hroadvice.pdf

Agency for Healthcare Research and Quality (AHRQ) – Patient
Safety Surveys
www.ahrq.gov/legacy/qual/patientsafetyculture

"From Tears to Transparency" Series: "The Story of Lewis Blackman"
DVD Learning Program
http://transparentlearning.mybigcommerce.com/
products/%E2%80%9CFrom-Tears-to-Transparency%E2%80%9D-
Series%3A-%E2%80%9CThe-Story-of-Lewis-Blackman%E2%80%9D-
DVD-Learning-Program.html

Institute for Healthcare Improvement (IHI)
www.ihi.org/IHI

Institute for Safe Medication Practices (ISMP)
www.ismp.org

Institute of Medicine (IOM)
www.iom.edu
Institute of Medicine Health Care Quality Initiative:

- To Err is Human: Building A Safer Health System (1999)

- Crossing the Quality Chasm: A New Health System for the 21st
  Century (2001)

- Health Professions Education: A Bridge to Quality (2003)

- Keeping Patients Safe: Transforming the Work Environment of
  Nurses (2004)

- Preventing Medication Errors: Quality Chasm Series (2006)

The Joint Commission
www.jointcommission.org

National Patient Safety Foundation (NPSF)
www.npsf.org

Quality and Safety Education for Nurses (QSEN)
http://qsen.org/

Team Strategies and Tools to Enhance Performance and Patient Safety
(TeamSTEPPS)
http://teamstepps.ahrq.gov

TeamSTEPPS Pocket Guide
www.ahrq.gov/professionals/education/curriculumtools/teamstepps/
instructor/essentials/pocketguide.pdf

When Things Go Wrong: Responding to Adverse Events
www.macoalition.org/documents/respondingToAdverseEvents.pdf

Chapter 11
A New Framework for Creating a Resilient Organization Using Reflective Practices

Stephen M. Powell, MS
Richard Stone, MS

In recent years, we have come to see hospitals as the expression of the complex interaction of six fundamental dimensions that are grounded in human factors: culture, leadership, teams, learning, implementation, and patients and families (see Figure 11.1). We have learned that we have the opportunity to profoundly impact the vitality of each of these dimensions by implementing reflective practices, which leads to tangibly improved patient outcomes. Conversely, the absence of reflective practices inevitably leads to less-than-optimal performance as well as unhealthy relationships within and between organizational structures, resulting in high levels of preventable patient harm. Taking time to reflect can truly impact patient outcomes and make our healthcare systems a safer place for both patients and staff.

FIGURE 11.1

The Healthy Organization

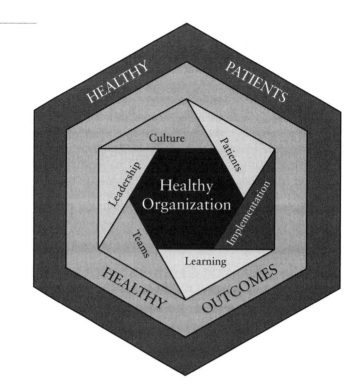

This chapter endeavors to shed a new light on performance improvement, quality, safety, change management, and how we can accelerate learning by applying the lens of reflection. We believe that reflective practices can enhance nearly every facet of your leadership effectiveness and clinical practice, and these reflective practices can then have, in turn, an extraordinary impact on the health of your organization.

We start by laying some groundwork and create a shared mental model about what we mean by "reflection." We discuss why reflective thinking is so integral to human learning and to the success of organizations, and more specifically, how healthcare leaders can support organizational practices so that their hospitals and clinics benefit from reflective practices, thereby providing better, safer care.

WHAT LIMITING ASSUMPTIONS STOP YOUR THINKING AND REFLECTIVE POWER?

It is virtually impossible to live without assumptions about the world, ourselves, and our organizations. These assumptions deeply inform our thinking and actions. Unfortunately, these assumptions frequently are simply untrue, leading at times to disastrous consequences. The essential antidote for untrue, limiting assumptions is reflection, which can help individuals and organizations recalibrate their sense of themselves and the world, and in the bargain become increasingly more effective in making decisions and delivering care.

Background

To begin our journey of understanding, reflection should rightfully be considered as a form of thinking that is directed, focused on a goal, and most importantly, a means for us to create a feedback loop to evaluate our actions and thoughts. In that sense, reflection is a form of course correction as well as a means of deducing from the given facts and circumstances a new perspective or interpretation that had been occluded from view before the reflective act.

In most respects, when it comes to our understanding of the important role reflection plays in our personal and organizational life, not much has changed over the centuries. Reflection, after all, has been a fundamental human activity from the dawn of human existence. Philosophers of old, including Plato and Aristotle in the West and Confucius in the East, all referred to the invaluable role of reflection. Here's what Confucius had to say on the subject more than 2,000 years ago: "By three methods we may learn wisdom: first, by reflection, which is noblest; second, by imitation, which is easiest; and third, by experience, which is the bitterest" (Muller, (2013).

Aristotle was also concerned with our ability to think reflectively about our experience and the untrue assumptions that often masquerade as truth that we are inclined to embrace. "It is the mark of an educated mind to be able to entertain a thought without accepting it" (Aristotle, n.d.). We could summarize that the unexamined, nonreflective life is one that is clouded by ignorance and small-mindedness, whereas the life of reflection and self-examination leads to wisdom, insight, and hopefully, better action and superior outcomes regardless of our goals.

In contemporary times, John Dewey (1993), the 20th-century philosopher, has probably informed educational thought on reflection more than any other writer. He defines *reflective thought* this way:

> Active, persistent, and careful consideration of any belief
> or supposed form of knowledge in the light of the grounds
> that support it, and the further conclusion to which it tends,
> constitutes reflective thought. It is a conscious and voluntary
> effort to establish belief upon a firm basis of reasons (p. 6).

Dewey goes on to get at the heart of the uneasy edge that reflective thinking creates within us, which may be why many people resist leading a reflective life:

> Reflective thinking is always more or less troublesome because
> it involves overcoming the inertia that inclines one to accept
> suggestions at their face value; it involves willingness to endure a
> condition of mental unrest and disturbance. Reflective thinking,
> in short, means judgment suspended during further inquiry; and
> suspense is likely to be somewhat painful (p. 13).

You can see Dewey's influence pervasively in contemporary educational thinking. Hatton and Smith (1995) identified four essential issues concerning reflection:

- It is important to look at complex problems and first ask ourselves whether our interpretation is correct. Test and retest your assumptions, and then modify your actions accordingly.

- After any action, take time to look back and think about what you did and what happened in a systematic way. Consider whether there is a way to extend your thoughts or thinking.

- Journaling and group discussions, while useful, aren't always acts of reflection undertaken for the purpose of solving a problem.

- When critically reflecting on a problem, it's important to include in our thinking the bigger context that includes historical factors, the impact of culture, and the politics of the day that subtly influence every conclusion we make.

Peter Pappas (2010) notes how important it is to consider Dewey's notion about reflection as linking together one idea after another in a chain—a key foundation for learning and teaching heuristics. Pappas developed a taxonomy of reflection that is useful for our understanding of how reflection can be invaluable for the purpose of our focus on reflective practices that are integral to high-functioning individuals and teams in healthcare (see Figure 11.2).

Taxonomy of Reflection	
Creating	What should I do next?
Evaluating	How well did I do?
Analyzing	Do I see any patterns in what I did?
Applying	Where could I use this again?
Understanding	What was important about it?
Remembering	What did I do?

FIGURE 11.2

Peter Pappas'
Taxonomy of Reflection
(Source: Pappas, 2010.)

Now, imagine yourself transposing these insightful questions to your organizational setting, regardless of whether you are a clinical or an administrative leader. This form of reflective thinking challenges you to move to higher-level approaches to understanding the complex world of a hospital. Reflective practices can have a host of other benefits as well, forcing you to move beyond stereotypic thinking about your problems and the structures of your organization, fostering a fresh perspective that will allow you to better see the needs of your organization and the people you serve. Invariably, reflection provides the ability to improve your sense-making of the myriad inputs and data streams that bombard and perhaps overwhelm you. Honest reflection can also challenge many deeply held beliefs that may be leading to faulty conclusions, helping you to become a more objective observer, always suspicious of your initial subjective responses and interpretations. In that sense, people who have mastered the art of reflection more often than not will be more keenly aware of their environment, will pick up on subtle cues that most would miss, and more likely will excel at active listening. The bottom line is that reflection almost always translates into more effective action.

ENHANCING THE SPIRIT OF ORGANIZATIONS

All too often, we think about organizations in mechanistic ways—linear organizational charts representing multifaceted, complex relationships, divisional maps, department structures, and so forth. This kind of thinking blinds us to the organic nature of human endeavors. Hospitals are no exception. Organizations, especially hospitals, are more akin to ecological systems than they are to industrial manufacturing facilities, and attempts to improve and change them as though they were machines too frequently have adverse consequences. As it turns out, the process of reflection shares many attributes of the feedback systems in complex ecological systems, providing us a means of participating in and amplifying organizational change and transformation. In fact, the process of reflection propels, enhances, and enriches the "spirit" of an organization. Without it, organizational spirit wanes with real consequences for financial and business indicators that we are most familiar with when assessing an organization's vitality.

You might be thinking that this all sounds idyllic; you have no time for reflection. Where will you find space in your busy schedule to even reflect for a minute? Perhaps even more challenging is the reaction that you might encounter from a hard-driving leader who measures your performance by your decisiveness and ability to make snap decisions. Taking time to reflect in the face of that managerial style could endanger your professional career, but without creating the spaciousness to pause and reflect, all the practices that we describe here will be of little value.

If we reflect on the deep assumptions that underlie the organizational cultures that we have unwittingly created in hospitals that do little to support reflective practices, it is easy to recognize practices that contribute to patient harm. The reality is actually counterintuitive. The more time we take to reflect on what we're doing, the more effective we become and the more time we will have because we will discontinue activities that truly add little value to the performance of our teams and hospitals.

Embracing reflective practices requires a courageous stance to interrupt unconscious cultural practices that are innately ineffective and perhaps self-destructive. For that reason alone, we don't create a reflective organization in one giant leap. Reflective organizations come by taking small incremental steps in your schedule and the schedules of your teams to embed this new discipline. Adopt only one of the following practices at a time. Practice it until it becomes routine, and you can't imagine doing business any other way. Then, assess which of the other practices will provide you the most value and add it to your repertoire in the same fashion. With time, reflective practice will become your most trusted ally to ensure that your organizational decisions are sound and sane, on target and meaningful, and, most importantly, examined from multiple perspectives, ensuring better personal, professional, and organizational outcomes.

THE PRECURSORS TO EFFECTIVE REFLECTIVE PRACTICES

There are important prerequisites for reflection. Without them, it's likely that this practice will not take root in an organization's life. Our colleague Nancy Kline (1999) has devoted most of her career to exploring how people think best and how effective thinking can produce significantly better outcomes. Without taking the time to think and reflect, you can be assured to arrive at less-than-satisfactory outcomes. The thing we hear more than anything else as the reason people in organizations don't take time to reflect is, "I haven't the time." This deeply embedded assumption will assuredly keep you stuck. So, consider these questions:

- *What is your relationship to time?*

continues

> - *What are the cultural forces in your organization that create messages that taking the time to reflect is a waste of time?*
> - *How do interruptions and the incessant inputs from your electronic devices impair your ability to listen to yourself and to the thinking and reflections of others?*
>
> *Kline suggests that our ability to reflect and think is directly commensurate with the quality of listening we receive from others. How do we encourage and develop this kind of capacity in our organizations, and what would the practical consequences be if we could enculturate profound listening in our meetings, regardless of whether it is with another individual or with larger teams?*

The Self-Knowing Organization

At this juncture we divert from the usual chapter pattern of background-project-outcomes format to follow a more narrative approach. Our chapter in truth closely follows the intuitive, reflective process we applied when invited to write this chapter.

In the realm of personal reminiscence, reflection is integral to self-knowledge. In some ways, we can posit that human beings are reflective beings, and we believe that reflection is an essential facet of what distinguishes human beings from other creatures. Perhaps Descartes got it wrong: Perhaps he should have posited, "I reflect; therefore, I am." A corollary for organizations would be, "We reflect; therefore, we learn and thrive."

The three kinds of personal reminiscence that are instructive to our endeavor to understand the potential role of reflection in organizational life are:

- **Instrumental.** The practice of sharing stories that tell of a time when the individual has faced similar challenges in the past with the hope of learning from, and even being empowered by, those previous challenges to overcome adversity and empower the individual to better meet the current circumstances with greater courage and vitality.

- **Integrative.** The practice of looking back on what might at first blush appear to be disparate and unrelated events and themes in one's life to find common threads and meaning.

- **Transformative.** The practice in which one looks upon the past and the present to assist in the transformation of what might have been difficult and even painful events, to see them anew in a light that allows us to embrace them fully, and even see their benefits in our life.

In all these forms of reminiscence, reflection is essential. Simply enumerating the events of the past is not enough: We must engage with them actively, and in so doing, something new is born that is more alive and more robust, unleashing new possibilities that were heretofore hidden from our consciousness.

We believe that a similar benefit can accrue to organizations if the individuals in the organization actively engage in reflecting on both the past and present. In the realm of individual life, reflection of the types enumerated earlier in this section leads to greater self-awareness, increased self-knowledge, and a deeper connection to ourselves and others. Similarly, organizations that engage in reflective practices have the potential to become "self-knowing" organizations that exhibit greater vitality, resilience, and the ability to succeed in a world of accelerating change where other organizations are more likely to fail. Such a movement toward organizational self-knowledge has the potential to accelerate performance across the organization, leading to greater productivity, improved teamwork, healthier relationships, and greater resilience.

Daily Practice Tools and Strategies

In our work through the years with healthcare teams, we have identified and even helped develop a range of evidence-based reflection tools that any practitioner can integrate into a personal behavioral repertoire and/or into the repertoire of teams and organizations. As we suggested earlier, given your current circumstances, choose one or two practices that make the most sense to you to integrate into your behavioral repertoire, regardless of whether you are a nursing student, faculty member, a nurse transitioning to practice, nurse change agent, nurse at the bedside, charge nurse, department head, or organizational leader. If you choose to make it your own, we can assure you that you and your teams will harvest the many benefits that reflection can provide.

WHERE ARE YOU?

Many questions can lead to important insight and course-correction in our personal lives and in the lives of organizations and their teams. In ancient Hebrew Midrash, there is a story that Adam is wandering in the Garden of Eden, and God calls out, "Adam, where art thou?" The rabbis struggled with this question. If God is omniscient, why would he have to ask Adam for a GPS bearing about where he was in the Garden? Wouldn't he already know? The rabbis responded that the question had little to do with geography, but rather was intended to engender in Adam a deep thoughtfulness—dare we say, reflection upon his circumstances emotionally and spiritually. These sages contend that we each must ask of ourselves periodically, "Where am I?" if we are to find our bearings, and make essential course-corrections in our lives. Likewise, organizations must have moments of reckoning in their lives. For many, this occurs during yearly strategic planning. We believe that this is just a place to begin. If organizations are to become truly healthy, everyone in the organization must be invited into this conversation on a regular basis asking, "Where are we?" and "Is it where we want to be?"

The Practice of Shared Decision-Making

Margaret Meade is famous for her quote, "Never doubt that a group of committed citizens can change the world; indeed, it's the only thing that ever has" (Brainyquote, n.d.). When members of your teams are truly committed to your mission as an organization and have a clear vision of where you're going, the need for top-down leadership not only becomes less relevant but also can be a huge impediment to team effectiveness, especially in times of crisis.

The scenario. At the time of writing this chapter, for example, the world's health organizations were facing a significant infectious disease crisis with the outbreak and spread of Ebola in West Africa and the inevitable impact on a world that is so interconnected, with individuals who were infected showing up within the borders of the United States. The first case that rocked the healthcare establishment occurred at Texas Health Presbyterian Hospital in Dallas, and it became clear in the there that one of the first things that broke down was effective, shared decision-making. The following is an account provided by many of the nurses involved in the case:

> When Thomas Eric Duncan first came into the hospital, he arrived with an elevated temperature, but was sent home.
>
> On his return visit to the hospital, he was brought in by ambulance under the suspicion from him and family members that he may have Ebola.
>
> Mr. Duncan was left for several hours, not in isolation, in an area where other patients were present.
>
> No one knew what the protocols were or were able to verify what kind of personal protective equipment should be worn, and there was no training.
>
> Subsequently, a nurse supervisor arrived and demanded that [Mr. Duncan] be moved to an isolation unit—yet faced resistance from other hospital authorities.
>
> Lab specimens from Mr. Duncan were sent through the hospital tube system without being specially sealed and hand delivered. The result is that the entire tube system by which all lab specimens are sent was potentially contaminated.
>
> There was no advance preparedness on what to do with the patient, there was no protocol, [and] there was no system. The nurses were asked to call the Infectious Disease Department. The Infectious Disease Department did not have clear policies to provide, either.

Initial nurses who interacted with Mr. Duncan nurses [sic] wore a non-impermeable gown front and back, three pairs of gloves, with no taping around wrists, surgical masks, with the *option* of N-95s, and face shields. Some supervisors said that even the N-95 masks were not necessary.

The suits they were given still exposed their necks, the part closest to their face and mouth. They had suits with booties and hoods, three pairs of gloves, no tape.

For their necks, nurses had to use medical tape, that is not impermeable and has permeable seams, to wrap around their necks in order to protect themselves, and had to put on the tape and take it off on their own.

Nurses had to interact with Mr. Duncan with whatever protective equipment was available, at a time when he had copious amounts of diarrhea and vomiting, which produces a lot of contagious fluids.

Hospital officials allowed nurses who had interacted with Mr. Duncan to then continue normal patient care duties, taking care of other patients, even though they had not had the proper personal protective equipment while caring for Mr. Duncan.

Patients who may have been exposed were one day kept in strict isolation units. On the next day, [those same patients] were ordered to be transferred out of strict isolation into areas where there were other patients, even those with low-grade fevers who could potentially be contagious.

Were protocols breached? The nurses say there were no protocols.

Some hospital personnel were coming in and out of those isolation areas in the Emergency Department without having worn the proper protective equipment.

CDC officials who [were] in the hospital and Infectious Disease personnel [had] not kept hallways clean; they were going back and forth between the Isolation Pod and back into the hallways that were not properly cleaned, even after CDC, infectious control personnel, and doctors who [sic] exited into those hallways after being in the isolation pods.

Advance preparation that had been done by the hospital primarily consisted of emailing us about one optional lecture/seminar on Ebola. There was no mandate for nurses to attend trainings, or what nurses had to do in the event of the arrival of a patient with Ebola-like symptoms.

This is a very large hospital. To be effective, any classes would have to [be] offered repeatedly, covering all times when nurses work; instead, this was treated like the hundreds of other seminars that are routinely offered to staff.

There was no advance hands-on training on the use of personal protective equipment for Ebola. No training on what symptoms to look for. No training on what questions to ask.

Even when some trainings did occur, after Mr. Duncan had tested positive for Ebola, they were limited, and they did not include having every nurse in the training practicing the proper way to don and doff, put on and take off, the appropriate personal protective equipment to assure that they would not be infected or spread an infection to anyone else.

Guidelines have now been changed, but it is not clear what version Nina Pham [a nurse who contracted the virus from this patient] had available.

The hospital later said that their guidelines had changed and that the nurses needed to adhere to them. [Confusion arose because] the guidelines were constantly changing. It was later asked which guidelines should [be followed]. The message to the nurses was it's up to you [sic].

It is not up to the nurses to be setting the policy, nurses say, in the face of such a virulent disease. They needed to be trained optimally and correctly in how to deal with Ebola and the proper PPE doffing, as well as how to dispose of the waste.

In summary, the nurses state[d] there ha[d] been no policies [for] cleaning or bleaching the premises without housekeeping services. There was no one to pick up hazardous waste as it piled to the ceiling. They did not have access to proper supplies and observed the Infectious Disease Department and CDC themselves violate basic principles of infection control, including cross contaminating between patients. In the end, the nurses strongly fe[lt] unsupported, unprepared, lied to, and deserted to handle the situation on their own.

Source: National Nurses United, 2014.

REFLECTION IN SENSE-MAKING

Karl Weick (1995) makes a compelling argument in his seminal book Sensemaking in Organizations *that organizations cohere through the sharing of stories. The organization's past exists only through the representation of it through a shared narrative, and its future is nothing more than a story projected into that time frame in the minds of the players within the organization. These stories coupled with sense-making ensure that the organization maintains a sense of cohesion. We would suggest that without the practice of regular reflection on these stories of the past and future, critically exposing the flawed assumptions that underlie these stories, sense-making will often be misguided and off the mark, leading to organizations pursuing stultifying strategies that can become the seeds of their demise.*

Outcomes. In reviewing these events, imagine if these teams were operating with a shared decision-making model, and if they were taking the time to pause and reflect at each of the important junctures of the events that unfolded. How would the outcomes have been different? Would the nurse supervisor have succumbed to the voices that resisted having the patient put in isolation immediately if she had paused and reflected on the situation? Would the nurse or tech who decided to send the lab specimens through the hospital tube system have acted as though this were a status quo event, or would that person have wondered whether it was a wise decision and taken a different course of action? Would hospital staff have allowed nurses to continue their normal patient care duties after interacting with the patient? Would the nurses themselves have paused and wondered whether that was a prudent decision and insisted on an alternate course of action?

We could continue to deconstruct this case from this perspective, but we challenge you to reflect on the lessons that you could learn about leadership and reflection as you transpose this story to your own circumstances.

REFLECTING ON ... USING REFLECTION IN LEADERSHIP

- *How can you bring the power of reflection to bear on your day-to-day work?*

- *How could you amplify the effectiveness of your decision-making and empower your teams to step up and participate in the decision-making process?*

The Practice of Debriefing

In our work with teams, we have witnessed that the most significant addition to their practice that spurs learning and improvement is debriefing, especially after any emergent event. Although on the surface this seems to be a simple process, there are fine nuances to facilitating an effective debrief. We detail some of those key techniques in this section.

The scenario. A number of years ago as our company was rolling out TeamSTEPPS® training (Team Strategies and Tools to Enhance Performance and

Patient Safety), we were facilitating the training at a large U.S. Navy medical facility. Following is an account of an event that occurred.

We first met Bruce Gillingham in 2007. He had returned the year before from his deployment with a Forward Surgical Team (FST) embedded with the U.S. Marines in Iraq. He was now the Commanding Officer of a Naval Medical Center—an orthopedic surgeon by training. Bruce had seen his share of trauma during his tour in Iraq as the FST leader during the infamous battles for Fallujah. The FST was managing significant casualties day and night. The teams got very little sleep, and resources were dwindling due to the op's tempo. Although patient-survival rates during the Iraq war were the highest they'd been in any previous armed conflict, the FST patients who were transported by helicopter suffered unusually poor outcomes after surgery as a result of hypothermia. Blankets had been in short supply for weeks, so the fix wasn't easy; supply lines were being impacted by the intense fighting.

The FST had adopted the practice of daily debriefs at the end of shift, led by Dr. Gillingham and his leadership team, to serve as a rapid-cycle improvement session given that the team was facing new challenges like the hypothermia problem almost daily now. During the debrief, the leader would pose the question for the team. In this instance the question was, "How can we keep these patients from getting hypothermic during airborne transfers to larger, more-equipped medical centers?" As was the practice, the junior team member always went first to reduce the hierarchy present in rank and medical profession.

Private First Class (PFC) Alonzo Scales knew the drill because he quickly realized he was low man on the totem pole. He was a transporter. At 18 years old and only 10 months since his high school graduation, he had already seen more than most experienced trauma nurses would see in 10 years, although he didn't have any formal clinical training. He was conscientious and a keen observer. The hardest part for him was transporting those killed in action (KIAs). Fortunately for the FST, their superior performance had helped to keep the KIA rate low. Scales pondered the question while others took their turn brainstorming around ideas, and the corpsman took notes with his smartphone. No silver bullet here, they thought. Getting more blankets really was the only answer, and that might take another week.

Then Scales spoke up: "What if we used the body bags?" Either it was going to be the dumbest idea ever or the most innovative yet. It was the latter. The team had an ample supply of body bags, and others quickly iterated on the design, including slits in the heavy plastic and painting red crosses on the bags to indicate a living patient.

In one debrief, the team solved a nagging clinical problem and nicknamed the modification the "Hot Pocket." The FST rate of hypothermic patients during transport fell to zero.

Outcomes. Debriefs or after-action reviews are powerful process-improvement events. Teams use debriefing to reflect on data—here, the rate of hypothermic patients during air transport—as well as other key performance indicators. Engaging all members of the team produces the best results because you never know who possesses the best information or solution. Asking simple reflective questions such as, "What went well?" and "What can we do better in the future?" can get the reflection process started. After asking Dr. Gillingham about the key to conducting effective team debriefs, he responded: "We as the senior leaders have to empower our team to speak up no matter rank, specialty, education, or role. Those closest to the patient usually have all the best ideas."

The evidence for the efficacy of debriefing is substantial (Fanning & Gaba, 2007). In one study, in-house cardiac arrest outcomes were significantly improved (Edelson et al., 2008). More recently, we have been involved with a collaborative of hospitals which instituted debriefing after emergent C-sections. After the hospitals went from zero debriefings to debriefing approximately 70% of the time, the outcome has been dramatic—a 20% decrease in infant mortality. If there was only one practice you consider adopting, debriefing has our top recommendation.

The Practice of Situation Monitoring

A broad awareness of others, constantly reflecting on each others' practices and their impact on patients, is a key clinical team practice that can protect patients from harm. Questioning authority and physician orders becomes an essential safety activity, and without a reflective mindset, this practice is likely to fail.

THE PRACTICE OF LEARNING FROM ERROR

Industry has long embraced the lessons of quality improvement and learning from defects. Healthcare is just beginning this journey, and for the most part, struggling with the challenges posed by improving human care delivery systems. A colleague of ours once told us that the real gold is in the near-misses—that these data points can be powerful predictors of where the next sentinel event could occur, and therefore can be the "canary in the coal mine" that helps us avert a human tragedy. Whether it is near-misses or good catches, or actual harm, without reflection, there can be no learning—and without learning, we will be destined to repeat history over and over again.

Situation monitoring is the process of actively scanning behaviors and actions to assess elements of the situation or environment. We are constantly validating information as we process it: "Are we sure it's accurate?" This reflective step creates a healthy skepticism in our daily management of risk. Looking both ways before crossing the street requires the instantaneous estimation of whether we can make it safely across before the next car reaches our location. It's these mini-reflective loops or cognitive questions that automatically inform our next action.

The scenario. Here is an example of situation monitoring in action:

Chad Carlson was riding his bicycle one morning in the dark when a car plowed into him at 30 miles per hour and tossed him into the air, after which he hit the car's windshield. After surgery, Chad was faced with a stay in the Intensive Care Unit (ICU).

One evening, Diane Richmond, the day nurse, impulsively knocked on the door of Chad's ICU room while bringing Carol Fisher, the night nurse, with her for a beside handover at shift change. The first thing Diane did was check all the equipment to be certain that everything was functioning properly. "This is our miracle patient. By all accounts, he shouldn't have made it, but Dr. Jackson thinks we should have him off the ventilator by Friday," Diane said. After a quick review of other key patient information, Diane said her goodbyes to Chad and Carol.

Carol continued at Chad's bedside, looking over the chart and rereading the doctor's notes. The doctor had ordered a reduction in the ventilator, but he had simultaneously ordered an increase in a key medication from 15mg to 20mg. In her mind, something didn't add up.

She called Diane on her cell phone. "Sorry to bother you, but I was looking over Mr. Carlson's chart. Did you know that Dr. Jackson is increasing his meds from 15 to 20mg?"

Diane paused trying to picture the chart in her mind. "That's not right. Are you sure?"

Carol was emphatic. "It's in black and white. What's odd is that he had reduced the med down to 15mg yesterday from 20 when they reduced the ventilator from 40 to 30%. Why would he be increasing it when we're going down further? What do you think we ought to do?"

Diane didn't hesitate. "I think we need to call Dr. Jackson."

Carol took a deep breath. "You know how he hates being interrupted at night, especially for minor things. He can be a real bear."

Diane responded, "Let him growl. I've got three-way conferencing on this phone. What's his number? Let's get him on the line."

A minute later they had tracked him down. Diane took the lead. "Dr. Jackson, sorry to bother you, but we have a question about your orders for Chad Carlson."

He was irritated. "This better be good. I was just getting ready to read my kid a bedtime story."

"Well, your orders indicate a reduction in ventilator settings to 20% while at the same time increasing his meds from 15mg to 20mg. That didn't seem to make sense to us?"

There was a long pause on the other end of the line. He said, "You're sure that's what I wrote?"

Diane replied, "Afraid so, Dr. Jackson."

There was another long pause as he attempted to retrace in his mind through the afternoon, and see whether he could think of what had distracted him to make such a significant error. He couldn't think of a thing. Taking a deep breath, he said, "You're right, that's not correct. Something must have distracted me. Great catch! It should be 10mg. Thanks. You did the right thing by calling."

Carol, the night nurse, was gracious. "I thought that that's what happened, but figured I should just check with you to be doubly sure."

Outcomes. Reflection takes on a multiplicative effect when others reflect with you, as during this example of a "good catch" by the bedside nurse. By involving others to validate your reflections on the situation, you can help to refine complex information like a ventilator-weaning process that includes multiple medications. Reflection alone didn't prevent patient harm in this situation; instead, it was reflection coupled with further questioning of the day nurse and the doctor—even if it meant that the nurse had to put her reputation on the line by questioning the doctor's orders. In a team environment where trust has been developed, questioning the "what" is more important than questioning the "who," especially when the action is critical to patient safety.

THE PRACTICE OF I'M SAFE

Awareness of your own condition to ensure that you are fit and ready to fulfill your duties is essential to delivering safe, quality care. Team members should assess and report if there is a personal situation affecting their ability to perform. The mnemonic I'M SAFE is a simple checklist that should be used daily (or more frequently) to determine both your co-workers' and your own ability to perform safely. I'M SAFE stands for:

- *I — Illness. Am I feeling so bad that I cannot perform my duties?*

- *M — Medication. Is the medication that I am taking affecting my ability to maintain situation awareness and perform duties?*

- *S — Stress. Is there something (such as a life event or situation at work) that is detracting from my ability to focus and perform my duties?*

- *A — Alcohol/drugs. Is my use of alcohol or illicit drugs affecting me so that I cannot focus on the performance of my duties?*

- *F — Fatigue. Will my tiredness affect my work? The effects of fatigue should not be ignored. Team members should alert the team regarding their state of fatigue (e.g., "Watch me a little closer today. I only had three hours of sleep last night.").*

- *E — Eating and elimination. Has it been 6 hours since I have eaten or used the restroom? Many times, we are so focused on ensuring our patients' basic needs that we forget to take care of our own. Not taking care of our elimination needs affects our ability to concentrate and stresses us physiologically.*

REFLECTING ON ... SITUATION MONITORING

- *When you are fatigued or feeling drowsy when driving a car but do not pull over and rest for a few minutes, what risks are you taking?*

- *When you do not take the time for food because of work demands, what is the impact on your effectiveness?*

- *If you have ever abused alcohol and/or drugs, how did that impact your decision-making and effectiveness?*

The Practice of STEP

How do you acquire a trained eye as you "monitor the situation" on your unit? What are relevant components of the situation that provide clues about impending complications or contingencies? The STEP process is a mnemonic tool that can help you monitor the situation and the overall environment. The STEP process involves ongoing monitoring of the:

- **Status of the patient**

- **Team members**

- **Environment**

- **Progress toward the goal**

In Mezirow's levels of reflectivity (2008), discriminant reflectivity involves a series of "how" questions for developing a patient care plan. The care plan is carried out by a team, even if the team is only a patient and one other person—say, a family member during at-home care. Having a reflective process to develop a comprehensive care plan helps to build a shared mental model for the patient and his care team.

Think about approaching a four-way stop sign at a street intersection. We automatically begin processing a strategy for safely navigating the situation. First, we apply the existing rules of the road from memory. Next, we assess the other drivers' actions, asking ourselves, "Are they going to follow the rules?" Using a reflective feedback loop based on the movement, positioning, and estimating, we make a calculated decision to proceed through the intersection while continually monitoring the result of our decision until we are assured of our safe navigation. This mental processing all happens in a matter of seconds for the experienced driver. Now consider how this process might be different for an inexperienced driver, a distracted driver, a foreign visitor unfamiliar with the rules, or a risk-taker. Is this skill teachable? Of course it is. The rules are studied, the process of evaluating your position is practiced, and distractions are limited while other passengers provide additional backup. But, there is a learning curve for creating this common heuristic.

The same is true in a healthcare delivery setting, especially when one is inexperienced or new to the environment. How do we come to know what we know? Obviously, someone else taught us, and we have experienced the situation. Our autonomic system takes over from there. In the context of healthcare delivery, using the STEP process is a reflective way to develop this skill of assessing a situation. Here is an example.

> **Status:** A post-surgical patient is placed on a Foley catheter while recovering on the medical/surgical ward. The timing of the removal of the catheter impacts the likelihood of the patient developing an infection.

> **Team members:** It's the weekend, and staffing is low. The nurse is unsure of the plan for removal because physician responsibility for the removal orders has shifted from surgeon to surgical resident to hospitalist due to weekend coverage.

> **Environment:** The physical environment lacks sufficient cueing, such as status boards to create visible reminders of key actions. Additionally, distractions and interruptions are frequent due to some renovations of the nursing station.

> **Progress toward goal:** The plan for removal of the catheter has been poorly articulated or is completely nonexistent, resulting in the patient experiencing a common bacterial infection that extends the hospital stay and adds increased costs, more pain, and a lengthier recovery time.

If the team used the STEP process as a continuous series of reflective questions, could the infection have been prevented? The simple answer is, possibly yes. Reflection itself is not sufficient to protect this patient. Instead, the team must be able to effectively mitigate the gaps in the process including communication, coordination, planning, and system improvements, such as limiting distractions, creating visible action cues, and providing adequate staffing. Just "knowing" the situation alone may be insufficient for managing the situation, requiring another full complement of reflective actions.

Final Reflections

We believe that reflection has measurable real-world consequences. The return on investment (ROI) for organizations to invest in reflective practices is significant and may be the difference between surviving in the competitive landscape of healthcare delivery and going out of business. We have seen the power of debriefs, for example, actually lead to a reduction of early elective deliveries by 50%. In another hospital system, the adoption of these practices led to the system's insurance carrier reducing its premiums by millions of dollars because preventable fetal harm had decreased to nearly zero over a 3-year period. In another large urban hospital, nearly three-quarters of a million dollars was recovered in reimbursements.

The research supports this view. Of the many crises facing healthcare, perhaps one of the most significant is staff engagement. The costs for replacing a nurse have been well established through a number of national studies, ranging from $22,000 to $64,000 (Geisz, 2010). Building a reflective organization may be one of the best pathways to engagement and improved retention.

In a UK research study by MacLeod and Clarke (2009), the authors found significant correlations to employee engagement:

- Companies with low engagement scores earn an operating income 32.7% lower than companies with more engaged employees.

- Similarly, companies with a highly engaged workforce experience a 19.2% growth in operating income over a 12-month period (Hibbard, Greene, & Overton, 2013).

There is also a growing body of literature that engaging patients with their own care can lead to improved outcomes, offering a direct economic benefit of healthcare institutions and the public as a whole. Many of the reflective practices described in this chapter can play a key role in patient engagement. Patient engagement is more than inviting patient participation; it is providing the knowledge, skills, tools, and opportunities to take an active role in their own care. For a family member, patient engagement includes patient advocacy for safe, effective care.

An example of patient engagement is the bedside handover or report. Shift changes create a handover of patient responsibility from one provider to another, including the transfer of essential patient information. Asking the patient or family member to share concerns or questions is essential to ensuring everyone is on the same page related to the patient care plan. When patients and families are actively involved in the handover at the bedside, patient safety and patient satisfaction improves (Maxson, Derby, Wrobleski, & Foss, 2012). Physician rounding is another opportunity for patient engagement to manage concerns, assess effectiveness of current therapies, make shared decisions, and manage future patient/family expectations. This practice is especially important for pediatric patients and any patient unable to make independent decisions.

Organizations that are more resilient in changing times are more likely to adjust to the challenges they confront, and bend rather than break when the business and regulatory climate becomes turbulent. Once again, reflective practices can move an organization from a reactive stance strategically to a more proactive stance that will allow it to weather the difficult times predicted in the years ahead.

Finally, organizations that build reflective thinking environments will be more likely to innovate and discover new and better ways to provide excellent, safe care. They will be the market leaders, attracting the best and brightest employees, thereby safeguarding their financial future.

References

Aristotle (n.d.). *Metaphysics*. Retrieved from https://ebooks.adelaide.edu.au/a/aristotle/metaphysics/

Brainyquote. (n.d.). Margaret Meade Quotes. Retrieved from www.brainyquote.com/quotes/quotes/m/margaretme100502.html

Dewey, J. (1933). *How we think: A restatement of the relation of reflective thinking to the educative process*. Boston, MA: D.C. Heath.

Edelson, D. P., Litzinger, B., Arora, V., Walsh, D., Kim, S., Lauderdale, D. S., ... Abella, B. S. (2008). *Archives of Internal Medicine*, *168*(10), 1063–1069. doi:10.1001/archinte.168.10.1063

Fanning, R. M., & Gaba, D. M. (2007). The role of debriefing in simulation-based learning. *Simulation in Healthcare: Journal of the Society for Simulation in Healthcare*, *2*(2), 115–125. doi:10.1097/SIH.0b013e3180315539

Geisz, M. B. (2010). *Wisdom at work: Retaining experienced nurses*. Princeton, NJ: Robert Wood Johnson Foundation. Retrieved from www.rwjf.org/content/dam/farm/reports/program_results_reports/2010/rwjf65925

Hatton, N., & Smith, D. (1995). *Reflection in teacher education: Towards definition and implementation*. The University of Sydney: School of Teaching and Curriculum Studies. Retrieved from http://www2.edfac.usyd.edu.au/LocalResource/Study1/hattonart.html

Hibbard, J. H., Greene, J., & Overton, V. (2013). Patients with lower activation associated with higher costs; delivery systems should know their patients' "scores." *Health Affairs*, *32*(2), 216–222. Retrieved from http://content.healthaffairs.org/content/32/2/216?=right

Kitchenham, A. (2008). The evolution of John Mezirow's transformative learning theory. *Journal of Transformative Education*, *6*(2), 104.

Kline, N. (1999). *Time to think: Listening to ignite the human mind*. UK: Cassell Illustrated.

Kolb, D. A. (1984). *Experiential learning: Experience as the source of learning and development*. Englewood Cliffs, NJ: Prentice-Hall.

MacLeod, D., & Clarke, N. (2009). *Engaging for success: Enriching performance through employee engagement*. Retrieved from www.engageforsuccess.org/wp-content/uploads/2012/09/file52215.pdf

Maxson, P. M., Derby, K. M.,Wrobleski, D. M., & Foss, D. M. (2012). Beside nurse-to-nurse handoff promotes patient safety. *Medsurg Nursing, 21*(3), 140–144.

Muller, A. C. (Trans.) (2013). *The analects of Confucius.* Retrieved from www.acmuller.net/con-dao/analects.html

National Nurses United. (2014). *Statement by RN's at Texas Health Presbyterian Hospital as provided to National Nurses United.* Retrieved from www.nationalnursesunited.org/blog/entry/statement-by-registered-nurses-at-texas-health-presbyterian-hospital-in-dal/

Pappas, P. (2010). *A taxonomy of reflection: Critical thinking for students, teachers, and principals (part 1).* Retrieved from www.peterpappas.com/2010/01/taxonomy-reflection-critical-thinking-students-teachers-principals-.html

Weick, K. (1995). *Sensemaking in organizations.* Thousand Oaks, CA: Sage Publications.

Chapter 12
QSEN Into Practice at Southwest General Hospital

Mary Jo Krivanek, RN, BSN, MPA
Mary Ellen Campobasso, MSN, RN, ACNS-BC
Beth M. Weese, MSN, RN, GCNS-BC
Sheila Blackmur, MSN, RN-BC, CMSRN

Quality and Safety Education for Nurses (QSEN) (Cronenwett et al., 2007) into practice at Southwest General Hospital (Middleburg Heights, Ohio) was launched into practice at Southwest General Hospital after the nursing clinical educators performed an assessment of the state of nursing and then attended the May 2013 QSEN Conference in Atlanta, Georgia. At the conference, Karen Drenkard, who at that time was Director of Magnet Recognition for the American Nursing Association Credentialing Center (ANCC), spoke about nurses being at the center of healthcare and that a feeling of safety is an intuitive part

With appreciation to Mary Dolansky, RN, PhD, Associate Professor in the Frances Payne Bolton School of Nursing, Case Western Reserve University.

This chapter has been written with appreciation to the QSEN Institute.

of our profession. She encouraged us to infuse QSEN into job descriptions, job evaluations, continuing education, and so forth. The conference also inspired us to embed QSEN into orientation, curriculum, leadership, reflective journaling, resources, teach-back, and whiteboards. Last, the conference encouraged us to evaluate our outcomes through the National Database of Nursing Quality Indicators (NDNQI) Nurse and Patient Satisfaction and patient harm reports.

This chapter is about how a group of clinical educators were motivated to bring the QSEN competencies directly to the nurses in our organization. In particular, our goal was to influence their practice at the bedside.

Background

In general, nurses will openly agree that they want to provide patient care that is safe, effective, efficient, timely, and patient-centered. Unfortunately, the patient care–delivery process in many healthcare organizations fails to provide nurses ample time to provide such care. Nurses then begin to feel that the quality of care delivery becomes eroded, resulting in nurses feeling frustrated and inadequate. Eventually, nurses may have difficulty finding satisfaction in the workplace and may begin to look elsewhere for employment.

Current healthcare delivery systems have a goal to improve the quality and safety of healthcare. To meet this goal at Southwest General, a 358-bed suburban hospital, the nursing clinical educators are at the foreground of implementing QSEN. QSEN, when incorporated into bedside nursing practice, has the potential to keep nurses focused in the workplace and empowers nurses to feel that they can provide safe, quality care to their patients that is effective, efficient, timely, and patient centered.

At Southwest General, the nursing clinical educators (and the authors of this chapter)—Mary Jo Krivanek, Mary Ellen Campobasso, Beth Weese, and Sheila Blackmur—heard the nurses' plea to be able to provide safe and competent delivery of patient care. We recognize the importance of blending our current bedside nursing practice with evidence-based nursing resources and emphasizing the QSEN Core Competencies as being essential to our nurses' orientation and skill performance process. In January, 2013, the nursing clinical educators established a team to support bedside nurses in their daily practice. Each nursing clinical educator was assigned to various nursing departments (units) as a clinical resource educator.

A driving force compelling us to bring forth change was our attendance at our bi-monthly Interdisciplinary Quality Risk (IQR) Review Committee meetings. This committee reviews hospital patient safety events reported through the electronic risk event–reporting system. The committee reviews all event reports, including those that involve injury to the patient. Members review the event reports and identify potential process improvements related to anesthesia, burns, emergency, equipment, falls, intravenous procedures, blood, medication, patient, security, surgery, treatment, procedure, skin, and other related incidents. The meetings are co-chaired by the Director of Quality Management and the Insurance and Operations Risk Manager.

Preparation

During the first quarter of 2013, the Southwest General Chief Nursing Officer (CNO), Martha Bauschka, granted us the time to conduct a needs assessment in the department of nursing. To begin, we interviewed nursing directors, nursing managers, nursing assistant clinical managers, pharmacy, risk, quality, specialty nurses, and staff of ancillary departments, using a standardized data collection tool. We observed General Orientation and Nursing Clinical Orientation. We performed a Nursing Council Review and a Staff Needs Assessment in the form of an online survey. We used a separate assessment for patient care assistants (PCAs) and RNs/LPNs. The assessment included 25 questions that used a Likert scale using Benner's rating from novice to expert. The assessment results showed a disconnect with what staff reported and what our quality indicators reported. For example, staff rated themselves very high with obtaining a patient's correct height and weight, yet pharmacy often reported that weights were incomplete or inaccurate. We also made observations while walking through the halls, riding elevators, sitting in on meetings, and attendance at daily check-in (DCI).

Some of our experiences came from simply listening to staff, patients, and visitors. Our nurses expressed the many challenges and barriers that they encounter on a daily basis. For example, nurses were confused about policies versus protocols, some standards were outdated, and references from nursing were reported as "confusing." In another example, our clinical managers felt that new staff, after attending general and clinical nursing orientation, come to their units "overwhelmed and confused."

At the end of the 3 months, we had an enormous amount of information to review, analyze, and sort into repeating themes. We used the QSEN framework to organize our observations. The underlying theme of the data collected was that change in the form of formalized education was needed. The ways and means of how newly hired nurses prepared and transitioned from orientation to the units needed extensive refurbishing. Preceptors needed a structured education program led by the nursing clinical educators. Although we perceived this as a huge undertaking, we embraced the challenge.

The Project

We presented our assessment findings to the Nurse Executive Team in April 2013 and recommended that the QSEN competencies guide Southwest General's entire healthcare system in the delivery of safe and effective quality care. The top three focus items we identified were:

1. Electronic health record (EHR) analysis

2. Skills fair

3. Update clinical nursing orientation

The Nurse Executive Team gave us their full support. In May 2013, we attended the National QSEN Conference, which provided us with concrete ideas that we could place into practice.

The educators at Southwest General have been integrating the QSEN competencies into practice since the second quarter of 2013. The competencies, described in the following sections (accessible from http://qsen.org/competencies/pre-licensure-ksas/), have been infused into clinical nursing orientation,

orientation checklists, annual competence/skill evaluations, education programs, Scope of Service documents, nursing policies, and guidelines. We have committed to moving from a personal effort to a systems-oriented effort. For example, a nurse who turns her patient has demonstrated a personal effort to maintain skin integrity. A nurse displays a systems-oriented effort when she compares her unit skin incident rates with other units and with national benchmarks.

Patient-Centered Care

The following sections describe examples of how Southwest promotes patient-centered care.

Teach-back. Patient-centered care is enhanced through the teach-back methodology for all patient education. *Teach-back* occurs when nurses ask patients to repeat in their own words what they need to know or do, in a nonintimidating way. Yes/no questions are not asked. Teach-back is *not* a test of the patient, but rather a verification of how well the nurse explained a concept to the patient. For more than one concept, two to three main points are taught, there is a check for understanding using teach-back, and then the nurse moves on to the next concept. Teach-back is a chance to check for understanding, and if necessary, reteach the information. At Southwest General, teach-back is used for all patient education.

Cultural diversity. Patient-centered care with sensitivity and respect for the diversity of the human experience was highlighted with cultural diversity resources made available for nursing. Our Case Management department developed a community provider list, posted online for all staff to access. The community provider list includes 31 items. There are lists of facilities for adult day care and assisted living,

PATIENT-CENTERED CARE

Recognize the patient or designee as the source of control and full partner in providing compassionate and coordinated care based on respect for patient's preferences, values, and needs (Cronenwett et al., 2007).

bereavement resources, chemical dependency resources, cleaning services, home health agencies, LGBT resources, Meals on Wheels, and more. The cultural diversity resources also include culture clues, information on interpreters, and nurse-to-patient communication sheets for patients who speak foreign languages.

Communication boards. Patient-centered care involves communicating care provided and needed. At Southwest General, every patient room includes communication dry erase boards (whiteboards). Nurses and PCAs update information on these boards every shift and as needed. Staff is directed to add:

- Unit name (example: "Welcome to 1 North")

- Patient's preferred name

- Room number, day of the week, and date

- Primary/admitting physician

- First name of the RN who has primary responsibility of the patient, and other nurses, with credentials (example: "Nancy RN, Bob LPN")

- First name of PCA or STNA (State Tested Nursing Assistant)

- Anticipated date of discharge, updated by case managers or other staff

- Today's plan (examples: daily goals, diet change, activity, testing, physical therapy, teach-back, dressing changes)

- Current level of pain and last time when analgesia was administered

- Special considerations, addressing personal needs of the patient:

  - "Home care instructions with: include daughter Rose"

  - "Visual impairment" or "Hears best in right ear"

  - "BP and lab from right arm only"

  - "Dietary or nutrition education," "Thicken liquids," or "Nectar"

Patient portal. Patient-centered care guides each transition of care. A patient portal facilitates better communication between patients and their physician's office by providing convenient access from the comfort and privacy of the patient's own home. The patient portal provides online access via the Internet for hospitalwide services, patient medical records, community resources, and eventually the patient education videos. If patients do not have Internet access, they may refer to the hard-copy discharge instructions. These instructions contain information on discharge instructions, medications, physician follow-ups, physician contact information, and appropriate specialty nurses. Postdischarge follow-up phone calls are made to all patients going home or to assisted livings.

Patient Education Committee. Patient-centered care involves engaging the patient in the care process. The Patient Education Committee is co-chaired by two nursing clinical educators and comprises approximately 20 members from various backgrounds: nursing, pharmacy, diabetic education, hospital education, patient representative, and others. This multidisciplinary approach allows all members to work as a collaborative team. The committee reviewed numerous online videos to identify those relevant to our current patient population's education needs. The use of these videos is extremely popular with our maternity patients. The committee is actively soliciting new ad hoc members from other disciplines to make recommendations for future online content. Reaching out to other disciplines has been met with positive feedback and recommendations.

In the first quarter of 2015, it is anticipated that this committee will have a promotional campaign throughout the hospital, helping our nursing staff and other bedside caregivers engage in promoting the online video system. The committee is currently reviewing the probability of having the online video system interfaced with our electronic health record (EHR) so that when a patient watches a video, that event is archived in the medical record. The committee is also investigating the possibility of patients and their caregivers accessing videos from home via the patient portal. This access will not only allow patients to receive education during hospitalization but also aid in reinforcement of the content after discharge. As an organization, Southwest General recognizes that standardizing and ensuring up-to-date patient education content promotes patient safety and quality healthcare delivery. Ultimately, this process will help ensure that our patients are able to actively participate in their care and prevent unnecessary hospital re-admissions.

The Patient Education Committee is also pursuing the best content for patient education purposes. Patient information is available from our Lexicomp Resources about medications. In addition, Southwest General's implementation of online Lippincott has provided the opportunity for easily understood patient education printouts. The educational content is now available for nurses to access and distribute to their patients. This too will be marketed more assertively in 2015.

TEAMWORK AND COLLABORATION

Function effectively within nursing and interprofessional teams, fostering open communication, mutual respect, and shared decision-making to achieve quality patient care (Cronenwett et al., 2007).

Teamwork and Collaboration

Teamwork and collaboration involves respecting the perspectives and expertise that each member of the team contributes (http://qsen.org/competencies/pre-licensure-ksas/). This competency is described in more detail in the following sections.

Nursing Standards Committee. Teamwork and collaboration is evident in the Nursing Standards Committee. The Nursing Standards Committee impacts safety and quality of care by facilitating the development of nursing policies, procedures, and workflows that serve to define and communicate appropriate clinical/operational practice. The Nursing Standards Committee includes a clinical nursing educator as the chairperson; a nursing director; a clinical manager; and nurse representation from Medical/Surgical, Surgical Services, Critical Care, Emergency Department, Post-Acute Care, Geriatric Behavioral Health, Labor and Delivery, and Post-Partum. We have ad hoc membership from Mental Health, Oncology, Home Health, Hospice, Dialysis, Endoscopy, cath lab, PACU/Pain Management, and Nursing Quality.

Nursing councils. Teamwork and collaboration is supported through the nursing councils with front-line staff, including the Clinical Informatics Council, the Nursing Engagement Council, the Nursing Operations Council, the Nursing Practice Council, the Nursing Quality Council, and the Patient Care Council.

Medication resources. Our online medication resources include the IV Drugs Approved Administration Resource created by Pharmacy and Nursing. Other online resources include Lexicomp and Micromedex. Nursing and Laboratory are working together to ensure correct collection, labeling, and processing of specimens.

Preceptor Café. Teamwork and collaboration is evident by demonstration of a commitment to team goals. The nursing clinical educators identified a need to "start over" with our preceptors. A literature search about preceptors brought us to Nelson's article "A Preceptor Café" (2010). Southwest General held a Preceptor Café in September of 2013 to renew commitment, refresh vision, and develop strategies for successful orienting of new hires. QSEN competencies were introduced to all preceptors. Groups of five to six preceptors moved through five stations, each lasting 30 minutes. The five stations, modeled after Nelson's article, included:

- **Universal value: security.** Preceptors were asked to remember their own first few days at the hospital and their first days on the unit. What were your big concerns? What kept you awake at night? Of these worries, which proved to be groundless? Which remained real challenges? Stories from new nurse graduates were shared.

- **Belonging.** Preceptors were asked to write inside a big circle what makes people on the unit feel belong and valued. A discussion of how people are drawn into the circle of belonging and ideas were shared on how to welcome new staff members.

- **Skill and power.** A discussion of how a preceptor can look for evidence of a new staff nurse's connections among assessment, planning, and interventions.

- **Transformation.** This discussion centered on how a preceptor uncovers the hidden talents of the new nurse and assesses for areas that need skill building. Preceptors were encouraged to discuss things before going into the patient room, instructing as-you-go and debriefing afterward.

- **Higher values of intuition, purpose, and unity.** Recognizing that the higher levels of intuition, purpose, and unity may not come during the first year of nursing, preceptors were encouraged to have new nurses reflect on how care is driven by vision and values, not just task check-offs.

In summary, 24 RNs attended the Preceptor Café with five instructors. Comments on the evaluations included:

- "Very helpful material that will help me to refocus the way I think about things."

- "This was very helpful in taking new techniques and thoughts back to my unit to apply to my preceptorship."

- "Now I will include not only being professional in our role, but also nurturing, compassion, and leading by example."

- "Nice refresher that the patient is always the focus of care. I will reprioritize the focus of the computer documentation *after* patient care and safety."

- "I feel that this program has highly impacted the orientation process. I feel I can be a better leader and include new staff members in a variety of ways to make them feel welcome and confident."

Upon exit, the participants received a continuing education unit (CEU) certificate for 3.0 contact hours and a nursing pin.

Interdisciplinary team rounding. Teamwork and collaboration involves acknowledging the potential to contribute to effective team functioning. The nursing clinical educators participate in interdisciplinary team rounding on their clinical units. While participating in rounds, the educators are observing educational needs and offering clinical expertise.

Teamwork and collaboration involves valuing the perspectives and expertise of all health team members. QSEN competencies are infused into our Scope of Service documents. Table 12.1 shows an example.

Table 12.1: Patient Care and Services Plans: Regional Spine and Pain Center

Hours of operation	Days of operation every Tuesday and Wednesday.
	Staffing hours vary according to patient volume. Staff works 8- and 12-hour shifts.
Types and ages of patients served	The staff provides compassionate, patient-centered care to adult inpatients and outpatients for management of chronic pain in various treatment modalities. Care is based on the patient needs and values. Treatments may include pain blocks with and without fluoroscopy and/or radiofrequency ablations.
Methods used to assess and meet patient care needs	Utilizes the nursing process in accordance with patient care standards and physician orders.
	Utilize AORN* and ASPAN** Standards and Recommended Evidence-Based Practices.
Scope and complexity of patient care needs	Nurses in the unit are driven to determine the best clinical practice evidenced by researching unit-specific performance improvement projects. Following ASPAN standards, patients are discharged when they meet set criteria using a modified Aldrete score. The three principal components of the Universal Protocol, including a time-out, are completed pre-procedure. Discharge instructions are given to patients both pre- and post-procedure.
Required number and mix of staff members to provide for patient care needs	Staffing: eight RN/LPNs (combined), two-three PCAs, one radiology tech
	Staffing is adjusted to volume.

continues

Table 12.1: *Continued*

	RNs, LPNs, and PCAs work as a team collaboratively with the physician caring for the patient throughout the continuum from admission through discharge. Nurses work as admitting, recovery, or circulator in collaboration with radiology for fluoroscopy. SBAR*** is utilized post-procedure for effective handoff to the recovering nurse.
Plan for improving the quality of care	Plan, Do, Check, Act Data collection, education, and review of reportable incidents are part of continuous quality improvement. Pain management staff values their own role in preventing errors. Discharge phone calls are made to follow up with patients and to encourage physician follow-up.

*Association of periOperative Registered Nurses
**American Society of PeriAnesthesia Nurses
***Situation, Background, Assessment, Recommendation
Sources: Southwest General Health Center, 2014; QSEN Institute, n.d.

Evidence-Based Practice

Evidence-based practice (EBP) has been adopted through the use of Lippincott Procedures online. Lippincott instantly delivers concise, evidence-based content entries directly to the bedside nurse. Lippincott educates nursing staff on the latest procedures and skills. Southwest General obtained this online resource in January 2013. The clinical nursing educators have promoted the use of this resource through scheduled educational offerings and as needed right at the bedside. Our Lippincott usage rates continue to climb (see Figure 12.1).

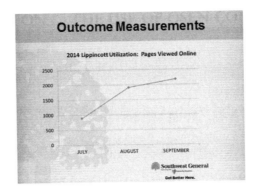

FIGURE 12.1

*Lippincott Pages
Viewed by Staff*

Evidence-based practice values the concept of EBP as integral to determining best clinical practice. The Nursing Practice Manual includes only evidence-based resources in the creation of Clinical Policies and Nursing Guidelines (see Figure 12.2).

Nursing Practice Manual	Table of Contents	
Nursing Practice/Patient Care Standards	CP–006	NEW
Pain Management	G–014	
Patient Icon Signage	G–027	
Patient Safety Huddle	G–036	NEW
PCA Patient Controlled Analgesia	M–007	
PCEA Patient Controlled Epidural Analgesia/Epidural Analgesia	M–008	
Peritoneal Dialysis Baxter Ultrabag™ Exchange Procedure	CP–PD–001	
Physiological Insulin Dosing/Insulin Management	M–002	
Point of Care (POC) ACT Activated Clotting Time	Procedure	
Point of Care (POC) Gastroccult Procedure	G–029	
Point of Care (POC) Glucose Meter Telcor Nova Statstrip	G–005	
Point of Care (POC) Hemoccult Procedure	Lippincott	
Point of Care (POC) i-STAT Procedure	G–031	
Point of Care (POC) Nitrazine Procedure	Lippincott	
Pre-Post Surgical Obstructive Sleep Apnea Management Procedure	CP–011	Revised

FIGURE 12.2

*Excerpt From Online
Nursing Practice
Manual*

EBP helps to structure new evidence into standards of practice. At Southwest General, the Graduate Nurse Residency Program supports the newly licensed nurse by providing various avenues of development and self-reflection. Evidence shows that journaling provides nurses the opportunity to clarify their thoughts and feelings and dissect challenges and situations in order to process and learn from them. The Graduate Nurse Resident (GNR) is provided a monthly journal topic associated with a QSEN theme. For example, the QSEN definition of teamwork describes the traits of mutual respect, open communication, and shared decision-making as paramount. With this definition, the GNR is asked to think about, reflect on, and write about four situations in which quality teamwork and collaboration had a direct impact on the care provided to the patient. The journal exercises are shared when the group meets quarterly. Discussion around the QSEN topics develops the GNRs' ability to see the care they provide on a broader continuum.

QUALITY

Use data to monitor the outcomes of care processes and use improvement methods to design and test changes to continuously improve the quality and safety of healthcare systems (Cronenwett et al., 2007).

Quality

Quality is appreciating that continuous quality improvement is an essential part of the daily work of all health professionals (http://qsen.org/competencies/pre-licensure-ksas/). The following sections describe our quality initiatives.

Core Competencies for Organizational Performance. Quality is evident in our standardized RN orientation checklists for every nursing area and contains the six QSEN competencies. By the end of 2013, all RNs, LPNs, and PCAs had newly revised orientation checklists. The checklists focused on such broad categories as scheduling and attendance; patient care populations; use and maintenance of equipment; skills performance; documentation; medication administration; and safety and infection control. The clinical educators took the checklists one huge step forward. They incorporated the six QSEN Core Competencies at the end of each checklist and titled this category *Core Competencies for Organizational Performance* (see Figure 12.3) to include these competencies as a way to strengthen the commitment that our Chief Nursing Office and clinical nursing educators had to our nursing staff. QSEN allowed us to make the orientation checklists professional yet personal to each and every individual nurse.

Southwest General

ORIENTATION: Medical Surgical Care Unit RN

Position Title: ____________ Employee Name: ________________________ Unit:

Method of Evaluation/Instruction Key: PS = Policy, Standards, Procedure Review; EC = Education/ Classroom Session SL = Self Learning Package; D = Demonstration O = Observation (in clinical setting); RD = Return Demonstration T = Written Test; DV = Discussed/Verbalized Understanding NA = Not Applicable * = SKILLS; **= Competency; *** = Core Competencies (QSEN)	Self-Assessment by Employee				Validation of Competency		
	Never Done	Needs Review/ Practice	Competent	Method of Instruction (Use Instruction Key on Left)	Date	Initials	Evaluation Method (Use Evaluation Key on Left)
b. Certification in unit specific/patient population specific specialty:							
c. Other:							
I. CORE COMPETENCIES for ORGANIZATIONAL PERFORMANCDE (QSEN)							
***Patient Centered Care:							
a. Recognizes the patient/family as the source of control & full partner in the patient's health care experience. b. Seeks opportunities to provide compassionate & coordinated care based on the respect for the patient's preferences, values & needs. c. Develops a patient-centered, individualized approach to coordinating patient care needs. d. Includes the patient/family in the decision making process of care coordination. e. Demonstrates cultural and age sensitivity during patient care. f. Demonstrates respect while maintaining patient privacy & confidentiality during patient care.							
***Teamwork & Collaboration:							
a. Functions effectively within nursing and interdisciplinary teams by fostering open communication, mutual respect & shared decision-making to achieve quality patient outcomes. b. Works effectively in advocating on behalf of the patient's/family's care needs. c. Works effectively with the patient/family to coordinate post discharge/home care needs. d. Develops a plan of care that reflects why the patient requires inpatient							

Initials	Signature	Initials	Signature	Initials	Signature

Developed/Released 9/19/13 Page 12 of 14

FIGURE 12.3

Sample Medical Surgical Care Unit RN Orientation Checklist

(Source: Southwest General Health Center, 2014.)

Daily check-ins. Nursing clinical educators participate in our daily check-in (DCI). An example of a quality-improvement project at Southwest General revolves around inspiration from Cincinnati Children's Hospital and encouragement from Southwest General's Lori Cihon, Nursing Director. DCIs began for the nursing department in May 2012 as a way to share focus and situational awareness in 15 minutes or less. In October 2014, DCI became hospital-wide.

Every day Monday through Friday, 19 department leaders come together to discuss patient safety events and employee safety events at 8:30 a.m. There is a conference call for those not reporting. Each day from 8:30 to 8:50 a.m. is a sacred time dedicated to safety and quality. Everyone, every day is expected to be on time. This is a high-level reporting led by a vice president of the hospital leading. For the senior leader, there is an awareness of what is happening at the front line. For the operational leader, there is an awareness of what is occurring in other areas.

DCI prevents risk from becoming "normal." A stoplight (red, green, and yellow) concept is used to identify risk issues related to staffing, volumes, and supplies. The concept is to look back, look ahead, and follow up with the patient as the center of the focus. The departmental leader says:

- What immediate actions they took

- What the impact is on the rest of the hospital

- How the situation impacts our ability to provide safe care

- What can be done to reduce the risk to patients, families, and caregivers

- How the leadership team can help improve the situation

- Whether the hospital is resourced appropriately for the situation

With DCIs, Southwest is able to link the priorities of our core values to the realities of what is happening at the front line of patient care.

Safety

Safety is the freedom from accidental injury (Institute of Medicine, 2001). Safety is also preventing harm to patients via vigilant patient monitoring, preventing patient harm, and striving to improve outcomes (National Academies Press, 2004).

Skills fair. Safety was recently promoted through our house-wide Nursing Skills Fair held in October 2013. The "Safety in Numbers" fair contained nine learning stations:

- **Social Media Guidelines:** The Social Media Guidelines for Nurses (2011) from the National Council of State Boards of Nursing (NCSBN) video was shown to kick off the fair. This 6-minute video summarizes key points of the NCSBN guidelines for nurses and nursing students for using social media responsibly. There is dramatization of potential scenarios of inappropriate social media use.

- **Safety with IV Therapy:** Vein preservation, IV extravasation, port identification, and documentation of care. Scrub the Hub! IM injections with No dorsogluteal IM poster.

- **NDNQI:** Safety in our Quality Indicators: Falls, Restraints, Skin Tear Prevention.

- **Heart Failure and Pulmonary Artery Hypertension:** Heart Failure and Weights, PAH, and Remodulin.

SAFETY

Minimize risk of harm to patients and providers through both system effectiveness and individual performance (Cronenwett et al., 2007).

- **Stroke and VTE:** VTE and stroke discussion.

- **Informatics:** Safety with our Patient-Centered Documentation: Readmit/ Discharge IPOC (Interdisciplinary Plans of Care), Discern Sepsis Alerts, Social Histories.

- **Safety with our Laboratory Procedures and Pharmacy:** Lab tubes, Nurse Collect, Specimens, High-Alert Medications.

- **Teach-back:** Safety with our Patient Education: Video and Role Play.

- **Safety in our Resources:** Lippincott, QSEN Competencies, Revised Clinical/Nursing tab on the intranet, New Nursing Practice Manual.

At each learning station, participants received a pocket card with useful reminders. Upon completion of all nine learning stations, participants received a key ring to hold all their pocket cards and a CEU certificate for 4.0 contact hours.

Patient safety huddle. All inpatient units at Southwest General conduct a Patient Safety Huddle every 12 hours. A Patient Safety Huddle is a communication method to identify patients who have a higher risk of falling. The charge nurse assigns the Safety Huddle captains. The Safety Huddle captain calls the Patient Safety Huddle prior to 8 a.m. on day shift and prior to 9 p.m. on night shift. All nursing staff must be present at the huddle before it begins. The huddle minimally includes:

- Identification of patient(s) at high risk to fall

- Identification of patient(s) confused/impulsive

- Patient with Falls Safe Monitors

- Sitters

- Medications ordered for patient(s) that may increase their risk to fall

- Use of ambulation assistive devices

Upon completion of huddle, it is the Safety Huddle Captain's responsibility to document a Fall Safety Huddle calendar. Unit leadership monitors the Fall Safety Huddle Calendars for compliance monthly.

Valuing the contributions of standardization to safety, Southwest General has a hospital intranet that includes an Equipment tab (see Figure 12.4) for nursing containing videos, quick reference guides, and instruction manuals for nurses.

Equipment Reference Material	
Alaris EtCO$_2$ Module Pocket Guide	
Alaris PCA Module Pocket Guide	
Arctic Sun Training Instructions	
Arterial Line Monitoring	
Atrium Chest Drainage	
Balloon Pump Training	
Bed Tower Technology Information	NEW
Bladder Scanner Instructional CD	
Capnography On-Line Training per Covidian	NEW
CareFusion Alaris IV Pump Training	
CareFusion Alaris EtCO$_2$ Module	NEW
CCE Technology Information	
Clinitron Comfort Controls	
DEFINITY Vialmix User's Guide	NEW

FIGURE 12.4

Excerpt From Online Equipment Tab

(Source: Southwest General Health Center, 2014.)

Intranet resource management. Safety involves reducing reliance on memory. The hospital intranet also has a Toolkits tab for nursing, which contains handouts from recent educational offerings (see Figure 12.5). Only classroom copies of educational materials are produced because staff is educated on how to find the resource when needed in the future.

REFLECTING ON ... PATIENT SAFETY

- *What interventions from Southwest General do you see as having the greatest impact on patient safety?*

FIGURE 12.5

Excerpt from Online Toolkits

(Source: Southwest General Health Center, 2014.)

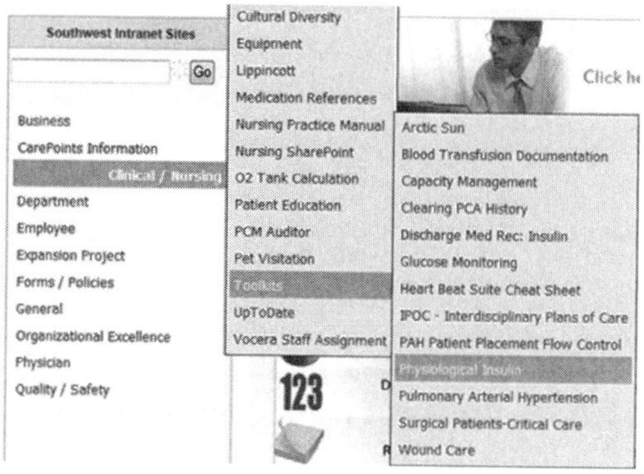

INFORMATICS

Use information and technology to communicate, manage knowledge, mitigate error, and support decision-making (Cronenwett et al., 2007).

Informatics

Admission tasks fire automatically when a patient is admitted to Southwest General. These tasks help to direct the nurse in the collection of a comprehensive history and assessment. There are various time parameters in place for these tasks to be completed. For example, the nurse will collect and document the objective and subjective physical data within two hours of admission along with obtaining the patient's allergies.

Nurses then review orders or contact the physician if orders have not already been received. Physicians must provide admission orders within 2 hours as per the Order Management Policy so that the care for the patient is not delayed. A complete medication history is obtained within 4 hours so that an Admission Medication Reconciliation can be performed by the ordering provider.

Additional information is obtained over the next 24 hours per the Nursing Documentation Policy, including a complete history and comprehensive plan of care. If a patient has been at Southwest before, the nurse can expedite care by reviewing previous medications and medical/social history. The nurse reviews previous information with the patient and updates any items that have changed. This process ensures continuity of care.

Nursing, Physician, and Ancillary Departments have been key in the development of the EHR and the standards to ensure consistency in the use of the system.

The RN initiates the appropriate individualized plan of care (IPOC), which is an individualized medical or surgical plan for the patient. Unit-specific IPOCs are in place for Behavioral Health and Maternity Services. Injury and Discharge Plan of Care is universal for all patients. The RN "accepts" plans of care according to patient needs and initiates additional plans of care for other nursing problems (e.g., altered nutrition). Free text goals and interventions can be added to plans of care to further individualize them. Nurses initiate and communicate the nursing plan of care at handoff and shift report. The plan is reviewed and updated by the RN every 12 hours. A task fires as a reminder at 2:00 a.m. and 2:00 p.m. Nurses have been instructed that individualizing plans of care and comprehensive discharge plans can assist in decreasing readmissions.

The Medical, Procedural, Family, and Social Histories are obtained. Required questions have rules to automatically consult social work or other ancillary referrals. The review of the orders will display automatic orders for the ancillary consults. The RN can order consults to certain ancillaries as needs are identified during both admission and throughout the hospital stay. The information in the histories can be easily displayed for future reference.

Informatics is promoted through Pyxis Workflows created for nursing, barcode medication administration, restructuring of Hospital Intranet Resources for Nursing, Enhanced Tracking Guide in our Emergency Department, and Sepsis/SIRS Discern Alerts house-wide. Front-line staff is working with IT on the following initiatives: VTE Prophylaxis, Nurse Lab Collection, EMR Documentation Enhancement, Physician Orders, and the New Patient Portal.

Nursing clinical educators are easily accessible on Vocera (wireless communicator) to support nursing with evidence-based resources.

REFLECTING ON ... REFLECTIVE PRACTICES

- *What reflective practices did Southwest General use to implement QSEN into practice?*

Outcomes

In reflecting back on our identified needs, EMR documentation, skills fair, and nursing orientation, we have received feedback that is positive. Feedback has been received from both formal and informal sources.

EMR initiatives such as order management and the documentation of critical items such as blood transfusion procedures have met organizational benchmarks.

A housewide skills fair for all of nursing provided an opportunity for staff to perform hands-on training. It also ignited a passion for additional knowledge of nursing practice.

Our new clinical orientation produced positive evaluations from newly hired staff. Clinical managers and our preceptors provided invaluable feedback and recommendations during our planning phase. As a result of this collaboration, they have reported that the new orientees are prepared and have a readiness to engage. However, our work with clinical orientation continues as we align with our organization's goals to meet staffing and fiscal needs.

REFLECTING ON ... INTERVENTIONS AT YOUR OWN ORGANIZATION

- *What specific interventions from Southwest General do you see your healthcare organization adopting?*

- *What interventions from Southwest General do you see taking a step further?*

Final Reflections

In 2014, the dialogue among nursing clinical educators, preceptors, nursing managers, and nursing leadership centered upon how to introduce new nursing staff to Southwest General Health Center. The underlying concept of orienting a nurse—whether a new graduate or seasoned nurse—has to be strategic, structured, standardized, and personalized while allowing the new hire to envision that the organization was genuinely investing in her success as a hospital employee. The nursing clinical educators reinforced the importance of integrating QSEN principles as a vital part of the continuum of professional nursing development for the new graduate nurse. However, seasoned nurses needed to understand the importance of holding themselves accountable for their own behaviors in the performance of current practice habits at the bedside. Regardless of whether the new hire was a new graduate or seasoned nurse, the implementation of QSEN in orientation reinforces that change is always imminent in the field of nursing. As nursing professionals, they are integral in supporting changes that impact patient care and patient outcomes.

QSEN Into Practice facilitates a focus on quality and safe delivery of patient care at Southwest General. The competencies promote the elevation of nursing practice and promote a culture of improvement to achieve optimal clinical outcomes. The support of our CNO, Nursing Directors, and our Nursing Councils facilitated the movement of QSEN into practice. Barriers to implementation included staffing and budget reporting. When staffing is short, nurses are unable to attend council/committee meetings, preceptor meetings, and GNRP education. Communication of changes in policy and practice are difficult to get to the bedside nurse. Nurses struggle with completing mandatory education and finding the time to keep up with all the informational updates.

The nursing clinical educators look forward to 2015 and the measurement of QSEN efforts. Patient satisfaction, nursing job satisfaction, nursing turnover, incident reports, and Lippincott usage reports will glean the feedback necessary to support our efforts or guide our enhancements to curriculum for staff education.

2015 Clinical Nursing Orientation is completely under revision, incorporating the Total Joint Commission and CMS training and education requirements.

References

Carney, D. M., & Bistline, B. (2008). Validating nursing competencies using a fair format. *Journal for Nurses in Staff Development, 24*(3), 124–128.

Cronenwett, L., Sherwood, G., Barnsteiner, J., Disch, J., Johnson, J., Mitchell, P., ... Warren, J. (2007). Quality and safety education for nurses. *Nursing Outlook, 55*(3), 122–131.

Johnston-Hanson, K. Nursing department education needs assessment: Implementation and outcome. *Journal for Nurses in Staff Development, 28*(5), 222–224.

Longo, A. (2012). Presentation skills for the nurse educator. *Journal for Nurses in Staff Development, 28*(1), 16–23.

National Academies Press. (2004). Keeping patients safe: Transforming the work environment of nurses. Washington DC: Author.

Nelson, J. (2010). A preceptor café: Serving up universal values for preceptors. *Journal for Nurses in Staff Development, 26*(4), 178–184.

Pre-licensure KSAs. Retrieved from http://qsen.org/

QSEN Institute. (n.d.). Pre-licensure KSAs. Retrieved from http://qsen.org/competencies/pre-licensure-ksas/

Part IV

Reflective Learning Environments Expanding Partnerships Across Boundaries

Chapter 13

Colorado QSEN Faculty Workshops—Facilitating Reflection for Curricular Development

Amy J. Barton, PhD, RN, FAAN
Gail E. Armstrong, DNP, ACNS-BC, CNE
Katherine Foss, MSN, RN

What do a herd of buffalo, a bed sheet duct-taped to a cabin wall, and a manic trip through a rural grocery store have in common? They are all situations that the Colorado Quality and Safety in Education for Nurses (QSEN) team faced in an effort to provide focused faculty-development workshops that were designed to facilitate organizational reflection and bring a vital, national initiative home to colleagues. The seemingly unconnected clues represent project challenges that involved dealing with adversity, which eventually enhanced the team's flexibility and creativity. These situations also provide clues as to why the Colorado QSEN team refers to this state-wide project as our "excellent adventure." This chapter outlines processes the authors used to facilitate faculty reflection on curricular updating that resulted in faculty ownership and excitement for schools of nursing across the state of Colorado.

Background

The project's purpose was to facilitate organizational reflection in schools of nursing across Colorado that would enable effective statewide dissemination of updated quality and safety content. The core team's experience with the national QSEN initiative fueled our desire to raise the bar for nursing education across the state and engage our colleagues from both baccalaureate and associate degree programs in curriculum reform. "Colorado QSEN" was a statewide dissemination effort generously funded by the Colorado Trust. The purpose of this initiative was to provide faculty development workshops for Colorado nursing faculty within their home institutions.

During the numerous road trips that the project availed, the authors—Amy Barton, Gail Armstrong, and Katherine Foss—grew deeper in our commitment to disseminate the work and visited a number of unique and interesting places. Wildlife was a common theme to our travels. While traveling to Colorado Northwestern Community College in Craig, CO in the northwest corner of the state, we encountered a herd of buffalo. While traveling to Trinidad State Junior College in Alamosa, we encountered a herd of Rocky Mountain sheep. Our project assistant thought we were traveling to Trinidad for the workshop and ordered catering for that location—hence, the manic trip through the grocery store in Alamosa where we each had a grocery cart: one for beverages, one for pastry, and one for fruit. We even bought serving bowls and spoons, plates, and napkins. We explored the depths of rurality, spending hours on two-lane highways (see Figure 13.1). One college invited us to their retreat that was being held at a dude ranch, accessible only by dirt roads. We projected our slides on a sheet that we duct-taped to the cabin wall. When we traveled to Pueblo, we thought our directions were erroneous when we landed in a strip mall. It turned out that the strip mall was home to one of our community colleges (located between a HoneyBaked Ham store and a local bead shop). Table 13.1 provides a complete list of sites we visited.

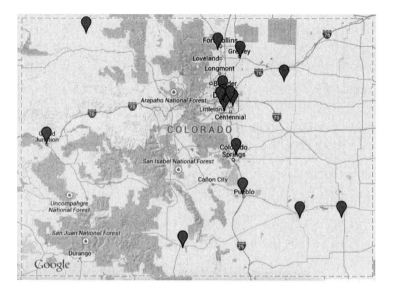

FIGURE 13.1

Colorado QSEN Faculty Workshop Sites

Table 13.1: Colorado QSEN Faculty Workshop Schools

Adams State University, Alamosa
Arapahoe Community College, Littleton
Colorado Christian University, Lakewood
Colorado Mesa University, Grand Junction
Colorado Northwestern Community College, Craig
Colorado Technical University, Pueblo
Community College of Denver, Denver
Front Range Community College, Fort Collins

continues

Table 13.1: Colorado QSEN Faculty Workshop Schools

Front Range Community College, Westminster
Lamar Community College, Lamar
Metropolitan State University of Denver, Denver
Morgan Community College, Fort Morgan
Otero Junior College, La Junta
Platt College, Aurora
Regis University, Denver
Trinidad State Junior College, Alamosa campus
University of Colorado, Colorado Springs
University of Northern Colorado, Greeley

WHOLE-SCALE CHANGE (WSC)

"A methodology used in a variety of applications such as strategic planning, work design, and culture change in which the whole system engages in the change process at a specific point in time" (Arena, 2004, p. 3). A fundamental understanding of WSC is that the strategies assist groups to uncover and engage the combined knowledge, wisdom, and hearts of their people to meet shifting demands and challenges (Shirey & Calarco, 2014)

Upon reflection of the experience and outcomes of Colorado QSEN, we realized that whole-scale change (WSC) methodology was a fitting model to frame our work. *WSC* is a methodology in which a whole system engages in the change process at a specific point in time (Shirley and Calarco, 2014). "A fundamental premise of WSC is that the techniques used help organizations to uncover and engage the combined knowledge, wisdom and hearts of their people to meet the challenges of a changing world" (Shirey & Calarco, 2014, pg. 564). The following list outlines the four cornerstones of WSC methodology (Shirey & Calarco, 2014):

1. Purpose drives choices made.

2. Whole system involvement leads to discovery of preferred outcomes.

3. Ownership and commitment come from involvement.

4. Past and present are valued as the future is created.

REFLECTING ON ... QUESTIONS FOR FACILITATORS

- *How can my questions uncover the existing knowledge?*

- *Is my facilitation creating a reflective space where participants can share what is important to them?*

- *Is my facilitation flexible enough to respond to the products of the group reflection?*

Purpose-Driven Choices

Colorado QSEN was an extension of our experience with the QSEN project funded by the Robert Wood Johnson Foundation, led by Dr. Linda Cronenwett. Phase II of the QSEN initiative began in 2007 (Cronenwett et al., 2007). Fifteen schools of nursing, representing diploma, associate degree, and baccalaureate degree programs from across the United States were selected to participate in a learning collaborative to facilitate integration of competencies and teaching strategies in nursing curricula (Cronenwett, Sherwood, & Gelmon, 2009). The University of Colorado (CU) was selected as one of the pilot schools. Our contribution to the national collaborative was the implementation of a Delphi study to developmentally level the QSEN knowledge, skills, and attitudes (KSAs) into beginning, intermediate, and advanced stages of the curriculum

THE DELPHI TECHNIQUE

Developed by the RAND Corporation in the 1950s, this is a structured group communication process that allows a group of experts to anonymously respond to questionnaires in an iterative manner, with feedback between rounds. When group feedback is considered in subsequent rounds, variability of responses decreases and consensus develops.

(Barton, Armstrong, Preheim, Gelmon, & Andrus, 2009). Ongoing reflection about how to "spread the QSEN word" resulted in the vision of Colorado QSEN.

During Phase III, which began in February 2009 and continued through February 2012, the American Association of Colleges of Nursing (AACN) joined the dissemination efforts to provide 10 regional train-the-trainer faculty development workshops. Members of our team (Armstrong and Barton) participated as faculty in these institutes. The decisions that guided Colorado QSEN were directed by ongoing involvement with the national QSEN dissemination efforts, and a sense of urgency about spreading the innovation of this vital initiative to our home state.

Whole System Involvement and the Discovery of Preferred Outcomes

We chose an individualized approach for each school because there is no effective generic formula for facilitating organizational reflection. This individualized approach allowed for important learning, reflection, and implementation variations. A high priority for Colorado QSEN was to effectively engage the whole nursing faculty at each school of nursing. Thus, Colorado QSEN's process was to literally take our workshops out on the road. It was our desire to meet with as many faculty as possible, and to do so, we needed to travel to them. Meeting with faculty colleagues on the participants' "home turf" accentuated that ownership of the reflective process was that of the home faculty; we as visitors were facilitators of the reflective process. This road-trip approach enabled nursing faculty to be fully involved at their own school, and engage in grounded, organizational reflection about their quality and safety curricula.

Engaging the entire nursing faculty in ongoing reflection during the QSEN workshop was top priority. Thus we gathered baseline data from the first few schools to identify a germane starting point for each faculty group. Table 13.2

contains examples of baseline data that were collected prior to planning the workshops. We contacted the dean or director for each program and provided options for a 4-hour or an 8-hour workshop. We also asked baseline questions to determine whether a particular area of emphasis would be valued over others. All programs preferred learning about incorporating QSEN activities into the clinical learning environment as well as the half-day workshop approach. Hence, after the first few surveys, we standardized our approach and made sure to validate our planned content before scheduling the workshop.

Table 13.2: Examples of Baseline Data Collected Before Colorado QSEN Workshops

Baseline Data Questions	Representative Responses
Which two of the competencies listed are you most interested in learning about?	Evidence-based practice Patient-centered care Informatics
What types of learning activities are you most interested in?	High interest in classroom and clinical activities Moderate interest in simulation activities
How familiar are you with the QSEN initiative?	Somewhat (I've done some reading) Not at all

The Development of Ownership and Commitment

An important aspect of Colorado QSEN's approach was having the participating nursing faculty guide the direction of the actual curricular revision work of the workshop. Our approach was to offer "theory bursts" of content around QSEN, using examples of curricular work from CU to demonstrate application, and then provide opportunities for participating faculty to identify how to proceed in their own curriculum (Armstrong, Spencer, & Lenberg, 2009). Table 13.3 offers snapshots of content presented with examples of reflective questions.

Table 13.3: Examples of Content Areas Presented With Reflective Questions

CONTENT AREA	REFLECTIVE QUESTIONS
Institute of Medicine background of QSEN	How familiar are your students with the background on current Quality & Safety (Q&S) initiatives?
The development of QSEN	What Q&S competencies describe what it means to be a respected nurse?
QSEN's six competencies and Knowledge, Skills, and Attitudes (KSAs) Strategies to update clinical teaching (in lab, in simulation, in clinical rotations)	What teaching and learning strategies will prepare graduates with the KSAs to continuously improve the healthcare systems in which they work?
Traditional concepts of QSEN's six competencies compared to updated concepts of these competencies	Are traditional or updated concepts of these six competencies being taught in your classes?
Crosswalk (a chart of overlapping criteria between two models) of QSEN and accreditation standards	How will this curricular work contribute to your accreditation self-reports?
Sharing of National Delphi Study results	Is there a systematic way to address the KSA elements of the six competencies in your courses?
Exemplars of QSEN content taught in nursing courses, examples of learning activities	What might updated Q&S look like in your curricula?
Review of plethora of QSEN teaching resources on QSEN website and related links	Where can you go to find quality content and teaching strategies for integrating QSEN into your course/ program?

Each QSEN faculty workshop was clearly owned by the participating faculty as they guided the pace, direction, and development of each workshop. Some smaller programs had only a handful of faculty, with limited exposure to QSEN. (One school had five nursing faculty around the table and had minimal exposure to QSEN.) Other schools had larger faculty with more experience with QSEN. We were able to adjust our approach and presentations based on the surfacing needs of each school.

How to incorporate QSEN into clinical teaching and clinical rotations were common points of reflection for participating faculties. Many faculty reflected on how a complex healthcare system and fast-paced, high-acuity patient care environment is often the learning context that nursing students encounter during their clinical courses.

Clinical instruction in this environment necessitates the need to illustrate and put into practice, for the student, systems management, methods of effective communication and teamwork, recognition of shifting priorities and actions to deliver safe patient care, and metrics used to evaluate care for the common goal: best outcome for the patient/family.

All faculty spoke about how students commonly point out the discrepancies between content presented in the classroom and what happens in the practice environment. Herein lies the opportunity, using QSEN as a framework, to create the bridge to teach components of quality, safety, and collaborative care. The primary linking question posed was

> What teaching and learning strategies will prepare graduates with the KSAs to continuously improve the quality and safety of the healthcare systems in which they work?

Discussion with faculty at nursing programs across Colorado included initiating discussion with practice partners to examine the gaps between what is being taught and current practice, with the idea of creating a "clinical syllabus" as a resource to link classroom content to actual nursing practice. One method used to create a clinical syllabus was to examine the patient care environment through a QSEN framework lens and develop crosswalks between standards of care and use of nursing process. Collaboration with a clinical partner was essential to accomplish this work. Figure 13.2 provides an example of such a crosswalk for rotations in perioperative services. This approach allowed faculty to contextualize a concept taught in the classroom, such as infection control, and create focused teaching activities for the perioperative environment, for students to observe, gather information, and practice infection prevention in real time with an interprofessional team.

FIGURE 13.2

Crosswalk of Perioperative Concepts with QSEN Competencies

Quality Improvement	Patient Safety
Operative site and side verification	Medication labeling
Operating room time-out	Surgical counts
Surgical site preparation	Antibiotic protocol
Patient satisfaction	Immediate use sterilization
Sharps safety	
Informatics	**Evidence-Based Practice**
Documentation	Patient/family involvement
Tracking/audits/billing	Skin integrity
Incident reporting	Pain management
First-time starts	Normothermia
Patient care technologies	Glucose management
Practice factors "preference cards"	Deep vein thrombosis protocol

The Value of Past and Present in Creating the Future

An important element of all workshops was sharing the abundance of QSEN resources available for nursing faculty so that participants had ready-to-use tools as they planned their curricula. All the resources that were reviewed in the workshop were linked with the QSEN website (http://qsen.org/), and familiarizing participants with that website proved a facile starting point. Table 13.4 offers examples of the wealth of resources shared at Colorado QSEN workshops, which moved participants quickly from new information to implementable ideas about updating their own curricula.

Table 13.4: Examples of QSEN Resources Reviewed in Colorado QSEN Workshops

QSEN website teaching strategies www.qsen.org	Peer-reviewed teaching strategies for classrooms, learning lab, simulations, and clinical rotations
Institute of Medicine reports www.iom.edu	Reports written by The Institute of Medicine to identify and address quality and safety issues in healthcare
The Joint Commission Safety Solutions www.jointcommission.org	Evidence-based solutions for identified patient safety problems in healthcare
The Picker Institute Resources on Patient-Centered Care www.pickerinstitute.org	Resources developed by The Picker Institute
Ending the Document Game http://endingthedocumentgame.gov	Narratives on the importance of accurate timely information to ensure patient safety
AHRQ Patient Safety Network http://psnet.ahrq.gov/classics.aspx/	Research tools and models for measuring and improving the safety of healthcare systems
Quality Grand Rounds Series in the Annals of Internal Medicine www.chcf.org/publications/2006/11/quality-grand-rounds-series-in-the-annals-of-internal-medicine	Thirteen ready-to-use case studies on patient safety
Committed to Safety www.commonwealthfund.org/publications/fund-reports/2006/apr/committed-to-safety--ten-case-studies-on-reducing-harm-to-patients	"Ten Case Studies on Reducing Harm to Patients" by The Commonwealth Fund
Institute for Healthcare Improvement's Open School Courses www.ihi.org/education/IHIOpenSchool	Online courses about quality improvement and patient safety for health professionals
Team Strategies and Tools to Enhance Performance and Patient Safety (TeamSTEPPS) http://teamstepps.ahrq.gov/	An evidence-based, federally funded, free training toolkit for enhancing healthcare team communication

> **REFLECTING ON ... SHARING RESOURCES**
>
> - *Flexibility to respond to reflection can be connected to proper preparation. As a facilitator, bring an up to date list of relevant resources for your participants.*
>
> - *How can you as the facilitator have a systematic method for participants to review available resources and easily determine which are most relevant to their own work?*
>
> - *How do you keep your own resources up to date? Share these mechanisms with your participants.*

Faculties' reflective processes culminated in a final faculty activity, which was a "gap analysis" to identify next steps. The strength of this cumulative activity was to explicitly draw on the strong points of current curricula and integrate the emerging emphasis on quality and safety content in a purposeful fashion. We were able to adjust facilitation of this activity based on each school's emerging needs. Some faculty chose to focus on the threading of one QSEN competency across their curriculum. Others used the National Delphi Study results to target introduction of QSEN into their beginning-level classes. Other schools focused on use of deliberate practice to introduce progressive QSEN learning activities across courses. Each workshop finished with faculty reflection on how QSEN would enhance what they were currently doing while augmenting students' understanding of quality and safety in their nursing practice.

Outcomes

Evaluation of Colorado QSEN was important given that we wanted to quantify the value of the statewide initiative for The Colorado Trust. There were 211 faculty participants from 70% (7 of 10) of the BSN programs and 66.67% (12 of 18) of the Associate Degree in Nursing (ADN) programs in Colorado.

At the conclusion of our 2-year project, we sent a program evaluation survey to all participating schools. We received responses from 86 faculty, almost 80%

of whom attended one of our workshops. The faculty indicated where many of the QSEN KSA elements were covered in the curriculum. Some that remain uncovered included:

- Impact of perceived power differences among the healthcare team roles on teamwork and patient safety

- Healthcare organization characteristics that influence effective team functioning

- Methods for determining how care quality in a local setting compares to national benchmarks

- Processes used in analyzing causes of error

Clearly, these findings support the need for additional work to be completed at the nexus of clinical and classroom education and require further development of clinical sites to incorporate student learning activities in quality and safety.

With regard to perceptions of being prepared to teach the various competencies, about 30% of faculty rate themselves at least somewhat unprepared to teaching informatics. Thus, faculty expressed more comfort in safety, teamwork and collaboration, patient-centered care, and evidence-based practice. Approximately 85% of faculty reported being prepared to find resources to add quality and safety content to their classes, with 60% specifically using the QSEN website to incorporate learning activities. Faculty members have added a number of strategies to update courses in quality and safety, including:

- Adding an article

- Including a learning activity

- Using an unfolding case study

- Adding quality and safety elements to a simulation

- Adding quality and safety elements to clinical rotation evaluations

- Assigning paper topics to students with explicit quality and safety foci

We were also interested in determining impact of curricular innovation on students. Because we were unable to access students directly, we asked deans and directors to send surveys to graduating students. We received responses from 207 students. Students indicated the following topics were not covered in their curricula:

- Effective strategies for communicating and resolving conflict among healthcare providers

- Impact of perceived power differences among the healthcare team roles on teamwork and patient safety

- Healthcare organization characteristics that influence effective team functioning

- Strategies for learning about the outcomes of care in a clinical setting

- Methods for determining how care quality in a local setting compares to national benchmarks

- Processes used in analyzing causes of error

Clearly, these results mirror those of the faculty and provide further support for pursuing integrative teaching strategies with clinical agencies. When asked about specific skills, students reported feeling at least somewhat unprepared to:

- Consult with clinical experts before deciding to deviate from evidence-based protocols

- Use quality-improvement tools, such as flow charts or cause/effect diagrams

- Identify gaps between actual care in their setting and best practice

- Evaluate the effect of practice changes, using quality-improvement methods and measures

- Use organizational systems for near-miss and error reporting

Lessons Learned

Facilitating ownership and reflection for nursing faculties across Colorado included many lessons for the authors. The three of us agreed that we learned a tremendous amount about ourselves as individuals and us as a group. Increased collegial respect and esteem for each other was a wonderful by-product. We continue to enjoy working together. Flexibility at all times was probably our key to success. We also learned much about the value of using a reflective approach to teaching, and the balance between "telling" and letting the faculties we worked with "discover" their own priorities in their quality and safety curriculum.

Home Field Advantage Is Important

An important success of Colorado QSEN was the ownership of the work by participating nursing faculties. Choosing to conduct workshops at each nursing school's home location provided opportunities for the teaching team to learn about the nursing school's culture, reality, and challenges. The nursing faculties were the experts about their own curricula and their own students. Location of the workshops contributed to faculties' commitment to engage in the reflection process and own the workshop outcomes.

Travel Breeds Reflection

The core team employed travel time between workshops for continual process improvement and their own reflective process. Each school instructed us in how to improve and hone our approach. Reflection encourages reflection, and the teaching team modeled this reflective process for participating schools.

Reflection Requires Flexible Processes

Because the teaching team could never know where each school's reflective process would take a workshop, we always built in flexibility for activities, workshop modules, and time allotments. The team was in constant, real-time consultation with each other and the participants about best use of workshop time. This flexibility enabled individually specific approaches to best meet the needs of each faculty.

Share Ideas and Resources

The bulk of the activity during Colorado QSEN workshops was the sharing of ideas and resources. Examples from CU demonstrated how curricular updates *might* be done and helped participants move quickly from updated information to application. After participants saw examples of how a Medical/Surgery course had been updated with quality and safety content, they were quick to think about their own classes and then develop their own QSEN vision. Resources gave participants ready-to-use tools so that they could exercise their own creativity and tailor the quality and safety content for their own school, class, and students.

Final Reflections

Reflective practice is often taught in nursing curricula as an individual practice or process. The Colorado QSEN project is a good example of a reflective team facilitating organizational level change for schools across the state, using a collaborative approach. The effectiveness of this approach is apparent as many faculty members continue to report on their continued QSEN curricular work. In so doing, they often speak about this work as a "journey," indicating their own ongoing reflection and growth.

References

Arena, M. J. (2004). Enhancing organizational awareness: An analysis of whole scale change. *Journal of Organizational Development, 22*(1), 9–20.

Armstrong, G., Spencer, T., & Lenburg, C. (2009) Using quality and safety education for nurses to enhance competency outcome performance assessment: A synergistic approach that promotes patient safety and quality outcomes. *The Journal of Nursing Education, 48*(12), 686–693.

Barton, A. J., Armstrong, G., Preheim, G., Gelmon, S. B., & Andrus, L. C. (2009). A national Delphi to determine developmental progression of quality and safety competencies in nursing education. *Nursing Outlook, 57*(6), 313–322.

Cronenwett, L., Sherwood, G., Barnsteiner, J., Disch, J., Johnson, J., Mitchell, P., ... Warren, J. (2007). Quality and safety education for nurses. *Nursing Outlook, 55*(3), 122–131.

Cronenwett, L., Sherwood, G., & Gelmon, S. B. (2009). Improving quality and safety education: The QSEN Learning Collaborative. *Nursing Outlook, 57*(6), 304–312.

Shirey, M. R., & Calarco, M. M. (2014). Whole scale change for real-time strategic application in complex health systems. *Journal of Nursing Administration, 44*(11), 564–568.

Chapter 14

Leading Transformation to Learning Organizations: Educating for Patient Safety, Quality, and Interprofessional Practice

Jan Boller, PhD, RN
Karen Hanford, EdD, MSN, FNP
John H. Tegzes, BSN, MA, VMD, Dipl. ABVT

The evidence is more compelling than ever that healthcare must be transformed to become safer, more effective, and more affordable (Institute of Medicine, 2013). And the need for healthcare reform is urgent. As of this writing, the United States spends more per capita for healthcare than any country (OECD, 2014)—2.5 times that of the average for the 40 Organisation for Economic Co-operation and Development (OECD) countries ($8,508 in the United States compared with $3,322 in OECD countries). Still, the United States continues to report poor outcomes in terms of healthy lifestyle practices, infant mortality, chronic illness management, and coordinated healthcare. Consider the following statistics:

- One of three hospitalized patients in the United States experiences adverse effects (Classen et al., 2011).

- The gap between new discoveries and transfer to practice spans decades (Morris, Wooding, & Grant, 2011).

- At an estimate of between 220,000 and 440,000 deaths per year, preventable healthcare errors are among the top three causes of mortality annually in the United States, following heart disease and cancer (James, 2013).

Although the Affordable Care Act (ACA) has begun to shift the focus to the Triple Aim of better care, better health, and lower cost-per-capita (Bisognano & Kenney, 2012), policy alone is not the answer. Strong transformational leadership at the point of care and in our communities is imperative.

Gaps also exist between how colleges and universities prepare new health professionals and what healthcare executives expect (Berkow, Virkstis, Stewart, & Conway, 2008). The Joint Commission identified leadership as among the top three root causes of sentinel events in U.S. hospitals between 2011 and 2013 (The Joint Commission, 2014). How will we better prepare health professionals to lead patient safety and quality efforts in meeting the Triple Aim? How are nurses taking the lead in healthcare transformation as social architects for patient safety, quality, and optimal health outcomes? Taking the advice attributed to Marcel Proust (1923)—"the real voyage of discovery lies not in seeking new landscapes but in seeing with new eyes"—nurses and other health professionals must shift perspectives and attitudes to recognize their power and responsibility as transformational leaders—from the very start of their career—with the ability to continuously rediscover the healthcare landscape as they lead transformation from the bedside to the boardroom to the community.

This chapter provides stories of three nurse leaders on three converging paths to transform one university—Western University of Health Sciences (WesternU)—

into a learning organization well positioned to transform healthcare. The university was founded with the values of humanism, science, and education, but had to learn new ways to break out of the older traditional model of higher education to bring these core values from vision to reality. These three stories eventually converge into one shared journey to integrate interprofessional collaboration and reflective practice into the preparation of health professionals as leaders and advocates in patient safety, quality, and the Triple Aim.

Developing a Learning Organization Within a Traditional University

Karen Hanford, EdD, MSN, FNP

In reflecting on my journey of starting a new college of nursing (1997) in a private nonprofit health science university, the memories and lessons learned are noteworthy. I share this story so that others whose unit is within an organization that operates in a different paradigm can achieve the same success.

Our university, WesternU, was founded as an osteopathic medical school that had been in existence for 20 years. And as anticipated, nursing wasn't exactly welcomed with open arms. However, as the founding dean of the College of Graduate Nursing (CGN), my vision was clear, and I was passionate about creating a college of nursing excellence.

In guiding and launching a new academic unit, I embraced the theoretical framework for organizational learning (OL). According to Levine and Prietula (2013), OL is constructed of four principles common

LEARNING ORGANIZATIONS

"Organizations where people continually expand their capacity to create the results they truly desire, where new and expansive patterns of thinking are nurtured, where collective aspiration is set free, and where people are continually learning how to learn together (Senge, 2006, p. 5).

Organizational learning is characterized by the ability of organizations to both quickly adapt (cope) and generate (create and expand capability) in the face of changing environments. Beyond adaptation, generative learning requires new ways of looking at the world (Senge, 2007, p. 101).

to learning organizations. These four principles validate the dynamic roles of faculty and staff that worked toward a common vision:

- **Purposeful goal.** Faculty and staff felt that they were creating cutting-edge curriculum combined with a new delivery model of education.

- **Collaboration.** The exchange of ideas was valued and encouraged.

- **Adaptive and flexible structure and processes.** Work was purposeful without a high level of structure.

- **Dynamic feedback.** Students, faculty, curriculum designers, and consultants were encouraged to contribute to improving and sharing new learning.

This operating model created a culture of excitement for all team members to solve complex problems by co-creating solutions. This model would serve us well in the coming years given that our first nursing program was the first web-based (hybrid) master's-level family nurse practitioner (FNP) program in the United States (1997).

In the late 1990s, the pervasive opinion by educators and the public was that web-based education was of poor quality. However, as a graduate of a traditional distance learning advanced practice registered nurse (APRN) program, I had a favorable experience, so I knew that distance education did not equate with poor quality. Although many believed that web-based learning was to be the way of the future, I certainly experienced many doubters. Fortunately, our charter students were up for the challenge and embraced this new educational delivery model. Faculty and staff learned as much as our students did that first semester. Students and faculty found that web-based education provided an excellent venue of learning for graduate-level professional nurses. We felt rewarded for our efforts, and there was no turning back.

As expected, the addition of distance learners required a paradigm shift for all university departments whose processes and structures were designed for campus-based students. In navigating the obstacles, new adaptive systems and processes were required (Porter-O'Grady & Malloch 2015). I knew that this change was possible because I had graduated from a distance-based FNP program that had developed student centered processes from admission to graduation. As a passionate nursing educator, I embraced the challenge. To better prepare myself for this opportunity, I enrolled in classes to learn Microsoft Office (my previous university used WordPerfect). The other significant blessing was that an expert team of faculty and a recognized expert in distance education and web-based education had developed the curriculum. The nursing consultant had many years of experience and served as my mentor for more than a year. Expert faculty that developed the curriculum chose to teach the courses initially, so my job was to fully direct and lead the program, hire staff and faculty, recruit students, and develop the infrastructure for the CGN.

Leading to the Gestalt

Many of you who are reading this narrative have probably read Jim Collins' book *Good to Great* (2001). If so, you are familiar with his famous phrase "getting the right people on the bus" and understand how critical this concept is to an organization's success. I had experienced a peak experience of guiding and working with a highly functioning team when I was a supervisor of an intensive care unit (ICU). It was truly a life-enhancing experience to be part of this team that transformed care, creatively solved problems, completed high-level training for new nurses, and produced positive outcomes for patients. Why couldn't a college of nursing achieve this? In reflecting on my leadership style, I aspire always to be an authentic "level five" leader (Shelton & Darling, 2003) who has the ability to envision a new reality, and I am blessed with a boundless determination to improve nursing education.

Turning Theory Into Practice Through Teamwork

To manage a distance-learning nursing curriculum, a different mix of professionals is needed. These include a webmaster and a curriculum designer, as well as a business professional to manage contracts and the daily operations of the college. As the CGN grew and became established, additional professional roles were added to provide leadership for increasingly complex processes. New professional roles were needed to support nontraditional students and distance faculty. To assist in this process, care was given to hire individuals with problem-solving skills as well as high-level interpersonal skills. During the ramp-up period, many processes were done in-house (writing of brochures, recruitment, and web page design), which I feel helped create a team environment.

Over time, the established university department took over many of these responsibilities. There were tense communications on a few dark days, but I understood much of the resistance related to employees' workload and that the university made its decisions top-down. Many employees felt a college of nursing was not needed, particularly without additional resources to support the infrastructure. Knipfer, Kump, Wessel, and Cress (2013) acknowledge that bottom-up organizational learning occurs when modifications are adopted by the organization. Researchers find that learning transfers from the individual to the collective and then to the organization. Organizational experts state that the process of reflection is one of the driving forces for bottom-up learning (Knipfer et al., 2013). Thus, collective inquiry results in "reflective learning at work," which is needed for continuous improvement, new thinking, and expanding mental models (Hilden & Takkamaki, 2013).

REFLECTING ON ... REFLECTION AS A LEARNING TOOL

How do we use reflection within and across professions as a tool for organizational learning?

How do leaders cultivate reflective teams?

How does reflection guide change in roles and processes to advance our mission?

Managing the Online Environment

In 1997, most universities did not have learning management platforms or online systems for course delivery. The curriculum designer designed the template for courseware, and faculty created the content for courses. We designed all courses in a similar fashion to eliminate frustration for students by standardizing how each faculty member organized the content. Further we developed instructional manuals to assist faculty to transition from the "sage on the stage" to that of facilitator. Because the university did not have servers to host web-based courses, we contracted with a service provider. Another important team member was the webmaster, who assisted faculty and students. In the early days, Internet connections were slow and not always reliable, so the webmaster was a key partner in this venture to problem solve technology challenges.

Creating Success Through Innovation and Interprofessional Learning

Now, looking back on these past 15 years, other important reflections seem pertinent to this discussion. How did quality and safety and interprofessional education (IPE) become part of our core? Centrally, we hired champions on these topics; and in 2009, the university began a university-wide IPE program for all students, but the IPE culture (Interprofessional Education Collaborative ([IPEC], 2011) was not part of the culture for faculty, particularly in several of the colleges. What I observed was an example of Rogers' (2003) *Diffusion of Innovation*, with the early adopters being individual faculty from several colleges. A benefit to this culture shift was leadership modeling as all deans trained and participated in the first year of IPE cases. For the next 5 years, faculty in the nine health colleges have progressed along the "diffusion" continuum. Today, IPE is now part of the footprint for the university. Initially, faculty from our Family Nurse Practitioner program had been guest lecturing in the medical program, now other faculty members from our Entry-Level Masters (MSNE), Health Systems Leadership, and Doctor of Nursing Practice programs are teaching Quality and Safety, Epidemiology, Population Health, and Evidence-Based Practice in the first semester of the medical program. We found that team teaching by nursing, medicine, and other health professions' faculty is a collaborative practice that we hope will not be so novel in the future.

Nursing is not only recognized as a leader in our state and beyond, but also we are now highly valued in the greater university. Faculty members from the CGN are helping to shape the knowledge, skills, and attitudes of other health professionals. Our nursing faculty and staff are highly sought after for guest lectures, joint research projects, and assisting with grants, and are leaders on high-level university committees.

The CGN has contributed to the infrastructure for the university by developing new staff roles, including Director of Operations, Director of Assessment, and Director of Student Services, Assistant Dean of Student Affairs, held by professionals who possess a baccalaureate or graduate degree. Many of the other colleges have created these staff roles for their colleges as well.

Building a Village: Ambassadors Create Change

The ambassadors include—clinical partners, advisory board members, students, faculty, staff, members of the faculty community, administration, university departments, and more; they are simply too numerous to list. The reflective learning here is that we are all connected, our university community is proud of our collective accomplishments, and good work is contagious. As well, our university is evolving, and the diversity of other health disciplines has positively altered the paradigm of a central decision-making university. Albeit far from perfect, I believe that the institution has moved forward on the continuum of the diffusion of innovation. The deans across the nine WesternU colleges work collaboratively and eagerly embrace the challenge to prepare the 20th-century health professional. I do believe that nursing was a catalyst for change, pushing the boundaries of a traditional university.

Over the years, successful external reviews provided added respect for our college, both internally and externally. Regional (WASC), state (BRN), and professional (CCNE) reviewers applauded our accomplishments. I am most proud of our most recent Commission on Collegiate Nursing Education (CCNE) site visit (2010) when the lead evaluator shared with me that our college was truly unique in its structure (more professional staff members). In addition, he shared that faculty and staff were highly engaged and also our student-centered culture was palpable. Although we were relatively young as a college, the reviewers were impressed and documented compliance with all standards and shared positive comments in their exit summary to the university.

Leading Excellence

Being an early adopter is not an easy path: Leading, expanding, and transforming a college of nursing has proven to be challenging. As the profession of nursing has a social contract with society, our discipline is not static and must meet the healthcare needs of our society. This requires reflection and openness to change as the profession must be forward-thinking. New nursing standards, new terminal degrees, change in senior leadership, difficult personalities (faculty, staff, students), recessions, and so forth are all part of our work. New organizational models and mental models are needed to do this complex work (Crowell, 2011; Porter-O'Grady & Malloch, 2015). Thus, our college team uses reflection as part of our "fuel" to advance our learning organization. Although there is consensus among educators that reflection is at the core of adult learning and contributes to professional growth and transformation, we ask ourselves whether we use reflection as a tool for organizational learning. Organizations that learn, engage in dialogue, and have a purposeful vision are found to be more successful (Casey, 2005; Collins, 2001).

> **REFLECTING ON ... TRANSFORMATION THROUGH REFLECTIVE DIALOGUE**
>
> - *How can faculty members and students inspire organizational leaders to engage in reflective dialogue to transform healthcare?*
>
> - *What are essential dimensions of effective reflective dialogue?*
>
> - *How does an organization's capacity for reflective dialogue evolve over time as teams mature?*

Creating Organizational Space for Expert Caring Practices

Jan Boller, PhD, RN

My story about leading reflective organizations begins 27 years into my nursing career, which included positions as ambulatory care nurse, critical care

NOVICE-TO-EXPERT DEVELOPMENT

Described by Hubert and Stuart Dreyfus (Dreyfus & Dreyfus, 1996) and further developed in nursing by Patricia Benner and colleagues (Benner, 1984; Benner, Tanner, & Chesla, 1996; Benner, Hooper-Kyriakidis, & Stannard, 1999). This theory of development describes a five-stage process of skill acquisition in complex practices such as nursing, playing chess, driving an automobile, flying a plane, based on integration of theory and other forms of evidence with experience-based practical know-how. The five stages are Novice, Advanced Beginner, Competence, Proficient, and Expert (Dreyfus & Dreyfus, 1996, pp. 29-47). Estimates are that it takes 10,000 hours of experience in a specific practice area to reach expertise (Clark, 2003), which typically translates to three to 5 years for health professionals.

staff nurse, educator, clinical nurse specialist, and organizational leader. In the late 1990s, while I was a PhD student at the University of California–San Francisco School of Nursing, I accepted a position as Manager of Professional Development at a small community hospital in northern California. The Joint Commission was scheduled for a survey at that hospital just six months after I was hired. New accreditation standards called for policies, processes, and systems for assessing employee competencies to assure patient safety. No organization-wide system for competency assessment was in place at this hospital. Because of my extensive background in novice-to-expert development (Benner, 1984; Boller, 1980) and competency-based education (del Bueno, Barker, & Christmyer, 1981), I knew I was the right person for the job.

Cultivating Collective Wisdom

What I learned at that hospital was pivotal in my own development as a transformational leader. This is where I learned about what true reflective practice looks like. The nursing management team was like none other I had ever been a part of. The team included the Chief Nurse Executive (CNE) and nursing directors. This team of nurse leaders had an exceptionally mature level of camaraderie and mutual respect. Their ability to expeditiously move diverging perspectives and frank arguments to agreement and action was phenomenal. Even more important to me was the absence of the typical strategic manipulation in the interest of competition and counter movements typical of so many organizations. Was this collegiality real? Would it last? Why was this different? How was it that we could say what we were thinking and feel safe to disagree?

I learned that this level of collaboration and mutual respect had not always been the case. This team of leaders had transformed through intention. The CNE shared the story of what it was like when she first came to the organization. At that time, there were separate "camps" in the six nursing departments: Emergency, Critical Care, Medical/Surgical, Obstetrics, Perioperative Services, and Transitional Care. In meetings, the Nursing Directors spent most of their time in turf battles, competing with each other for scarce resources. That was about to change.

Shortly after accepting her executive position, the CNE contacted her leadership mentor, Alan Briskin, PhD, an organizational development consultant. The CNE asked Briskin to do some team-building with the nursing management group. Briskin advised, however, that he does not do team-building. Instead, he works with organizational leaders to develop their capacity to have *generative dialogue,* which according to David Bohm, is "Real dialogue ... where two or more people become willing to suspend their certainty in each other's presence" (Briskin, Erickson, Ott, & Callanan, 2009, p. 53). Generative dialogue cannot be accomplished by individuals alone. Dialogue helps break down fragmentation so that a group can generate effective solutions. Briskin taught the group about the practices of collective wisdom (Briskin et al., 2009), which includes creating safe spaces for

COMPETENCY-BASED EDUCATION (CBE)

An approach to preparing health professionals for practice that is fundamentally oriented to graduate outcome abilities and organized around competencies derived from an analysis of societal and patient needs. It de-emphasized time-based training and promises greater accountability, flexibility, and learner-centeredness (Adapted from Frank et al., 2010).

inquiry and reflection, deep listening, shifting the focus from individual to group expertise, and asking the central questions from which groups can move to actions with positive impact (Briskin et al., 2009, p. 175). Eventually, many of the hospital's executives and department leaders joined in regular meetings with Briskin with impressive results in terms of creating an organizational culture of respect, leading to timely and meaningful action. The practices of collective wisdom can be a leadership strategy to integrate reflective practice (Sherwood & Horton-Deutsch, 2012) into the culture of organizations.

REFLECTING ON ... GENERATIVE DIALOGUE AND COLLABORATION

- *How can we engage with communities in generative dialogue and collaboration for improving the health of our communities?*

- *How do teams cultivate the trust needed to have generative dialogue?*

- *How does reflection from generative dialogue and collaboration create new opportunities for new thinking?*

Even though it is hard to explain what actually happened in those meetings, Briskin's process was to have us start with our stories, paying attention to core values and principles that emerged, listening deeply, and tapping into the collective wisdom of the group as we addressed pressing issues. Briskin introduced us to writings of a variety of experts whose philosophy, research, and theories helped guide us as transformational leaders through the messy processes of organizational leadership and change. I refer to these authors as my "change mentors." And although I had had extensive training and experience as a group facilitator, nothing prepared me for facilitating generative dialogue as those years working and learning with our team of health professionals. We then collaborated to introduce this process to a group of nurse leaders throughout the hospital, resulting in the publication of a book, *Daily Miracles,* that described our collective work to bring excellence and compassion to the center of our nursing practices (Briskin & Boller, 2006). That brief golden era of collaboration came to an end as new leadership replaced old, and managers moved to other facilities. However, we all carried practices of collective wisdom with us.

Creating Organizational Space for Patient Safety

In the late 1990s, the Institute of Medicine (IOM) report *To Err is Human* (Kohn, Corrigan, & Donaldson, 2000) revealed the alarming statistics on deaths from medical errors. As Director of Clinical Effectiveness, responsible for leading the hospital's safety and quality efforts, this had a profound effect on me as I recognized the extent of death from preventable medical errors, which at that time was estimated to range from 44,000 to 98,000 deaths annually. At first, I thought I would be solving the problem of what was the equivalent of jumbo jets crashing into U.S hospitals, leaving behind no survivors, on a weekly basis (Leape, 1994). I would use what I was learning from the highly effective processes of Lean Six Sigma and Rapid Cycle Improvement (IHI, 2003, 2005). But because communication was identified among the top root cause of medical errors (The Joint Commission, 2014), improvement processes alone were not going to be enough. We had to create organizational space for reflection and dialogue to ensure patient safety.

At the next hospital I had moved to, I found it extremely hard to engage with my colleagues at the same level of generative dialogue that I had previously experienced. When I mentioned to one nurse executive that we needed to create space for expert caring practices through interprofessional dialogue, she replied that our five hospitals were already full to capacity, and we didn't have any more space or time for that. She wanted to focus on more pressing issues of patient safety, such as like medication errors, decubiti, and falls prevention. Interesting! I thought I *was* working on those problems! I knew then that we were speaking two different languages, and it was time to move on. I made the decision to transition into academia, recognizing that transformation in healthcare to patient safety and quality will not happen until a new generation of health professionals is prepared in a new paradigm of working together for patient safety with high-level capacities for communication and collaboration.

Collaborating Statewide to Redesign Nursing Education

As I was transitioning to academia as part-time faculty, I was invited to lead a statewide group of thought leaders in California to redesign nursing education to better prepare the future nursing workforce. This gave me the opportunity to use what I had learned about collective wisdom to guide 100 thought leaders to consensus around nursing education redesign. Similar to previous situations, there were different silos across the key stakeholders from education and practice: Associate Degree Schools of Nursing, BSN, Graduate Nursing Schools, Public Schools, Private Schools, Clinical Educators, Nurse Executives, Advanced Practice Nurses, and Professional Association Leaders. These professionals had been moving to collaboration over several previous statewide projects. They were motivated to work cooperatively.

We learned from our colleague from the Oregon Consortium of Nursing Education (OCNE) that we were all part of one community of practice (Wenger, McDermott, & Snyder, 2002). We began by answering the four central questions of appreciative inquiry (Cooperrider, Whitney, & Stavros, 2008). The four questions center on peak experiences about which individuals are most proud; what they value most about themselves and their work, and what they bring to the team or organization; core factors that give life to the organization; and three wishes to heighten the vitality of the organization (Whitney & Trosten-Bloom, 2003, p. 140).

1. Tell me about a peak experience or high point in your professional life...a time when you felt most alive, most engaged, and really proud of yourself and your work.

2. Without being humble, what do you most value about

   - yourself, and the way you do your work? What unique skills and gifts do you bring to this team and organization?

   - your team?

   - your organization, and its larger contribution to society and the world?

3. What are the core factors that give life to this organization when it is at its best?

4. If you had a magic wand, and could have any three wishes granted to heighten the health and vitality of this organization, what would they be?

Source: Whitney & Trosten-Bloom, 2003 (p. 140).

Through the processes and practices of collective wisdom, these dedicated nurse leaders collaborated to break down the silos and come to consensus on seven visionary recommendations for nursing education redesign (Boller & Jones, 2010; California Institute for Nursing and Health Care, 2008). Many of these recommendations paralleled recommendations of the subsequent IOM report on the *Future of Nursing* (National Research Council, 2011).

The seven recommendations for nursing education redesign in California included:

- Forge academic/service partnerships.

- Establish agreement on core competencies for new graduates.

- Develop and retain high-performing faculty.

- Foster seamless advancement in education.

- Provide transition to practice programs for new graduates.

- Integrate simulation and technology into the curriculum.

- Gather and disseminate data on outcomes.

This is where Quality and Safety Education for Nurses (QSEN) entered my life and the California nursing education redesign movement. Dr. Nancy Spector from the National Council of State Boards of Nursing (NCSBN) presented at one of the education redesign meetings and shared the NCSBN model for transition to practice, with the QSEN competencies at the core of the model (Spector & Echternacht, 2010). Dr. Spector recommended that California adopt these competencies as we moved forward with our recommendations—and that is what we did. Schools of nursing who were recipients of grants for ADN-to-BSN programs and those receiving grants for RN transition to practice programs were required to integrate the QSEN competencies into their curricula as a condition of the grant award. The California Simulation Alliance, which was established before the white paper was published, incorporated QSEN competencies into their simulation scenarios.

Advancing Patient Safety Through Academic, Service, and Community Partnerships

Soon after moving into academia, I realized that traditional classroom teaching methods of lecture and multiple-choice tests did not fit my style. Coming from clinical practice, I was used to experiential competency-based learning and interprofessional collaboration. Fortunately, Dean Karen Hanford, one of the thought leaders in the California Nursing Education Redesign project, invited me to take a look at WesternU, which had already implemented much of what was recommended in the California White Paper on Nursing Education Redesign. Founded in the values of humanism, the CGN program was student-centered and offered self-directed experiential learning in a hybrid format, which was one of the first in the country and highly successful. The CGN was launching a new Associate Degree-to-Masters Degree program and the Clinical Nurse Leader track, which focused on patient safety and quality leadership. WesternU was also establishing an IPE program across its nine health professions colleges.

I felt at home at WesternU with colleagues across the health professions who shared the same vision of a transformed health system. I was named director of the Health Systems Leadership (HSL) track, and from the very beginning, our small group of HSL faculty members embraced transformational leadership as a paradigm for leading patient safety and quality. Reflective practice, which incorporates practices of collective wisdom, is central to our effectiveness. Emphasizing the need for communication as the key to patient safety, we introduced the practices of crucial conversations (Patterson, Grenny, McMillan,

& Switzler, 2012) and collective wisdom (Briskin et al., 2009) into our own faculty practice as well as into the student curriculum.

In 2011, our college received an endowment to advance patient safety and quality. This endowment gave us the opportunity to move our work beyond our WesternU interprofessional curriculum and into the community, working in collaboration with our service and community health partners. Shortly after I was named Endowed Chair for Nursing Safety and Quality, we asked Dr. Gwen Sherwood to be our mentor as we explored ways to integrate quality and safety practices into our communities. Her advice was to "wrap QSEN around all we teach." She has been exceptional at guiding us to become a center of excellence in community-wide integration of reflective practices and cultivating collective wisdom for patient safety and quality.

The QSEN competencies have been integrated into both the prelicensure and graduate curricula as well as in curricula across the colleges. And now we are taking this education into the communities, working in collaboration with our clinical partners. Figures 14.1 and 14.2 present the two logos for Interprofessional Education and Community Engagement, illustrating our vision of the health professionals from our nine academic programs coming together to share different perspectives from our separate professions for a more collaborative approach to healthcare (Figure 14.1) and taking interprofessional collaboration practice into our communities, contributing to better health for the populations we serve.

CRUCIAL CONVERSATION
"A discussion between two or more people where (1) stakes are high, (2) opinions vary, and (3) emotions run strong" (Patterson et al, 2012, p. 3). Patterson and colleagues identify seven practices for effective crucial conversations leading to improved relationships and better results.

FIGURE 14.1

Western University of Health Sciences Interprofessional Education Logo: Nine Perspectives, One Focus

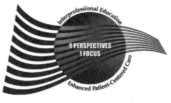

FIGURE 14.2

Western University of Health Sciences, College of Graduate Nursing Community-Based Quality and Safety Logo: Cultivating Healthy Communities

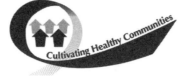

The process of integrating patient safety and quality curriculum across the health professions curriculum is expedited by a mature interprofessional education program, which is described in the next section.

Pioneering Interprofessional Education

John Tegzes, BSN, MA, VMD, Dipl. ABVT

Creating and fostering an environment of collaboration has always been near and dear to WesternU's founding President, Philip Pumerantz, PhD. As a champion for humanism in both education and clinical practice, Dr. Pumerantz established an IPE program before it was a national trend. Because of the scope of his vision, an IPE program was established to include all health professions' students, starting at the beginning of each program and continuing into the clinical phases of the curricula. The program was funded, and new positions and committees were created to develop and implement the program at a time before the Interprofessional Competencies (IPEC) existed and when few IPE programs existed in the United States. IPE coincided with the university's launch of three new health professions colleges. With this launch, the university grew to include nine health professions. These nine professions are diverse and are not all typical professions that work side-by-side. Thus, when the IPE program was created, it brought together professions and educators who were not familiar with collaborative practice.

Faculty Pioneers

A core group of enthusiastic and creative faculty volunteered to develop the program and to actualize the president's dream, not initially knowing what it would look like. Merely mentioning the professions included reveals the challenge. Compounding the challenge were varying program lengths, different academic schedules, and diverse accreditation standards. This brave group of pioneers and leaders defied conventional thinking and successfully created a dynamic, rigorous academic program that now includes learners from these professions: Dental Medicine, Graduate Nursing, Optometry, Osteopathic Medicine, Pharmacy, Physical Therapy, Physician Assistant, Podiatric Medicine, and Veterinary Medicine. Tremendous energy was instilled into the program that began with all first-year, first-

PROBLEM-BASED LEARNING (PBL)

"...an educational process where learning is centered around problems as opposed to discrete, subject-related courses. In small groups, students are presented with patient scenarios or problems, generate learning issues related to what they need to learn in order to understand the problem, engage in independent self-study, and return to their groups to apply their new knowledge to the patient problem" (Solomon, 2011, p. 137).

semester students from all nine professions working together in small teams exploring clinical cases using a problem-based learning (PBL) format. IPE cases were written and delivered through progressive disclosure in teams of 9 or 10 students, with each team led by a faculty facilitator. There were 94 teams created, requiring 94 faculty members to serve as facilitators.

IPE Program Implementation and Expansion

Each IPE case was delivered over three consecutive sessions. Five IPE cases were delivered over the course of the academic year. Faculty members across the university were trained to facilitate these IPE cases using PBL. It took more than 2 full years of time and effort before we were able to launch the program. We breathed a sigh of relief after the program was delivered during that first academic year. That sigh lasted only a second, however, before we realized that we also needed to create, develop, and implement an ongoing IPE program that spanned into year two, and later into year three of each program. After a moment of panic (yes, it was panic), we discovered the Agency for Healthcare Research and Quality (AHRQ) TeamSTEPPS program (United States Department of Health and Human Services, AHRQ, n.d.). This program was the impetus for the inclusion of safety and quality in our IPE curriculum.

IPE for Patient Safety

The IPE curriculum has evolved to fully embrace safety and quality as a core focus. When we started our IPE program, national competency domains for safety and quality had not been fully developed. We soon embraced safety and quality as guiding principles. Each of our five core competency domains emphasizes safety and quality components. We believe strongly that by focusing on these concepts early in the education of our learners, we will build a culture of collaboration that will pervade how our learners practice in the clinical years and throughout their careers.

In our IPE program, our goal is not only to provide educational experiences that foster a culture of safety and quality, but that also build leadership skills in these areas—and not just at the bedside with traditional in-patient health professions, but across the landscape of health professions that not only passes through out-patient and in-patient services, but also spans species.

The Best of Both Worlds: An Interprofessional Career

My own personal journey as a healthcare professional began in nursing. As a nurse, I worked in a variety of healthcare settings, eventually settling in home care and hospice. Later, I returned to school to fulfill a personal dream of becoming a veterinarian. As a veterinarian, I consistently got feedback from my clients and co-workers that I was different from most vets they had encountered before. I always smiled broadly and exclaimed that it was because I was also a nurse! My nursing education and practice experience built communication and compassion skills that I never learned during my veterinary education, and I put these skills to use every day.

After working as a veterinarian for a few years, I missed my nursing practice, so I returned to working as a nurse in a large academic health center on a part-time basis while I continued my full-time work as a veterinarian. Similarly, while working as a nurse, I would receive comments about how I was different from most other nurses. I would smile and respond that it was because I was also a vet! Just as my nursing education provided me skills that I used as a vet, my veterinary education provided other skills that were useful in my nursing practice.

As a veterinarian, I honed my nonverbal and physical exam and observation skills that are necessary when our patients are animals. These same observational skills used in my nursing practice gave me insights into providing safe and quality patient care that I did not previously use. I often brag that the gems I learned from each of my professions are what make me most effective in clinical practice, and knowing how to harness these gems when necessary. Now as an educator in an IPE program, I challenge learners from nine diverse professions to recognize their profession's gems and then to maximize them to enhance the safety and quality of patient care. I teach them to recognize the gems in one another so that as interprofessional teams, the synergy they create is magnified to enhance the safety and quality of care, and to improve outcomes.

Final Reflections

Just as the separate paths of health professions are merging to provide better health outcomes through collaborative practice, leaders must also come together across organizations, systems, and communities to create the conditions for excellence to happen. We believe that we are moving closer to the ideal of the reflective learning organizations. Challenges remain, but our faculty and students are driving change. The next chapter continues this discussion with four vignettes of transformation in action.

References

Benner, P. (1984). *From novice to expert: Excellence and power in clinical nursing practice.* Menlo Park, CA: Addison Wesley Publishing Company.

Benner, P., Hooper-Kyriakidis, P., & Stannard, D. (1999). *Clinical wisdom and interventions in critical care: A thinking-in-action approach.* Phladelphia, PA: W. B. Saunders Company.

Benner, P., Tanner, C. A., & Chesla, C. A. (1996). *Expertise in nursing practice: Caring, clinical judgment, and ethics.* New York, NY: Springer Publishing Company.

Berkow, S., Virkstis, K., Stewart, J., & Conway, L. (2008). Assessing new graduate nurse performance. *Journal of Nursing Administration, 38*(11), 468–474.

Bisognano, M., & Kenney, C. (2012). *Pursuing the Triple Aim: Seven innovators show the way to better care, better health, and lower costs.* San Francisco, CA: Jossey-Bass.

Boller, J. (1980, December). Observations on the development of the ICU Nurse. *Focus on AACN, 7*(6), 24–27.

Boller, J., & Jones, D. (2010, April). Change California? Reflections on leading statewide collaboration on nursing education redesign. *Nurse Leader,* 40–46.

Briskin, A., & Boller, J. (2006). *Daily miracles: Stories and practices of humanity and excellence in health care.* Indianapolis, IN: Sigma Theta Tau International.

Briskin, A., Erickson, S., Ott, J., & Callanan, T. (2009). *The power of collective wisdom and the trap of collective folly.* San Francisco, CA: Berrett-Koehler Publishers.

California Institute for Nursing & Health Care. (2008). *Nursing education redesign for California; White paper and strategic action plan recommendations.* Berkeley, CA: California Institute for Nursing & Health Care. Retrieved from http://cinhc.wpengine.netdna-cdn.com/wp-content/uploads/2009/12/5_Nursing-Ed-Redesign.pdf

Casey, A. (2005). Enhancing individual and organizational learning. *Management Learning, 36*(2), 131–147.

Clark, R. (2003). *Building expertise: Cognitive methods for training and performance improvement.* (2nd ed.). Silver Spring, MD: International Society for Performance Improvement.

Classen, D. C., Resar, R., Griffin, F., Frederico, F., Frankel, T., Kimmel, N., ... James, B. C. (2011). "Global Trigger Tool" shows that adverse events in hospitals may be ten times greater than previously measured. *Health Affairs, 30*(4), 581–589.

Collins, J. (2001). *Good to great.* New York, NY: Random House.

Cooperrider, D., Whitney, D., & Stavros, J. (2008). *Appreciative inquiry handbook* (2nd ed.). San Francisco, CA: Berrett-Koehler.

Crowell, D. M. (2011). Complexity leadership: Nursing's role in health care delivery. Philadelphia, PA: F.A. Davis Co.

del Bueno, D. J., Barker, F., & Christmyer, C. (1981). Implementing a competency-based orientation program. *Journal of Nursing Administration, 11*(2), 24–29.

Dreyfus, H. L. & Dreyfus, S. E. (1996). The relationship of theory and practice in the acquisition of skill. In P. Benner, C.A. Tanner, & C.A. Chelsa. *Expertise in nursing practice: Caring, clinical judgment, and ethics.* (pp. 29-47). New York, NY: Springer Publishing Company.

Frank, J. R., Mungroo, R., Ahmad, Y., Wang, M., De Rossi, S., & Horsley, T. (2010). Toward a definition of competency-based education in medicine: A systematic review of published definitions. *Medical Teacher, 32*(8), 631–637.

Hilden, H., & Tikkamaki, K. (2013). Reflective practice as a fuel for organizational learning. *Administrative Science, 3,* 76–95. doi:10:3390/admsci3030076

Institute for Healthcare Improvement (IHI). (2005). *Going lean in healthcare.* Cambridge, MA: Institute for Healthcare Improvement. Retrieved from http://www.ihi.org/resources/Pages/IHIWhitePapers/GoingLeaninHealthCare.aspx

Institute of Medicine (IOM). (2013). *Best care at lower cost: The path to continuously learning health care in America.* Washington, DC: National Academies Press.

Interprofessional Education Collaborative (IPEC). (2011). *Core competencies for interprofessional collaborative practice: Report of an expert panel.* Washington, DC: Interprofessional Education Collaborative. Retrieved from http://www.aacn.nche.edu/education-resources/ipecreport.pdf

James, J. T. (2013). A new, evidence-based estimate of patient harms associated with hospital care. *Journal of Patient Safety, 9*(3), 122–128.

Knipfer, K., Kump, B., Wessel, D., & Cress, U. (2013). Reflection as a catalyst for organizational learning. *Studies in Continuing Education, 35*(1), 30–48.

Kohn, L. T., Corrigan, J., & Donaldson, M. S. (2000). *To err is human: Building a safer health system.* Washington, DC: National Academies Press.

Leape, L. (1994). Error in medicine. *Journal of the American Medical Association, 272*(23), 1851–1857.

Levine, S., & Prietula, M. (2013). Open collaboration for innovation: Principles & performance. *Organization Science, 22*(5), 1414–1433.

Morris, Z. S., Wooding, S., & Grant, J. (2011). The answer is 17, what is the question: Understanding time lags in translational research. *Journal of Research in Social Medicine, 104*(12), 510–520.

Organisation for Economic Co-operation and Development (OECD). (2014). *Society at a glance. OECD Social indicators.* Paris, France: OECD Publishing. doi:10.1787/soc_glance-2014-en.

National Research Council. (2011). *The future of nursing: Leading change, advancing health.* Washington, DC: National Academies Press.

Patterson, K., Grenny, J., McMillan, R., & Switzler, A. (2012). *Crucial conversations: Tools for talking when stakes are high* (2nd ed.). New York, NY: McGraw-Hill.

Porter-O'Grady, T., & Malloch, K. (2015). *Quantum leadership: Building better partnerships for sustainable health* (4th ed.). Sudbury, MA: Jones & Bartlett Learning.

Proust, M. (1923). Remembrance of Things Past_ [1913—1927] Vol. V, _The Captive_ [1923], ch. II "The Verdurins Quarrel with M. de Charlus" (1929 C. K. Scott Moncrieff translation).

Quality and Safety Education for Nurses (QSEN). Retrieved from http://qsen.org/

Rogers, E. M. (2003). *Diffusion of innovations* (5th ed.). New York, NY: Free Press.

Senge, P. M. (2006). *The fifth discipline: The art and practice of the learning organization.* New York: Currency Doubleday.

Senge, P. (2007). The leaders' new work: Building learning organizations. In J. S. Osland, M. E. Turner, D. A. Kolb, & I. M. Rubin. *The organizational behavior reader.* (8th ed.) 100–122).

Shelton, C., & Darling, J. (2003) From theory to practice: Using new science concepts to create learning organizations. *The Learning Organization, 10*(6), 353–360.

Sherwood, G. W., & Horton-Deutsch, S. (2012). *Reflective practice: Transforming education and improving outcomes.* Indianapolis, IN: Sigma Theta Tau International.

Solomon, P. (2011). Problem-based learning. In M. J. Bradshaw and A. J. Lowenstein. (Eds). *Innovative teaching strategies in nursing and related health professions.* (5th ed., pp. 137–145). Sudbury, MA: Jones and Bartlett Publishers.

Spector, N., & Echternacht, M. (2010). A regulatory model for transitioning newly licensed nurses to practice. *Journal of Nursing Regulation, 1*(2), 18–25.

The Joint Commission. (2014). *Sentinel event data: Root causes by event type.* Retrieved from http://www.jointcommission.org/assets/1/18/Root_Causes_by_Event_Type_2004-2Q_2014.pdf

United States Department of Health and Human Services; Agency for Healthcare Research and Quality. (n.d.) TEAMSTEPPS: National Implementation. Retrieved from http://teamstepps.ahrq.gov/

Wenger, E., McDermott, R., & Snyder, W. (2002). *Cultivating communities of practice: A guide to managing knowledge.* Boston, MA: Harvard Business School Press.

Whitney, D., & Trosten-Bloom, A. (2003). *The power of appreciative inquiry: A practical guide to positive change.* San Francisco, CA: Berrett-Koehler Publishers.

Resources

Argyris, C. (1991, May). Teaching smart people how to learn. Reprinted from *Harvard Business Review, Reflections, 4*(2), 4–14. Retrieved from http://www.ncsu.edu/park_scholarships/pdf/chris_argyris_learning.pdf

Arrien, A. (1993). *The four-fold way: Walking the ways of the warrior, teacher, healer, visionary.* San Francisco, CA: Harper San Francisco.

Bass, B. M., & Riggio, R. E. (2006). *Transformational leadership* (2nd ed.). Mahwah, NJ: Lawrence Erlbaum Associates Publishers.

Brookfield, S. (2000). Adult cognition as a dimension of lifelong learning. In J. Field & M. Leicester (Eds.), *Lifelong learning: Education across the lifespan* (pp. 89–101). New York, NY: Routledge Falmer.

Brown, J., & Isaacs, D. (2005). *The world café: Shaping futures through conversations that matter.* San Francisco, CA: Berrett Koehler.

Gardner, H., (2008). *5 minds for the future*. Boston, MA: Harvard Business Press.

Herrmann, N. (1996). *The whole brain business book*. New York, NY: McGraw-Hill.

Kotter, J. (2012). *Leading change*. Boston, MA: Harvard Business Press.

Mezirow, J. (1991). *Transformative dimensions of adult learning*. San Francisco, CA: Jossey-Bass.

Mezirow, J., & Associates (Eds.). (2000). *Learning as transformation: Critical perspectives on a theory in progress*. San Francisco, CA: Jossey-Bass.

Needleman, J. (1997). *Time and the soul*. New York, NY: Doubleday Business.

Palmer, P. J. (2000). *Let your life speak: Listening for the voice of vocation*. San Francisco, CA: Jossey-Bass.

Scharmer, C. O. (2007). *Theory U: Leading from the future as it emerges*. Cambridge, MA: Society for Organizational Learning.

Scharmer, C. O., & Kaufer, K. (2013). *Leading from the emerging future: From ego-system to eco-system economies*. San Francisco, CA: Berrett-Koehler.

Senge, P., Scharmer, C. O., Jaworski, J., & Flowers, B. S. (2004). *Presence: An exploration of profound change in people, organizations, and society*. New York, NY: Currency/Doubleday.

Wheatley, M. J. (2006). *Leadership and the new science*. San Francisco, CA: Berrett-Koehler.

Chapter 15

Reflective Organizations: On the Front Lines to Transform Education and Practice

Pat Callard, DNP, RN, CNE, CNL
Linda S. Flores, MSN, RN
Marci Luxenburg-Horowitz, DNP, RN, CNL
Patricia Salazar Shakhshir, PhD, CNS, RN-BC
Dawn Salpaka Stone, RN, ANP-BC, COHN-S
Jan Boller, PhD, RN

The previous chapter provided insights from three leaders on converging pathways to transform an academic organization to a learning organization. At Western University of Health Sciences (WesternU), health professionals are moving out of their individual professional specialties to learn and practice in an interprofessional collaborative environment to improve health outcomes. This chapter features four vignettes providing examples of how faculty members along the education pathway at WesternU, from prelicensure through graduate (MSN and DNP) education levels have designed learning experiences for reflection around patient safety, interprofessional practice, human diversity, and professional role development. These are a few examples of innovative education taking place in this university and across the country. Collectively, health professions faculty are reshaping role formation of the health professions through reflection and interprofessional practice.

Background

Reflective practice is a vital competency for translating the best evidence into practice and involves a spirit and stance of continuous inquiry and critical evaluation (Freshwater, 2012). By reflecting on knowledge, practice, and outcomes simultaneously, practitioner/scholars become leaders of change, not only for improved quality of care but also for a transformed healthcare system. Reflective practice requires a high degree of self-awareness, situation awareness, awareness of others, systems awareness, and engaged relational comportment. Developing skills in reflective practice prepares health professionals to navigate the most tumultuous circumstances and ethical challenges, bringing the best evidence to guide practice improvement and transformation (Sherwood & Horton-Deutsch, 2012).

Gwen Sherwood and Sara Horton-Deutsch (2012) view reflective practice as foundational to healthcare redesign, led by nurses who will move healthcare out of the current dysfunctional box of medical errors and ineffective care and into a future where the U.S. healthcare system is a model for excellence and efficiency. Freshwater (2012) identifies cornerstones of reflective practice as the ability to step back, explore with others, reflect on what is happening, and determine where one wants to go—with responsibility, accountability, self- and collective-awareness, and openness. Reflective practice deepens learning and enhances the ability to translate vision and knowledge into action.

Reflective practice requires some time to think: thinking before action, thinking in action, and thinking after action. Lee Shulman, President Emeritus of The Carnegie Foundation for the Advancement of Teaching, offers a model for learning that incorporates reflective practice as a key element for learning in action (Shulman, 2002). Shulman's model incorporates the practice of reflection along an interrelated continuum of engagement/motivation, knowledge/ understanding, performance/action reflection/critique, judgment/design, and commitment/identity (Shulman, 2002). In the journey to clinical expertise, without reflective practice, something vital is missing.

Freshwater (2012) suggests that the reflective practitioner questions rather than commands—collaborates rather than orders. Reflective practitioners are open to others' views rather than judging others; are honest and willing to admit they are wrong; are accountable as lifelong learners to find the best evidence and the best solutions; and take full responsibility for their actions.

In the sections that follow, take time to consider the dimensions of reflective practice as five health professions educators discuss their approaches to incorporate reflection as an approach to improve learning outcomes.

Reflections on Integrating QSEN Into the Prelicensure Nursing Curriculum

Linda Flores, MSN, RN
Patricia Shakhshir, PhD, CNS, RN-BC

In 2009, Patricia Shakhshir and Linda Flores created an annual "Lab of Horrors" simulation for Halloween. The entire mini-hospital simulation lab is transformed into safety failures from active to latent failures for the pediatric and adult populations. Groups of first- and fourth-semester nursing students, dressed in Halloween costumes, walk from the rooms of horror to spooky Halloween themed stations. Students identify and list the 50 to 70 active and latent observable patient safety failures.

The Project

One week after the safety infraction simulation, during their fundamentals clinical rotation, the students' knowledge of the Quality and Safety Education

5 WHY'S

The 5 Why's is a technique used in the Analyze phase of the Six Sigma Define, Measure, Analyze, Improve, Control (2015) methodology. Write an observable safety infraction and describe it. Ask "why" the problem happens and write the answer. Repeat 3–5 more times—ask "why" the "new" problem happens until a root cause is identified.

JUST CULTURE

High-reliability organizations create a positive working environment utilizing evidence-based care and transparency to improve safety and quality of care. Within a just culture, when an adverse event occurs, analysis of the root cause or system starts with the 5 Why's, not "who" is the problem. Concentrating on "who" perpetuates shame and blame. Concentrating on the root cause will prevent future errors (AHRQ, 2012; Barnsteiner, 2011b).

for Nurses (QSEN) based safety competencies is measured. In this test, first-semester students complete another safety list, surveying hospital clinical units for adherence to safety. They identify any areas of safety non-adherence. Postconference discussion debriefing includes a reflection process using the "Five Whys" (Six Sigma, 2015) is used, and following the processes of Just Culture (Khatri, Brown, & Hicks, 2009), students learn a blameless communication technique to identify sources of the problem (Agency for Healthcare Research and Quality [AHRQ], 2012; Barnsteiner, 2011b). Students observe Just Culture and blameless communication as faculty share results with the unit educator. The unit educator may elect to share the results with the unit manager and staff.

Fourth-semester students complete the same survey at their preceptor sites. A class assignment requires them to conduct a literature review of the problem and best practices. A group research poster presentation is then presented at the College of Graduate Nursing research day. Peers and faculty judge and award outstanding safety and quality of care research.

The Process

WesternU supports and promotes faculty development on current practices and trends in education. Several faculty members attended the 2011 QSEN faculty development conferences. At the Seattle QSEN conference, Patti Shakhshir and Linda Flores realized that their "Lab of Horrors" was a best practice activity for active and latent failure simulation. The original objectives included recognition of safety infractions, but the 2011 QSEN conference provided the inspiration to include the concepts of Just Culture and blameless communication (AHRQ, 2012; Barnsteiner, 2011a, 2011b). The language and spirit of QSEN (Barnsteiner, 2011a; Flores, Shakhshir, & Lopez, 2014; Johnson, 2011) is fully integrated into all CGN Masters of Science in Nursing-Entry (MSNE) clinical evaluation tools to further support the implementation and integration of quality and safety. The goal ultimately will result in a plan-do-study-act project during the student's master's portion of the program.

QSEN emphasizes strategies for making competencies efficient and conducive to learning (Conner, 2012). Hands-on experiences or simulations utilize Kolb's experiential learning theories, contextual learning, and constructivism learning theories (Jarzemsky, 2009). Through a simulation lab of "sharp end" at the bedside and "blunt end" organizational safety hazards, first- and fourth-semester students became more aware of maintaining a safe environment for patients. First, content on defining safety hazards is reviewed in didactic courses. Second, fundamentals lectures review patient safety risks from the environment and from healthcare agencies. Fourth-semester students focus on creating a Just Culture, functioning as change agents. Fourth-semester course work, focusing on leadership, research, evidence-based practice, and quality improvement begins the transition into the master's portion of the program.

BLAMELESS COMMUNICATION

Entails confidential and voluntary reporting of errors or potential latent conditions. An event analysis (5 Why's) prevents blame, attribution, and hindsight bias. Disclosures require truth telling on: What happened? Has it happened before? Could it happen again? What caused it to happen (root cause analysis using 5 Why's) and Who should be told (AHRQ, 2012; Barnsteiner, 2011b; Six Sigma, 2015).

IMPLEMENTING QSEN COMPETENCIES THROUGHOUT THE BSN ESSENTIALS CURRICULUM

Here are several ideas for how you can implement QSEN competencies:

- *Create a simulation lab where students identify active and latent failures (Conner, 2012).*

- *On a whiteboard, create the root-cause analysis diagram and ask the 5 Why's to the problem identified on the clinical unit (Six Sigma, 2015; AHRQ, 2012).*

- *Brainstorm on identifying the cause and what can be done to change the system, using a Just Culture and blameless communication approach (Barnsteiner, 2011b).*

- *Have students in clinical rotations identify safety adherence on the hospital unit and share the observational findings with the unit manager to reinforce positive behaviors exhibited by unit team members (Flores, Shakhshir, & Lopez, 2014).*

- *Share with the unit manager areas that need improvement; share the findings and be part of the solution by offering to complete a 1-minute update at pre-conference or conduct a lunch in-service.*

- *Implement QSEN language each semester. Thread QSEN concepts in lecture, labs, simulations, and language. Scaffold QSEN-izing processes first with identification; second with implementation; third with analysis and evaluation exercises as outlined in the QSEN competency-based clinical evaluation tools (Flores, Shakhshir, & Lopez, 2014).*

- *Engage the adjunct clinical faculty with 1-on-1 meetings on the concept of quality and safety. Include adjuncts in faculty development processes.*

- *Assign didactic points to safety- and quality-based papers, group projects, and exemplars.*

- *After the students possess the knowledge and practice the skills, have them serve as role models, change agents, and encourage others to be practice safety behaviors—resulting in improved patient outcomes.*

> ### REFLECTING ON ... THE USE OF QSEN COMPETENCIES
>
> - *What themes can be embedded within simulation to make learning QSEN competencies fun and applicable to practice?*
>
> - *How can your organization layer the QSEN competencies of safety, evidence-based practice, patient-centered care, quality improvement, and teamwork collaboration into the language of the curriculum?*
>
> - *How can students develop QSEN competence by collaborating with the clinical unit to improve safety and quality?*

Outcomes

The goal of Lab of Horrors and subsequent learning experiences throughout the MSNE curriculum was to enhance knowledge about a culture of safety and translate this knowledge to practice within context during clinical rotations. By instilling a broader view of rationales for maintaining patient safety, attitudes will be changed from a "laying blame" to a "system failure" attitude (AHRQ, 2012; Johnson, 2011). Originally, high-stakes testing solely demonstrated an increase in knowledge retention for safety hazards (presimulation versus postsimulation). Currently, the addition of clinical exemplars (an aspect of the QSEN clinical competency evaluation tool) also captures reflections of attitudes and reasoning in transition for safety and quality in the clinical setting (Benner, Sutphen, Leonard, & Day, 2010; Flores, Shakhshir, & Lopez, 2014; Tanner, 2006).

> ### REFLECTING ON ... BLAMELESS COMMUNICATION
>
> - *What measures of blameless communication will your students and clinical faculty use to convey safety concerns?*

After reviewing the first-year and second-year students' completed hospital safety surveys, we discovered that approximately 40% of the identified safety infractions fell into the infection control category. With the coordination of a nurse educator, a unit manager, and charge nurses, a campaign for breaking the chain of infection ensued on a unit of a hospital in southern California. Students identified unrestrained long hair of healthcare professionals as a route for infection. The students designed a poster in which information related to the reason hair should be secured, which they displayed on the unit. The observational study to measure outcomes is pending.

The nurse educator of a second hospital partner in southern California has created "Rooms of Horror" on different units, on a quarterly basis. The nurse educator sets up safety, infection control, and Health Insurance Portability and Accountability Act (HIPAA) violations. The nurse educator and hospital partner implemented this safety activity after having participated at our CGN's Lab of Horrors. The simulation is duplicable. Follow-up on creating a culture of safety, collaboration among unit nurse managers, nurse educators, staff, and nursing students will be needed to maintain sustainability of the safety intervention plans. Efficacy of safety interventions will entail another observational survey from the next cohort of nursing students assigned to the same unit. Since 2011, annual safety simulations and unit surveys have been embedded within the clinical practicum portion of the program.

REFLECTING ON ... OUTCOMES

- *How will your organization document or measure outcomes for knowledge retention, skill mastery, and attitudes?*

Final Reflections

With early introduction of the concepts of healthcare systems, the laying-blame stigma of infractions is alleviated (Johnson, 2011). To follow up on creating a culture of safety, the simulation activity would entail linking the safety infractions to a root-cause analysis and then developing a process plan for safety. This exercise can become a leadership project during the students' final semester. At WesternU's CGN, integration of QSEN core competencies begins in first semester. Quality, evidenced-based, safety, patient-centered care, teamwork collaboration, and informatics are concepts threaded in the entire curriculum, clinical evaluation tools, and simulation exercises. Taking the safety core competency one step further to increase adherence to infection control in our clinical partners will result in better patient outcomes. Promoting nursing students who analyze root causes for blameless communication and creating a thinking process and attitude for changing the system will result in better patient satisfaction and outcomes (AHRQ, 2012; Barnsteiner, 2011a; 2011b).

One major challenge relates to the unit managers at five clinical practice sites. Some experienced discomfort and became defensive during our safety debriefing. To avoid the "laying blame" culture, clinical partners are invited to celebrate the annual Lab of Horrors and are included in choosing the students' change project.

Plans are in process to determine what quality-improvement project the staff is working on for quality and safety, and then to integrate the advance medical/surgical clinical students into the unit's 1-minute update before shift begins or a lunch in-service. To warm the unit managers to the safety observational project, the conversation was begun with accolades for their safety compliance behaviors and culture. After acknowledging strengths, opportunities for improvement are identified, with rewording from the term "non-adherence" to "areas that need reinforcement." Inviting the unit managers and educators to the Lab of Horrors promotes openness and acceptance while experiencing a fun exercise with Halloween treats at the end.

Human Diversity: Improving Sensitivity Through Self-Reflective Practice

Dawn Salpaka Stone, RN, ANP-BC, COHN-S

Diversity characterizes the human experience and is essential to the development of identity. With a greater emphasis on international migration, the demographics in the United States are expected to change during the upcoming 50 years. According to the U.S. Census Bureau (2012), the Hispanic population and persons over the age of 65 will double by 2060. In contrast, the U.S. nursing workforce is currently 75% Caucasian with a recent growth in nurses under the age of 30 (Health Resources and Services Administration [HRSA], 2013). Nursing as a global occupation practicing in a heterogeneous society will need to be prepared to provide care for patients across a wide spectrum of cultures, with an emphasis on older adults (American Association of Colleges of Nursing, 2009).

WesternU's CGN is home to a distance program with students throughout the United States. With anticipation of the changes in American demographics and the expected interactions among various age and ethnic groups within healthcare settings, a need for deeper self-reflection among graduate nursing students in the CGN's Advanced Human Diversity course was identified. The goal was not only to recognize and appreciate differences among the patient populations and healthcare providers, but also to discover bias within the self that may hinder interactions during the provision of care, jeopardizing quality and safety.

REFLECTING ON ... DEMOGRAPHICS

- *What is the demographic profile in your practice arena among healthcare professionals, including nurses, and patient populations?*

- *What steps are taken by individuals and the institution to ensure sensitive care to prevent ageism and support cultural diversity?*

Background

The Advanced Human Diversity course is part of the Family Nurse Practitioner and Ambulatory Care Nursing curricula. Previously, this course was delivered in a hybrid format with online discussions and lively small group face-to-face seminar sessions. Curricular modifications required change to an exclusively online format driving the need to teach and promote reflective practice using different but equally effective pedagogy. Hence, the goal of this project was to modify Advanced Human Diversity to capture self-reflection about sensitive issues surrounding diversity topics online. This course is a one-semester unit prompting mindfulness of workload for students and faculty alike with the addition of self-assessments and reflection assignments.

The Project

A comprehensive review of the literature revealed that self-assessment is the first essential step to understand self-identification and the influences that shape values and biases (Welch, 2003). Given that conscious and unconscious values and beliefs impact acceptance and perceptions of others, the integration of published self-assessment or attitudinal tools using the test feature within an electronic learning management system (LMS) was launched. Self-assessments contained a variety of question formats using multiple choice (Likert scales) and true/false. Essay/short answer questions prompted synthesis of responses with the development of a plan for improvement. Unfortunately, the electronic LMS mandates one correct answer to auto-score, so students were ultimately given points for simply completing each of the self-assessments and reflective assignments.

Outcomes

The Advanced Human Diversity course is offered once during each academic year; this project has just finished its first round of completion. The response from students has been openly favorable. Some students shared what they learned about themselves in the online discussion forums, noting the value of recognizing bias/prejudices and the need to address impressions acquired and internalized during childhood. Because all students are practicing Registered Nurses, the value of reflective practice was also noted to be immediately useful in current roles. Additional feedback will be obtained through the anonymous course evaluation tool required at the end of every term.

Reflective Response

The project will improve quality of safe patient care by promoting self-reflection to enhance sensitivity to diversity during patient and provider interactions within healthcare settings. Surprisingly, some students expressed tremendous concern over low points earned on the self-assessments and how these scores would impact final grades. Gentle reminders were given to encourage reflection about what a low score means (bias and stereotyping). The importance of reviewing the self-assessments as a whole and creating a plan for improvement in the essay question was strongly encouraged.

Future course offerings could consider use of other features in the electronic LMS to eliminate concern about numerical scores. Faculty members could also explore adding "sensitivity to human diversity" into clinical evaluations for continuous awareness, application of knowledge, and reflective practice. For example, during precepted or mentored clinical experiences, if a student adds patient education to a care or treatment plan considering the impact of a specific cultural diet on a health condition, sensitivity to the patient's unique cultural needs has been demonstrated and addressed.

The Advanced Human Diversity course would benefit all specialties of graduate nursing students and should be considered part of the core curriculum. This course could also become available to all health science colleges through the Inter-professional Education Program at WesternU.

REFLECTING ON ... DIVERSITY

- *How can you develop awareness of attitudes to diverse situations in yourself and colleagues?*

- *What could you do to create a respectful culture of sensitivity to the differences among people in your healthcare facility or workplace?*

Interprofessional Student Teams and Developing Reflective Practice

Pat Callard, DNP, RN, CNE, CNL

The importance of teamwork in healthcare has been identified in the literature for many years. In 2003, The Institute of Medicine (IOM) released a report listing five proficiencies for healthcare professionals and students, one of which is participating in interprofessional teamwork (National Research Council, 2003). Collaboration and teamwork are supported by professional healthcare organizations and are integral parts of health profession curricula (American

Interprofessional Health Collaborative [AIHC], 2012; Blue, Mitcham, Smith, Raymond, & Greenberg, 2010). In 2009, several healthcare education organizations recognized the importance of interprofessional teamwork and collaboration and formed the Interprofessional Education Collaborative (IPEC). Core competencies for interprofessional education (IPE) were identified, including values and ethics for interprofessional practice, roles and responsibilities, interprofessional communication, and teams and teamwork (IPEC, 2011, pp. 15–16).

Background

During the past 10 years, I have worked with students as they completed the first and second year of their health professions education. These students worked hard to earn the best grades possible in their undergraduate program and went through a competitive admissions process to be accepted in the desired health profession program. Their focus was being the best individual student and candidate to reach their ultimate goal.

REFLECTING ON... TEAMWORK

- *How can educators transition students from focusing on individual success to the importance of team success?*

- *What can educators and clinicians do to promote interprofessional learning and collaboration in practice?*

Health professions curricula tend to be in silos, with students going to class, lab, and clinical experiences with students in the same profession. Many students continue in a competitive environment to score well in their professional courses, hoping to secure desirable positions in the workplace. Class sessions or experiences may include students in other professions, but those are few and far between. Occasionally, students participate in health and wellness events, but again these are primarily with students from their own profession.

This is where IPE can have an impact. At WesternU, students studying osteopathic medicine, pharmacy, nursing, physician assistant, physical therapy, veterinary medicine, dental medicine, optometry, and podiatry participate in IPE during the first year of their health profession education. Students meet in small teams with students from other professions to learn about each other's scope of practice and also how to communicate and work in a team while discussing health- or disease-related scenarios.

As students completed IPE assignments, faculty initially noticed that students often worked in a "divide and conquer" approach for team assignments, with each student taking a section to complete. Sometimes the assignment flowed smoothly; other times, it read like unrelated ideas with no connection. When students were asked about teamwork, most felt that they worked well in a team, often giving examples of debate teams and sports teams, which tend to be more competitive. Teamwork that benefits someone outside the team was seldom encountered in prior experiences.

The Project: Self Versus Team Reflection

With a shift to patient-centered care, health profession teams must be able to work with the patient or others to reach goals. This led faculty members to explore strategies to transition the thought process from a competitive individual to working on a team for a common goal. Students completed an individual self-reflection and other learning assignments. The self-reflection was designed to integrate and synthesize course material including the team learning experience. Once again, students reflected on their own learning experience rather than how the team worked together.

Recently, the decision was made to change to a team reflection with questions that encouraged synthesis of individual comments as well as evaluating team effectiveness. After discussing a public health case, students were asked to reflect on the following questions:

- What are the team and individual perceptions of situations in the last session? What different perceptions did team members have?

- What went well in your team? What did you learn about team interaction and the effect on outcomes that you can apply to practice?

- Share your thoughts about how to effectively communicate goals with the patient, other affected individuals, and members of the healthcare team.

- Talk about the team interaction and include differences of opinion and how you overcame them. Given that there is always room for improvement, how could your team improve communication and interaction?

- What areas of concern did your team identify and discuss related to the environmental and/or public health conditions of human and animal populations for the topic?

Outcomes

Although there are still signs of the "divide and conquer" approach, some teams of students have been able to reflect on their performance and talk about what worked and what did not. Some are beginning to think as a group and expand on ideas and thoughts initiated by other professions.

The ability to reflect on what has been done and how it could be improved is not always easy. As students gain more experience with team reflection, our hope is that they will recognize the importance of communication and working together to meet patient goals through teamwork and collaboration.

Final Reflections

As I observe health profession students become more comfortable talking with one another, I notice they have also become more familiar with the roles and responsibilities of other professions. This adds to the thought that "learners must apply their experiences in interprofessional learning to their own practice and must reflect upon their own performance in an interprofessional context, in order to make change and to practice true collaboration" (Bainbridge & Wood, 2013, p. 133).

The value of interprofessional collaboration and teamwork may not become part of the health professional until they have more experience in professional practice. Anecdotal comments from colleagues in other professions show this may be true. We are beginning to hear comments about IPE from former students who are in advanced clinical training or professional practice. Comments include: "Now I understand why we had IPE," "I felt so much more comfortable working on a team," and "They really do use SBAR in hospitals." It seems that IPE in the early years of health profession education can influence how an individual thinks about patient care and interactions with others.

COMPLEXITY SCIENCE

A method to examine the various aspects of complex living systems often neglected or understated in traditional scientific inquiry. Greater understanding of the patterns of relationships, how these patterns are sustained, how the system self organizes, and how outcomes emerge provide opportunities to determine where small changes could have the greatest impact on organizational growth and evolution (Zimmerman, Plsek, & Lindberg, 2002).

Partnership for Quality and Safety

Marci Luxenburg-Horowitz, DNP, RN, CNL

Nurses across the continuum of care have a pivotal role in health system improvement. In order to improve care, enhance outcomes, and decrease costs, nurses must coordinate and collaborate within and between organizational systems. The shared professional commitment for quality and safety (American Nurses Association, 2001, 2010, 2011) can be utilized to bring nurses from all points along the continuum of care to work together for the greater good. This shared commitment to quality and safety can be the foundation of an academic-service partnership.

Background

As an experienced nurse leader who entered academia, I maintained a relationship with a local healthcare organization. Complexity science (Crowell, 2010) and appreciative inquiry

(Cooperrider, Whitney, & Stavros, 2008) guided my leadership practice. My dream was to develop an academic-service partnership with a shared focus on quality and safety. I worked closely with the Director of Clinical Services, who was a champion for change within the organization. She was working to enhance the culture of safety within the organization. Together, we identified areas within this complex system where small changes could have the greatest impact.

I began to attend shared governance council meetings. At the Professional Development Council meeting, an opportunity presented itself. A review of the nurses' job description and clinical ladder document revealed discrepancies between nursing education and service expectations. I shared the changes that had occurred in nursing curricula as a result of the QSEN initiative (Cronenwett et al., 2007). I also discussed the recent IOM reports (National Research Council, 2001, 2003, 2011) and nursing's role as leaders and facilitators of health system improvement. At the next meeting, I presented the QSEN documents (Cronenwett et al., 2007, 2009) and discussed how the documents could guide the leveling of the clinical ladder levels to ensure that all nurses were optimizing their role in quality and safety. After review of the documents, the team immediately and unanimously decided to align the QSEN competencies to the current ladder structure to identify gaps and areas of needed change.

The Professional Development Council comprised nurse leaders from the point of care, unit-based

APPRECIATIVE INQUIRY
A philosophy and strength-based approach to change that seeks to find the best in people and the organization. Asking appreciative questions uncovers the positive core as well as the dreams within the group. AI facilitates the system's capacity to heighten its positive potential. It is a co-creative and evolutionary process that enhances an organization's ability to achieve its most desired future (Cooperrider, Whitney, & Stavros, 2008).

educators, one administrative support person, and two nurse directors who acted in an advisory capacity. The group recognized that releveling the nursing job description and clinical ladder would result in changes to the expectations and competencies for nurses at all levels. A decision to take a two-phase approach was adopted. The group would first evaluate the presence of and/or add the appropriate quality and safety competencies of the first two levels of the clinical ladder. New nurses entering the organization would be oriented to the updated job description and clinical ladder. This first change would impact the new hires and would have limited impact on the nurses already practicing within the organization. The anticipated changes at levels 3 and 4 would increase the expectations for the nurses already working at those levels. Changing these levels would be far more disruptive, and greater resistance to the needed change was anticipated.

The Project

An all-day retreat was scheduled with support from the chief nurse executive. Participants included all members within the organization on the professional development council, the director/advisor, one administrative support person, and an academic member. Nurses were provided with the QSEN documents (Cronenwett, et al., 2007, 2009), the Scope and Standards of Practice (ANA, 2011), and the Code of Ethics (ANA, 2001). The entire process took close to a year and included two all-day, offsite retreats along with two half-day onsite meetings. The progress of the work was reviewed at each monthly council meeting.

For the nurses, this project was not business as usual. In past projects, nursing input was elicited; however, the nurses shared that it was their perception that executive decisions had been made before staff members had provided their thoughts and ideas. In contrast, the clinical ladder/QSEN alignment project emerged from the group. The nurses were engaged and highly passionate throughout the process. Nurse executive leadership has provided support and funding for the project. The use of an iterative, appreciative reflective process strengthened relationships and helped the group move forward. The synergy of our collective strengths and talents allowed the group to grow and move in directions that were not possible in the past.

Outcomes

Honoring the nature of complex systems and using an appreciative approach helped lay the foundation for the ongoing success of the group. The appreciative process provided multiple opportunities for individual and group reflections. Becoming partners for quality and safety has enhanced the relationship between the organizations. The outcomes of this project extend well beyond the initial group.

The review process resulted in the nurses examining their job description and clinical ladder in the context of several key documents including the Scope and Standards of professional practice (ANA, 2011), nursing's Code of Ethics (ANA, 2001), and the Healthy Work Environment initiative (American Association of Critical-Care Nurses [AACN], 2005). Nurses not only enhanced professional practice and accountability within the clinical ladder, but reviewing and discussing key documents within the profession reignited their passion, pride, and commitment for the practice of professional nursing. They are re-energized and have become positive forces for change within their units.

The integration of QSEN and the elevation of expectations for professional practice for clinical levels 1 and 2 are complete. The final approval by the management teams and the union for these changes is in process. The team is currently integrating QSEN and other related competencies in levels 3 and 4 of the clinical ladder. The clinical levels 3 and 4 nurses have been educated on the basics of QSEN.

More nurses at multiple levels between the organizations have become involved as a result of the enhanced connectedness between the various groups and the organizations. Partnering for quality and safety has resulted in several new projects between the two organizations. Quality and safety as a shared goal has created a solid foundation for this budding academic-service partnership.

REFLECTING ON ... PARTNERSHIPS

- *How can a reflective process be used to bring people together?*

- *How does a reflective process like appreciative inquiry facilitate teamwork and collaboration?*

- *How does individual and group reflection transform education and practice?*

Final Reflections

These four vignettes provide examples of how faculty at the CGN have used reflection on practice to advance patient safety and quality, diversity, interprofessional collaboration, and professional role development in both academic and clinical practice settings. Reflective practice deepens clinical wisdom in areas that matter the most to patients, families, health professionals, and healthcare organizations. Reflective practices led to changes in knowledge, competencies, and patient care improvements, translating vision and knowledge into action. These vignettes provide some answers to questions raised in the previous chapter. Other questions remain:

- How will we study and capture data on the outcomes of reflective organizations?

- What are the policy implications if research demonstrates that better patient care is linked to the use of reflective practices?

- What are the technology implications and how is reflective practice documented in electronic health records (EHR)?

The CGN faculty team at WesternU looks forward to finding answers to these questions. Working collaboratively across our organization, communities, and around the globe, nursing can take leadership to assure that the Triple Aim goal becomes a reality and a positive turning point in healthcare.

References

Agency for Healthcare Research and Quality (AHRQ). (2012, October). *Patient safety primers: Safety culture.* Retrieved from http://psnet.ahrq.gov/primer.aspx?primerID=5

American Association of Colleges of Nursing (AACN). (2009, November). *Establishing a culturally competent master's and doctorally prepared nursing workforce.* Retrieved from www.aacn.nche.edu/education-resources/CulturalComp.pdf

American Association of Critical-Care Nurses (AACN). (2005). *AACN standards for establishing and sustaining healthy work environments: A journey to excellence.* Alisa Viejo, CA: American Association of Critical-Care Nurses.

American Interprofessional Health Collaborative. (2012). What is AIHC? Retrieved from www.aihc-us.org/what-is-aihc/

American Nurses Association (ANA). (2001). *Code of ethics for nurses with interpretive statements.* Silver Spring, MD: American Nurses Association.

American Nurses Association (ANA). (2010). *Nursing's social policy statement: The essence of the profession.* Silver Spring, MD: American Nurses Association.

American Nurses Association (ANA). (2011). *Scope and standards of practice* (2nd ed.). Silver Spring, MD: American Nurses Association.

Barnsteiner, J. (2011a, September 15). *State of the science of safety and quality: Call to arms.* Podium presentation at the American Association of Colleges of Nursing, Quality and Safety Education in Nursing: Enhancing faculty capacity preparing nurse faculty to lead curricular change. QSEN Education Consortium, Seattle, WA.

Barnsteiner, J. (2011b, September 15). *Just culture and high reliability organizations.* Podium presentation at the American Association of Colleges of Nursing, Quality and Safety Education in Nursing: Enhancing faculty capacity preparing nurse faculty to lead curricular change. QSEN Education Consortium, Seattle, WA.

Benner, P., Sutphen, M., Leonard, V., & Day, L. (2010). *Educating nurses.* San Francisco, CA: Jossey-Bass.

Blue, A. V., Mitcham, M., Smith, T., Raymond, J., & Greenberg, R. (2010). Changing the future of health professions: Embedding interprofessional education within an academic health center. *Academic Medicine, 85*(8), 1290–1295.

Conner, S. (2012). *Strategies for making assessment of QSEN competencies efficient and conducive to learning: Module 8 [electronic resource].* Retrieved from www.qsen.org/modules/module8/content.php

Cooperrider, D. L., Whitney, D., & Stavros, J. M. (2008). *The appreciative inquiry handbook: For leaders of change* (2nd ed.). San Francisco, CA: Berrett-Koehler Publishers.

Cronenwett, L., Sherwood, G., Barnsteiner, J., Disch, J., Johnson, J., Mitchell, P., … Warren, J. (2007). Quality and safety education for nurses. *Nursing Outlook, 55*(3), 122–131.

Cronenwett, L., Sherwood, G., Pohl, J., Barnsteiner, J., Moore, S., Sullivan, D. T., … Warren, J. (2009). Quality and safety education for advanced nursing practice. *Nursing Outlook, 57*(6), 338–348. doi:10.1016/j.outlook.2009.07.009

Crowell, D. M. (2010). *Complexity leadership: Nursing's role in health care delivery.* Philadelphia, PA: FA Davis Company.

Flores, L., Shakhshir, P., & Lopez, M. (2014). *Clinical evaluation tools embodying AACN BSN essentials and 6 QSEN KSAs. QSEN Institute.* Retrieved from http://qsen.org/clinical-evaluation-tools-integrating-qsen-core-competencies-and-aacn-bsn-essentials/

Freshwater, D. (2012). Foreword. In G. W. Sherwood, & S. Horton-Deutsch, *Reflective practice: Transforming education and improving outcomes* (pp. xxiv–xxv). Indianapolis, IN: Sigma Theta Tau International.

Health and Human Services Administration: Health Resources and Service Administration, Bureau of Health Professions, National Center for Health Workforce Analysis. (April 2013). *The US nursing workforce: Trends in supply and education.* Retrieved from http://bhpr.hrsa.gov/healthworkforce/reports/nursingworkforce/nursingworkforcefullreport.pdf

Interprofessional Education Collaborative (IPEC). (2011). *Core competencies for interprofessional collaborative practice.* Retrieved from https://ipecollaborative.org/uploads/IPEC-Core-Competencies.pdf

Jarzemsky, P. (2009, June 29). *A template for simulation scenario development that incorporates QSEN competencies.* Retrieved from http://qsen.org/a-template-for-simulation-scenario-development-that-incorporates-qsen-competencies/

Johnson, J. (2011, September 15). *Change for quality and patient safety.* Podium presentation at the American Association of Colleges of Nursing, Quality and Safety Education in Nursing: Enhancing faculty capacity preparing nurse faculty to lead curricular change. QSEN Education Consortium, Seattle, WA.

Khatri, N., Brown, G. D., & Hicks, L. L. (2009). From a blame culture to a just culture in health care. *Health Care Management Review*, *34*(4), 312–332.

Mind Tools. (n.d.). *The 5 Why's: Getting to the root of a problem quickly*. Retrieved from www.mindtools.com/pages/article/newTMC_5W.htm

National Research Council. (2001). *Crossing the quality chasm: A new health system for the 21st century*. Washington, DC: National Academies Press.

National Research Council. (2003). *Health professions education: A bridge to quality*. Washington, DC: National Academies Press.

National Research Council. (2011). *The future of nursing: Leading change, advancing health*. Washington, DC: National Academies Press.

Sherwood, G. W., & Horton-Deutsch, S. (2012). *Reflective practice: Transforming education and improving outcomes*. Indianapolis, IN: Sigma Theta Tau International.

Shulman, L. S. (2002). Making differences: A table of learning. *Change*, *34*(6), 36–44.

Six Sigma. (2015). Determine the root cause: 5 Why's. Retrieved from www.isixsigma.com/tools-templates/cause-effect/determine-root-cause-5-whys/

Tanner, C. (2006). Thinking like a nurse: A research-based model of clinical judgment in nursing. *Journal of Nursing Education*, *45*(6), 204–211.

United States Census Bureau Newsroom Archive (December 12, 2012). *U.S. census bureau projections show a slower growing, older, more diverse nation a half century from now*. Retrieved from https://www.census.gov/newsroom/releases/archives/population/cb12-243.html

United States Health and Human Services Administration: Health Resources and Service Administration, Bureau of Health Professions, National Center for Health Workforce Analysis. (April 2013). *The US nursing workforce: Trends in supply and education*. Retrieved from http://bhpr.hrsa.gov/healthworkforce/reports/nursingworkforce/nursingworkforcefullreport.pdf

Welch, M. (2003). *Teaching diversity and cross-cultural competence in health care: A trainer's guide. Perspectives of differences diversity training and consultation services for health professionals*. San Francisco, CA: Perspectives of Differences Diversity Training and Consultation Services for Health Professionals (PODSDT).

Zimmerman, B., Lindberg, C., & Plsek, P. (1998). A complexity science primer. Plexus Institute Material - Adapted From: Edgeware: Lessons from complexity science for health care leaders. Dallas, TX: VHA.

Resources

Sigma Theta Tau International Honor Society of Nursing. (2014). *Diversity resources.* Retrieved from www.nursingsociety.org/GlobalAction/Initiatives/Pages/diversity.aspx

United States Health and Human Services Department of Minority Health. (2014). *Think cultural health.* Retrieved from https://www.thinkculturalhealth.hhs.gov/Content/ContinuingEd.asp

United States Health and Human Services Health Resources and Service Administration. (2014). *Culture, language and health literacy.* Retrieved from www.hrsa.gov/culturalcompetence/index.html

Part V

Sustaining Self and Interprofessional Partnerships: Guidance for Transformational Leaders

Chapter 16

Building Academic Cultures With Reflective Practice in Mind: Leadership Agility and Transformational Learning

Daniel J. Pesut, PhD, RN, PMHCNS-BC, FAAN
Sarah A. Thompson, PhD, RN, FAAN

Academic leaders are faced with complex and dynamic challenges: disruptive innovation such as MOOCs; budget cuts in many areas such as state support, research dollars, and philanthropy; changing student needs and expectations; and new educational competitors. Leaders are called to continually reflect upon and refine their skills to move their colleges and schools forward. The purpose of this chapter is to prompt reflection on the topic of leadership agility and skill sets that create, build, and sustain future-oriented academic cultures. To build and transform academic cultures, a fundamental challenge rests in understanding how leadership agility skills can be enhanced and developed in self and others.

The value of futures-literacy and futures-thinking is highlighted. Differences between change and transformation are discussed. Leadership agility is described and discussed as a function of professional insight and mastery of self, context, stakeholders, and creative reflective judgment. The nature of leadership agility skills and the importance of transformational learning to develop one's leadership skill set is described and discussed. Specific developmental lines of a leader's action-logics are outlined. The types of leadership skills needed to build and sustain an academic culture are recommended. Questions designed to prompt personal reflection of one's values, beliefs, and current levels of leadership are presented. Readers are challenged to reflect on and consider the leadership agility skill sets of self and others with whom they work in order to clarify one's contribution to the academic enterprise.

FUTURES-LITERACY

Having knowledge of future thinking research knowledge, methods and skills. Creating scenarios about the future that inform actions and decision in the present.

FUTURES-THINKING

Attention, understanding and insight related to the cross impact analysis of healthcare industry trends and cascading consequences that have social, economic, demographic, governmental and policy impact.

Futures-Literacy: Change Versus Transformation

Transformation and redesign of a 21st-century healthcare system requires understanding the differences concerning change and transformation. Strategist and consultant Chris McGoff (2011) observes that a *change* is a fix, whereas a *transformation* is a creation. Transformation is about responding to a desired future. Transformation is supported by futures-literacy (Miller, 2011). *Futures-literacy* invites people to create and share stories about the future to inform current practice and realities. Nurse educators who want to build innovations across educational programs must engage in futures-thinking (Pesut, 2000; Pesut & Pesut, 2010) and be knowledgeable about trends and consequences that are likely to impact strategic planning, curriculum development, and the future of academic enterprises.

For example, the National Center for Healthcare Leadership (http://nchl.org/index.asp) convened futurists to discern trends related to the state of health in the 21st century. The following list describes some of the identified trends:

- The United States will become part of a global system focusing on wellness and preventive care worldwide.

- Patients will receive care from "virtual" centers of excellence around the world.

- Deeper understanding of the human genome will create exciting new forms of drugs that will prevent disease. Treatment will evolve from disease management to prevention or minimization.

- As baby boomers become senior citizens around 2020, the issue of rising costs, resource allocation, and priorities will be exacerbated.

- Fueled by access to information through the Internet, people will take more self-management of their personal health decisions and demand that healthcare providers and healthcare systems treat them as customers rather than users.

- Most Americans will receive care from specialized centers for chronic diseases (cancers, women's health, cardiac issues, and others).

- Standard diagnostic health will largely be electronic, with people conducting their own "doctor visits" from home via miniature data collection and monitoring devices.

These and other such trends have consequences for the type of educational programs that will develop future workers' skill sets. A need exists to build academic cultures that support innovation and a futures-thinking mindset. Creating and sustaining such cultures requires transformational leadership skills on the part of all faculty, administrators, and community stakeholders. Because academic enterprises have a mission to prepare next generation, healthcare workers faculty and administrators would be wise consider the results of a recent report by the Institute of the Future, commissioned by the Phoenix Research Institute. This report identifies six drivers and 10 skills necessary for a 2020 workforce (http://cdn.theatlantic.com/static/front/docs/sponsored/phoenix/ future_work_skills_2020.pdf):

- **Extreme longevity.** Increasing global life spans will change the nature of careers and learning.

- **Smart machines and systems.** Such technology will influence work place automation, nudging human workers out of rote repetitive tasks.

- **Computational world.** Massive increases in sensors and processing power will make the world a programmable system.

- **New media ecology.** This evolution will evoke new communication tools and require new media literacies beyond text.

- **Superstructured organizations.** Such organizations will harness social technologies and drive new forms of production and value creation.

- **Globally connected world.** Global connectivity will put diversity and adaptability at the center of organizational operations.

The cross-impacts of these drivers' pinpoints and underscores 10 vital skills for a future workforce. These skills should be a part of future academic nursing curricula. The skills and abilities are:

- **Sense-making:** Determining the deeper meaning or significance of what is being expressed

- **Social intelligence:** Connecting with others in a deep and direct way in order to sense and stimulate reactions and desired interactions

- **Novel and adaptive thinking:** Proficiency at thinking and coming up with solutions and responses beyond that which is rote or rule-based

- **Cross-cultural competency:** Capability of operating in different cultural settings

- **Computational thinking:** Capability of translating vast amounts of data into abstract concepts and to understand data-based reasoning

- **New media literacy:** Capability of critically assessing and developing content that uses new media forms, and then leveraging these media for persuasive communication

- **Transdisciplinarity:** Literacy in and the capability to understand concepts across multiple disciplines

- **Design mindset:** Capability to represent and develop tasks and work processes for desired outcomes

- **Cognitive load management:** Capability to discriminate and filter information for importance, and to also understand how to maximize cognitive functioning using a variety of tools and techniques

- **Virtual collaboration:** Capability to work productively, drive engagement, and demonstrate presence as a member of a virtual team

Given the future trends and the vital work force skills described above, faculty and administrators in higher education contexts need to be mindful and appreciative of how these trends and work expectations impact and influence present day program planning, curriculum development, and evaluation. Such mindfulness requires attention to the development of leadership competencies that build academic cultures with a desired future in mind. It is no longer acceptable to replicate past programmatic successes given the demands of future expectations. Thus, nurse leaders in academic contexts must reflect and re-imagine the leadership competencies that are required to sustain success and advance the evolution and development of future-oriented academic cultures that meet the needs of next generation students and stakeholders.

Leadership Competencies That Build Academic Cultures

Reflecting on the drivers and the skills proposed, consider the following:

- To what degree do nurse leaders and educators have the knowledge, skills, and capabilities to create and sustain the academic enterprises that will produce the healthcare workforce of the future?

- How do current academic cultures support innovation and action in service of a desired future?

- What are the leadership competencies that support the creation of innovative academic nursing cultures?

- How does one exercise leadership influence to build academic cultures that are future-oriented?

Given the complexities of healthcare, nurse leaders in academic settings must be influential (Sullivan, 2013). Exerting influence requires leadership competence and agility. The National Center for Healthcare Leadership Competency Model was designed to provide the foundation and support the development of leadership skills for a 21st-century healthcare system. The model makes explicit three essential domains of leadership (transformation, people skills, and execution) and defines 26 competencies within those domains. The domains and competencies are applicable to leadership in academic contexts as well as in other areas of the healthcare enterprise.

The transformation domain involves skills in visionary thinking, energizing and stimulating change processes that engage people and communities in the design, and development of new models of healthcare and wellness. Competencies that support this domain are strategic orientation, innovative thinking, information seeking, analytic thinking, community orientation, financial knowledge management, and stakeholder concerns. Remember that change is a fix: Transformation is a creation with a desired future in mind (McGoff, 2011).

In the people domain, skill expectations and competencies relate to capabilities to engage and energize employees in service of valuing people's capabilities and appreciating the impact that and influence that people have on each other and stakeholders with whom they engage. Competencies that support this domain are relationship-building, interpersonal understanding, professionalism, self-confidence, self-development, talent development, team leadership, and human resources management.

In the execution domain, expected skills and competencies are concerned with translating vision and strategy into organizational performance. Additional competencies that support this domain are organizational awareness, change leadership, impact and influence, accountability, collaboration, communication skills, initiative, information technology management, performance measurement, process management/organizational design, and project management. The domains of transformation, people skills, and execution require understanding and development of leadership agility skills and academic cultures committed to full engagement and development of all stakeholders. It takes leadership agility to activate and realize the competency expectations of future healthcare leaders.

Developing Leadership Agility

Academic leaders need well-developed leadership agility skills to engage faculty and community stakeholders to co-create desired futures. The pace of change will continue to accelerate. With change comes uncertainty. Although there may be threats that one cannot see or predict, there are also opportunities that emerge when people are challenged to create a desired future. Leaders must invest in both creative thought and innovative action to discern what works and what does not work in given contexts (Pesut, 2013a, and 2013b). These leaders must challenge and support the development of healthy academic cultures in order to realize the benefits of full engagement of faculty, staff, students, and community partners.

Leaders who learn to adapt quickly, as well as those who learn how to design effective strategies for chaotic and uncertain environments, will be the effective leaders of the future. Such skills require leadership agility. We believe that the work of Joiner and Josephs (2006) provides a useful framework for reflecting, acknowledging, and building on the leadership competencies and skills sets necessary to succeed in the 21st century. Joiner and Josephs (2006) suggest that the leadership agility required to be successful consists of four competencies and eight skills, shown in their Leadership Compass (see Figure 16.1).

FIGURE 16.1

Leadership Compass with supporting capacities. Reprinted with permission from Leadership agility: Five levels of mastery for anticipating and initiating change, John Wiley & Sons (2006; page 39).

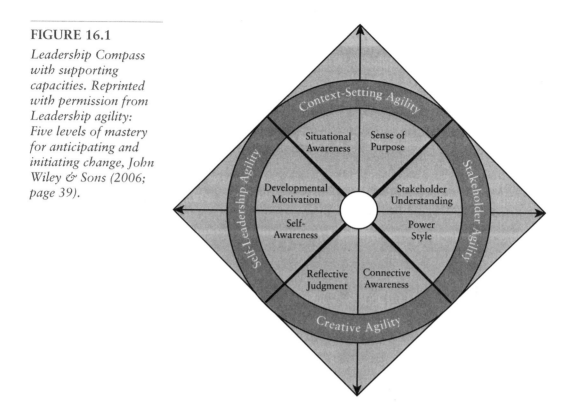

Capacities that support self-leadership agility include self-awareness and developmental motivation. Sense of purpose and situational awareness also support context-setting agility. Stakeholder understanding and appreciation of the influence and effects of power also support mastery of stakeholder agility.

Creative agility is supported by connective awareness and reflective judgment. As you read and reflect on the following skill sets, reflect on your own degree of personal mastery of these skills. Think of successful leaders whom you admire, and consider and reflect on the degree to which they enact the skills described here. Discern your current level of mastery with each skill and reflect on how, specifically, you can enhance the skill sets that you already possess in terms of leadership agility. Highly agile leaders use all four competencies and practice the eight skills. To what degree do you believe you have mastered these skill sets? Read the description and then use the four-point scale in Table 6.1 to assess the degree to which you possess the skills.

Table 16.1: Self-Assessment of Leadership Agility

	NEVER	RARELY	OFTEN	ALWAYS
Self-Leadership Agility				
How comfortable are you with feedback about your performance?	1	2	3	4
Do you actively seek feedback?	1	2	3	4
Are you aware of or do you assess your "shadow side"?	1	2	3	4
Is leadership an opportunity for you to grow personally?	1	2	3	4
Is leadership an opportunity to contribute to a meaningful purpose beyond yourself?	1	2	3	4
Context-Setting Agility				
When you make a decision or begin a new initiative, how often do you consider the impact on other units in your organization or external environment?	1	2	3	4
How often do you initiate decisions or actions while considering the organizational values and purpose?	1	2	3	4
Stakeholder Agility				
How often do you seek input from stakeholders?	1	2	3	4
Have you ever used the opinions of stakeholders to influence your decision-making?	1	2	3	4
Do you engage stakeholders before you have made up your mind?	1	2	3	4
How often have you made a decision without consulting others?	1	2	3	4
Creative Agility				
How often are you able to see multiple issues housed within one problem?	1	2	3	4
When examining opposing views, how often can you see merit in both?	1	2	3	4
How often do you reflect on others' perceptions, assumptions, and opinions?	1	2	3	4
How often do you question your own assumptions?	1	2	3	4

Examine the pattern of your responses. What are your areas of strength, and what areas can you intentionally develop?

Self-Leadership Agility

Self-aware leaders have the desire and ability to learn about their *shadow side*—the unknown aspects of themselves that others may or may not know (Pesut, 2015)—and regularly seek feedback on how others view them. Leaders who possess well-developed self-leadership agility have a keen awareness of how one's thoughts and assumptions shape their feelings and responses to complex problems. They have developed a deep reflective capacity regarding their strengths and limitations as a leader. They are intrinsically motivated to grow as a person and find meaning in their work.

Context-Setting Agility

Leaders who demonstrate context-setting agility have the ability to scan their environment and obtain a deep understanding of interrelated contextual factors that facilitate and impede organizational initiatives and how changes in organizational initiatives intersect with an external environment. Leaders are adept at simultaneously seeing the small and large picture—the forest *and* the trees. These leaders create an organizational sense of purpose based in core values and tied to outcomes. A deeply held purpose serves as a compass to guide decision-making.

Stakeholder Agility

Leaders who embody stakeholder agility actively engage stakeholders, firmly believing in the wisdom gained from diverse opinions. Stakeholders facilitate an understanding of diverse opinions and perceptions, influence decision-making, and are not *used* to achieve one's personal agenda. Stakeholder wisdom is a key source of support and power. Assertive power approaches are rarely used.

Creative Agility

Creative agility is reflected in a comfort with and acceptance of ill-structured, poorly defined, complex problems. These novel problems cross departments, organizations, and external constituencies. Leaders grasp the interconnections and are able to hold and understand two opposing views, realizing and appreciating that opposing views each have merit. Leaders seek and evaluate new untried solutions. Using well-developed self-reflection, creative agility enhances the ability to examine assumptions, self, and others. Leaders adept at creative agility reflect on diverse viewpoints and understand that perceptions are reality. Reflective ability leads to deeper insights and more thoughtful action.

Reflective Practice and Transformational Learning

Active development of leadership agility skills is likely to help leaders build and sustain transformational academic nursing cultures. Such development requires insight and understanding of reflective practices and transformational learning principles. Jack Mezirow (1991) defines learning as "the process of construing and appropriating a new or revised interpretation of the meaning of an experience as a guide to awareness, feeling and action" (p. 35). Mezirow (1991) cites three types of reflection:

- **Content reflection** is thinking about the actual experience.

- **Process reflection** is thinking how to handle the experience.

- **Premise reflection** involves examining long-held, socially constructed assumptions, beliefs, and values about the experience or problem.

Griffiths & Tann (1991) propose a five-level model of reflective process:

1. **Rapid reaction.** This first level is instinctive and immediate.

2. **Repair reflection.** The second level is more habitual and often activated on the spot.

3. **Review reflection.** The third type of reflection involves time out for reassessment and may take place over hours or days.

4. **Research reflection.** This level is systematic, is sharply focused, and takes place over weeks or months.

5. **Reformulation reflection.** This final level is abstract, rigorous, and clearly formulated, and it takes place over weeks, months, or years.

Whether academic leaders uses Mezirow's or Griffiths and Tann's reflective processes, reflective practice is an essential skill in their management and leadership toolkit.

One of many ways a leader can build and sustain transformation in academic cultures is to actively engage the various types of reflection among individuals, groups, and teams. Because, as Mezirow (1991) suggests, "[T]ransformative learning involves reflectively transforming the beliefs, attitudes, opinions and emotional reactions that constitute our meaning making schemes or transforming our meaning perspectives (sets of related meaning schemes)" (p. 223). Meaning-making is a function of the developmental achievements and stages of an individual's action logics. As individuals move through the states of concrete experience, reflective observation, abstract conceptualization, and active experimentation, learning insight occurs (Kolb, 1984).

Meaning-Making and Developmental Levels of Leadership

The developmental level of a leader or member of a team influences the nature of leadership, followership, team dynamics, and organizational culture in which they operate. From a constructivist cognitive developmental theoretical framework (Pruyn, 2010), individuals create and make meaning of situations based on experience, values, and beliefs, and grow and develop through time (Cook-Grueter, 1990; Rooke & Torbert, 2005). Consider the developmental levels described in Table 16.2 in light of building academic cultures and developing organizational leaders.

Building on the work of Bradford and Cohen (1997, 1998), Joiner and Josephs (2006) define and describe five distinct developmental levels of leadership mastery:

1. Expert

2. Achiever

3. Catalyst

4. Co-creator

5. Synergist

Each level has a signature view of leadership with associated talents and strengths for leading teams and organizations. Table 16.2 details the five developmental levels. Note that these five levels of developmental mastery build on the basic foundation of a pre-expert level of development. Joiner and Josephs suggest that that these levels can be placed in two other categories: *heroic* and *post-heroic* stages of leadership.

The sections that follow Table 16.2 include a brief discussion of the five developmental levels, each of which includes an illustrative example from academic nursing.

REFLECTING ON … HEROIC/POST-HEROIC LEADERSHIP

- *How can people in your organization develop along the heroic/post-heroic leadership path?*

- *How, specifically, do these people impact and influence the culture and sustainability of an organization dedicated to transformation and creating a desired future?*

- *What role do pre-expert followers play in an organization and how are they included in the strategic and tactical organizational planning?*

- *What sorts of cognitive, emotional and or developmental experiences do you think help leaders advance, grow and develop into later leadership categories?*

Table 16.2: Joiner and Josephs' Five Levels of Agility*

LEVEL OF AGILITY	VIEW OF LEADERSHIP	AGILITY IN PIVOTAL CONVERSATIONS
Heroic Levels		
Pre-expert (~10%)	May not see self as a leader but more of a follower.	Willing to follow and be a good citizen in support of formal lines of authority in regard to leadership.
Expert (~45%)	Tactical, problem-solving orientation. Believes that leaders are respected and followed by others because of their authority and expertise.	Style is either to strongly assert opinions or hold back to accommodate others. May swing from one style to the other, particularly for different relationships. Tends to avoid giving or requesting feedback.
Achiever (~35%)	Strategic outcomes orientation. Believes that leaders motivate others by making it challenging and satisfying to contribute to larger objectives.	Primarily assertive or accommodative with some ability to compensate with the less-preferred style. Will accept or even initiate feedback, if helpful in achieving desired outcomes.
Post-heroic levels		
Catalyst (~5%)	Visionary; facilitates orientation. Believes that leaders are articulate and innovative, inspiring vision and bring together the right people to transform the vision into reality. Leaders empower others and actively facilitate their development.	Adept at balancing assertive and accommodative styles as needed in particular situations. Likely to articulate and question underlying assumptions. Genuinely interested in learning from diverse viewpoints. Proactive in seeking and applying feedback.
Co-creator (~4%)	Oriented toward shared purpose and collaboration. Believes leadership is ultimately a service to others. Leaders collaborate with other leaders to develop a shared vision that each experiences as deeply purposeful.	Integrates assertive and accommodative sides in pivotal conversations and is agile in using both styles. Able to process and seriously consider negative feedback even when highly charged emotionally.
Synergist (~1%)	Holistic orientation. Experiences leadership as participation in a palpable life purpose that benefits others while serving as a vehicle for personal transformation.	Centered "within" not "with" assertive and accommodative energies, expressed as appropriate to the situation. Cultivates a present-centered awareness that augments external feedback and supports a strong subtle connection with others, even during challenging conversations.

AGILITY IN LEADING TEAMS	AGILITY IN LEADING ORGANIZATIONAL CHANGE
More likely to be loyal follower rather than a leader.	Committed to organizational goals and objective in support of authorizing agents or leaders.
More of a supervisor than a manager. Creates a group of individuals rather than a team. Work with direct reports is primarily one-on-one. Too caught up in the details of own work to lead in a strategic manner.	Organizational initiatives focus primarily on incremental improvements inside unit boundaries with little attention to stakeholders.
Operates like a full-fledged manager. Meetings to discuss important strategic or organizational issues are often orchestrated to try to gain buy-in to own views.	Organizational initiatives include analysis of industry environment. Strategies to gain stakeholders' buy-in range from one-way communication to soliciting input.
Intent on creating a highly participative team. Acts as a team leader and facilitator. Provides and seeks open exchange of views on difficult issues. Empowers direct reports. Uses team development as a vehicle for leadership development.	Organizational initiatives often include development of a culture that promotes teamwork, participation, and empowerment. Proactive engagement with diverse stakeholders reflects a belief that their input increases the quality of decisions, not just buy-in.
Develops a collaborative leadership team, where members feel full responsibility not only for their own areas but also for the unit or organization they collectively manage. Practical preference for consensus decision-making but doesn't hesitate to use authority as needed.	Develops key stakeholder relationships characterized by deep levels of mutual influence and genuine dedication to the common good. May create companies or organizational units where corporate responsibility and deep collaboration are integral practices.
Capable of moving fluidly between various team leadership styles uniquely suited to the situation at hand. Can shape or amplify the energy dynamics at work in a particular situation to bring about mutually beneficial results.	Develops and maintains a deep empathetic awareness of conflicting stakeholder interests, including the leader's own. Able to access synergistic intuitions that transform seemingly intractable conflicts into solutions beneficial for all parties involved.

Each level of agility includes and goes beyond the competencies developed at previous levels. The percentage figures refer to research-based estimates of the managers currently capable of operating at each agility level.

360-DEGREE PERFORMANCE FEEDBACK

Feedback is provided from one's peers and subordinates as well as supervisor. This approach facilitates a more comprehensive view of one's performance including such aspects as communication, interpersonal relations, teamwork, and basic job skills from multiple perspectives.

Experts

Expert leaders are task-oriented and have developed little capacity for self-reflection. They address problems one by one, without considering the larger context, such as how a problem or solution intersects with the larger organization. For experts, leadership is a formal title—one that should garner respect from subordinates. Expert leaders rely on authority and evaluate their success by running a highly efficient unit. They rarely seek others' opinions or feedback on their performance.

For example, consider John, who is the director of student services in a college of nursing. There are several process issues related to student recruitment, admissions, and progression, especially the tracking of student data. John has completed several courses in data management and is proud of his expertise. He implements problem-solving strategies in each area without viewing the interconnections among the three processes. He does not elicit the views of stakeholders such as potential applicants, current students, student service staff, or faculty. Because of his educational training, he believes he knows best. John creates a data management process but is unaware of how it could potentially intersect with the organization's other data systems. Several of his direct reports are annoyed that he did not seek their input into the development and implementation, and they complain to his supervisor. John is confused by their anger: He has little self-awareness, believing that he has done a good job and solved a problem.

Achievers

Achievers are more self-reflective regarding their values and beliefs: They have a greater awareness of context and some capacity for feedback. They use data to make decisions but lack awareness of how their own biases may influence decision-making. Achievers realize that they need stakeholder buy-in, but they have difficulty using stakeholder input to facilitate decision-making. They have moved from managing tasks to managing people, but believe that it is their role to bring stakeholders around to their viewpoint. Achievers believe they are effective leaders if they adhere to strategic plans and design sound organizational systems and processes.

For example, Sally is dean of a college of nursing, and she wants to cut programs that she believes are inefficient due to lower enrollment. She charges her directors of finance and academic programs to gather and display data in a manner that illustrates how the two programs are losing revenue. She brings stakeholders together for dialogue and uses the data to convince others that the programs need to be cut. Sally elicits others' viewpoints but does not use the information to seek or consider alternative solutions. Many of the faculty are frequently heard saying, "She has made up her mind before the meeting. Why do we go?" Sally meets target goals of efficiency and quality on an annual basis, but she doesn't understand why morale in the organization is low.

Catalysts

Catalysts seek solutions that are influenced by diverse viewpoints, moving from using stakeholders to gain buy-in to a deep awareness that complex problems benefit from multiple perspectives. Catalyst leaders create teams where input is essential and valued. They have a greater understanding of how context, internal and external, influences problems and shapes solutions. Catalysts are much more reflective and are able to use this skill in the present moment to enhance communication. They are able to see merit in diametrically opposed viewpoints. Catalysts have a deeper awareness of human behavior, and understand the intersection of assumptions, values, feelings, and relationships. They invest in the development of people and teams, seek feedback, and promote a culture of participation and teamwork.

For example, Henry is a new dean at a college of nursing located within a thriving academic health science center. Keenly aware of the rapidly evolving higher education and healthcare landscapes, he quickly develops relationships with multiple and diverse stakeholders, such as chief nursing officers, community leaders, and elected officials. Understanding that the wisdom gained from multiple perspectives is greater than his own, he creates a diverse advisory board to guide the college's response to potential initiatives and real challenges. Henry has considerable ability to engage in self-reflection and works to gain increasing awareness of his shadow side. He values feedback and uses a professional coach to continually increase his capacity as a leader and requests 360-degree performance feedback at the end of his first year. He fosters team development and organizational learning.

Co-Creators

At the co-creator level, the leader is service-oriented and purpose-driven for the common good. Motivated by a sense of interconnectedness, the co-creator leader fosters high-level collaboration and shared responsibility. The co-creator leader moves into a deeper understanding of others' needs and perceptions while maintaining an ability to make independent decisions. This leader has developed comfort with ill-structured, emotionally charged, and mentally complex challenges and is keenly aware of the mutual shaping of realities. The co-creator uses mindful attention and intention to stay with difficult feelings during complex encounters and can see simultaneously micro and macro perspectives. At the co-creator level, leaders embody a deep and complex awareness of self. Facilitated by the understanding that culture is created, the co-creator intentionally crafts a learning organization.

Another dean, Ann, works quickly to align her college's mission, vision, and values to a central purpose—that of improving the health and well-being of people. Under her leadership, the college develops programs that will extend its impact regionally and nationally. She uses techniques such as *Liberating Structures* (Lipmanowicz & McCandless, 2013), which is a rapid-paced, interactive process that unleashes organizations' or teams' creative potential by fostering diverse opinions, safety, engagement, dialogue, respect, trust, self-reflection, and discovery. Through processes such as Liberating Structures, Ann engages multiple constituents to create a dynamic vision and to design and transform the future of nursing.

Synergists

For synergists, leadership is about life-purpose. These leaders have a deep sense of meaning and purpose beyond themselves. For them, the organization has a greater purpose to influence the common good, but the magnitude moves from national to global. Synergists not only have deep and empathetic understanding of themselves and others, but also they use intuitive promptings to foster transformative approaches. Development of people and self is not about perfection, but rather a journey toward wholeness.

Given that these leaders represent approximately only 1% of all leaders (refer to Table 16.2), it is difficult to adequately illustrate this leader with an example. However, it is possible to speculate that two prominent nurse synergists' role models are Martha Rogers and Jean Watson.

REFLECTING ON ... LEADERSHIP MASTERY

- *How does an individual's level of leadership mastery influence the dynamics and cultures of the academic organizations in which they operate?*

- *What thoughts, feelings, or ideas does reflecting on each level of mastery bring up for you?*

- *What description/case study describes your leadership style?*

- *What sort of coaching or leadership development do you believe would help you reach a new level? How about your team or organization?*

Final Reflections

The intersection of complex and dynamic academic and healthcare environments calls for new leadership skills. Combining reflection, futures literacy, and leadership agility offers leaders skills to create, build, and sustain future-oriented academic cultures. Readers are urged to reflect on their own leadership agility and acknowledge their personal stage of leadership development; using this understanding of self, leaders can consider how to foster their own personal growth as well as that of their organization.

References

Bradford, D., & Cohen, A. (1997). *Managing for excellence: The leadership guide to developing high performance in contemporary organizations.* Hoboken, NJ: John Wiley & Sons.

Bradford, D., & Cohen, A. (1998). *Power up: Transforming organizations through shared leadership.* Hoboken, NJ: John Wiley & Sons.

Cook-Greuter, S. R. (1990). Maps for living: Ego-development theory from symbiosis to conscious universal embeddedness. In M. L. Commons, J. D. Sinnott, F. A. Richards, & C. Armon (Eds.), *Adult development: Vol. 2, Comparisons and applications of adolescent and adult developmental models* (pp. 79–104). New York, NY: Praeger.

Griffiths M., & Tann, S. (1991). Ripples in the reflection. In P. Loma (Ed.), *BERA Dialogues,* No. 5 (pp. 82–101). London, England.

Joiner, W., & Josephs, S. (2006). *Leadership agility: Five levels of mastery for anticipating and initiating change.* New York, NY: John Wiley & Sons.

Kolb, D. (1984). *Experiential learning.* Upper Saddle River, NJ: Prentice-Hall.

Lipmanowicz, H., & McCandless, K. (2013). *The surprising power of liberating structures: Simple rules to unleash a culture of innovation.* Seattle, WA: Liberating Structures Press.

McGoff, C. (2011). *The primes: How any group can solve any problem.* New York, NY: Victory Publishers.

Mezirow, J. (1991). *Transformational dimensions of adult learning.* San Francisco, CA: Jossey-Bass.

Miller, R. (2011). Futures literacy: Embracing complexity and using the future. *Ethos, 10,* 23–28. Retrieved from www.cscollege.gov.sg/Knowledge/ethos/Issue%2010%20 Oct%202011/Pages/Opinion%20F

Pesut, D. (2015). Avoiding derailment: Leadership strategies for identity, reputation and legacy management. In J. Daly, S. Speedy, & D. Jackson (Eds.), *Leadership & nursing contemporary perspectives* (2nd edition) (pp. 251–261). Chatswood (NSW), Australia: Churchill Livingston, Elsevier.

Pesut, D. (2013a). Book review of the innovation equation: Building creativity and risk taking in your organization, by Jacqueline Byrd and Paul Brown. *Creative Nursing, 9*(3), 164–165.

Pesut, D. (2013b). Creativity and innovation: Thought and action. *Creative Nursing, 19*(3), 114–121.

Pesut, D. J., & Pesut, E. Z. (2010). Future forces affecting 21st century health professions education: Mastering the knowledge, skills, and abilities to support 21st century learning. In L. Caputi (Ed.), *Teaching nursing: The art and science* (2nd Ed., Vol. 1) (pp. 198–228). Glen Ellyn, IL: College of Dupage Press.

Pesut, D. (2000). Looking forward: Being and becoming a futurist. *Nurses Taking the Lead. Personal Qualities of Effective Leadership* (pp. 39–65). Pennsylvania, PA: WB Saunders Company.

Pruyn, P. (2010). *An overview of constructive developmental theory (CDT).* Retrieved from http://www.developmentalobserver.blog.com/2010/06/09/an-overview-of-constructive-developmental-theory-cdt/

Rooke, D., & Torbert, W. R. (2005). Seven transformations of leadership. *Harvard Business Review, 83*(4), 66–76.

Sullivan, E. (2013). *Becoming influential: A guide for nurses* (2nd ed.). Boston, MA: Pearson Education.

The Institute of the Future for the University of Phoenix Research Institute. (2011). Future work skills 2020. Retrieved from http://cdn.theatlantic.com/static/front/docs/ sponsored/phoenix/future_work_skills_2020.pdf

The National Center for Healthcare Leadership (NCHL). Retrieved from http://nchl.org/ index.asp

Chapter 17

Partnering to Create Sustainable Futures: Organizational Leadership Strategies That Invite Engagement, Reflection, and Action

Sara Horton-Deutsch, PhD, RN, PMHCNS, FAAN, ANEF
Kathryn Kuehn, BA
Gwen D. Sherwood, PhD, RN, FAAN, ANEF

Throughout this book, we introduced reflective models and theories. Stories and practices relate how using these reflective approaches facilitates and embraces transformation. In each chapter, the authors demonstrated the reflective process of learning from experience to craft future transformations. Sherwood and Horton-Deutsch (2012) presented reflection as a systematic way of thinking about actions and responses to create a preferred future. In this chapter, we explore how organizational leaders—particularly those who work at professional and service organizations—reflect on and cultivate their own strengths to act in partnership with others to serve the greater good. Successful leadership within the organizational context requires self-knowledge and skills (Pesut, 2007), an appreciation of evolving trends in organizations (Coerver & Byers, 2011), and engaging members in intentional ways to create a sustainable future.

Strength-Based Leadership to Transform Organizations

Pesut (2007) states, "[U]nderstanding and intentionally using one's strengths in an organizational context are among the keys to successful organizational leadership and governance" (p.157). Knowing one's individual talents and strengths accelerates ability to work more efficiently and effectively with others. Strength-based leadership (Rath & Conchie, 2008) identifies and values the individual strengths of group members, recognizing the collective whole is greater than any part. Diversity among organization and/or team members increases the overall capacity; organizations gain strength through the collection of diverse talents of group members. The Gallup Organization has researched signature strengths of leaders for more than 30 years (Rath & Conchie, 2008), and its work is currently portrayed in 34 signature strengths that cluster into four domains: executing, influencing, relationship building, and strategic thinking.

Applying Leadership Domains

To become a more effective leader, Rath and Conchie (2008) advocate three approaches. First, leaders need to recognize their own strengths, and leaders must also invest in helping others develop their strengths. Second, leaders need to identify the strengths needed to accomplish the goals of the organization or team and then recruit people with the right strengths to meet those goals. Third, effective leaders must understand and ensure that the four basic domains of executing, influencing, relationship-building, and strategic thinking are well represented in the organization or team. The following list describes these domains:

- **Executing.** Leaders whose strengths lie in the executing domain make things happen. They are action-oriented and work tirelessly toward a goal.

- **Influencing.** These leaders ensure the larger organization is heard by reaching out to members.

- **Relationship building.** These leaders hold the team together and ensure that the organization is greater than the sum of its parts.

- **Strategic thinking.** These leaders keep everyone focused on what is possible. They constantly analyze information as it is gathered and help the team make good decisions.

The most effective teams have representation of strengths in each of the four domains. Complementary teams value all contributions and drive organizational growth.

REFLECTING ON ... LEADERSHIP DOMAINS

- *Consider a team/group/professional or community service board with which you currently are working. Can you identify characteristics of each domain among the members?*

- *How can you use your and your team members' unique strengths to maximize contributions?*

Transforming Organizational Culture

Transforming organizational culture is complex and challenges even high-functioning teams. Internal and external intersections impact organizations. Evolving trends in the external environment directly or indirectly affect internal organizational cultures, and long-established values, beliefs, and behaviors that characterize group members are often deeply embedded, and thus difficult to replace. Societal trends also influence culture. Coerver and Byers, in "Race for Relevance" (2011), identify how six marketplace realities that occurred over the past 25 years have significantly influenced the way people function in organizations:

- **Time.** Americans are working more and longer hours, and face increasing demands on their time, making "work/life balance" an elusive goal.

- **Value expectations.** The growth in products and services in the past two decades has fueled consumer demand and expectations. People want what they want when they want it—and if they don't get it, they turn elsewhere.

- **Market structure.** Consolidations, mergers, and buy-outs are the status quo—increasingly so, since the Great Recession.

- **Generational differences.** For the first time, Coerver and Byers maintain, there are five living generations: four of them working together in the workplace, and each with different values, styles, and expectations.

- **Competition.** Organizations are competing for an increasingly savvy consumer who is dictating the delivery channels of products and services.

- **Technology.** The birth of the Internet has forever changed how organizations operate and serve their employees, members, and markets, and influenced information management and distribution.

REFLECTING ON ... THE EFFECT OF MARKETPLACE REALITIES

- *Which of these marketplace realities impacts your team/group/organization?*
- *How do these realities affect your internal organizational culture?*

Most professional and service organizations have a passionate commitment to make their associations better, stronger, and more relevant to members. At the same time, most organizations are driven by tradition where change occurs slowly and members avoid risk. This traditional drive often results in a broad range of programs, services, and activities. Coerver and Byers (2011) recommend a sequence of radical changes that move from association governance, member market, program and product mix, to technologies to delivery of services. These sequential changes aim to ensure organizational relevance. And even though their work focuses on the structure and activities of nonprofit professional organizations, it can be applied broadly to organizational relevancy overall.

These recommendations include (Coerver & Byers, 2011):

1. Right-size the organization's governance structure to create a small, competency-based board or leadership team where members' presence and attention are essential. A board composed of members who know their strengths and collectively possess all four leadership domains helps to ensure the competencies needed to govern the organization.

2. Streamline committees and retain only those that do valuable and relevant work. Consider the mission of the organization, determine the committees really needed, and retain only those that are useful and productive.

3. Empower the CEO and enhance the contributions of the staff. Because professional organizations have become more complex through expanded programs, services, and activities, they require increased management competencies and the need to delegate responsibilities previously done by volunteers.

4. Focus on the needs of a definable group that helps members perform and succeed. This approach allows organizations to concentrate resources for maximum performance.

5. Concentrate resources on a tightly focused menu of services and member benefits so the organization can excel in a few key areas.

6. Embrace technology, including information, communication, delivery systems, and infrastructure. A comprehensive technology plan that improves efficiency and productivity and meets the needs of members is essential for an organization's relevance and performance.

REFLECTING ON ... ORGANIZATIONAL STRUCTURES AND GOVERNANCE

- *Consider your organization: What structures or processes need to be changed or adopted to address these challenges?*

GENERATIVE THINKING

The process of generating new ideas. Open-ended questions that explore possibilities and encourage exploration of a number of possibilities support generative thinking.

SENSE-MAKING

A reflective dialogue and conversation that aims to gather what members know, believe, and value.

After leaders establish the organization's strengths and clarify the need for changes to ensure relevance, they must engage members in intentional ways to achieve sustainable futures. According to Chait and colleagues (2005), three modes of governance together foster effective leadership: fiduciary, strategic, and generative. Although the first two may be more familiar, the latter is essential for organizational relevance and growth. Before an organization can strategically solve problems and make the most fiscally sound decisions, it must engage in sense-making. Taken together, generative thinking and sense-making—combined with thoughtful consideration of market trends and realities—provide the foundation for both strategic and fiscally sound decisions.

Therefore, the remainder of this chapter will visit ways to engage members of an organization in *sense-making*: a reflective dialogue and conversation that aims to gather what members know, believe, and value. The outcome of this exercise is used to both inform and guide leadership teams within an organization, as well as the iterative process of providing ongoing communication and gathering additional feedback from members to engage them in creating a preferred future. The overall approach to leadership for guiding this process is discussed with questions to facilitate personal reflection for transforming organizations in a way that is responsive to current members. Finally, readers are invited to reflect on ways to bring new life and new connections to their organizations to create relevant and desirable futures to positively influence health and healthcare.

Leadership Strategies That Invite Engagement, Reflection, and Action

Creating desired futures within organizations, as highlighted in the previous chapter, is about transformation that is supported by futures literacy (Miller, 2011). Members are invited to create and share stories about the future to inform current practices (see Chapter 16 of this book by Pesut & Thompson, 2015). *Futures-literacy* guides professional healthcare organizations on how to bridge from their current realities to a preferred future by reflecting on trends and consequences likely to impact forthcoming research, education, and practice affecting the organizational enterprise.

Liberating Structures: Complexity Science for Futures-Thinking to Transform Organizations

Organizations that want to remain relevant must engage in futures-thinking (Pesut, 2000; Pesut & Pesut, 2010) by considering how the past and present influence the future. *Liberating Structures* (Lipmanowicz & McCandless, 2013) are nonhierarchical methodologies based on complexity

FUTURES-THINKING
Refers to thinking about how the past and present influence the future.

LIBERATING STRUCTURES
Easy to learn micro-structures that enhance relational coordination and trust. They foster lively participation in groups and include everyone. Often referred to as disruptive innovation, liberating structures replace more controlling and constraining approaches with group processes that are more inclusive and invite creativity (Lipmanowicz & McCandless, 2014).

science designed to unleash futures-thinking and improve performance. Liberating Structures include and engage everyone in an organization to shift the pattern of interactions and unleash the collective wisdom. For example, at a recent International Society of Psychiatric Mental-Health Nurses interactive closing keynote address, "Creating Desired Futures" (Pesut, 2014), members were asked to engage in a Liberating Structure called *1-2-4-All* (Lipmanowicz & McCandless, 2013) and consider the following questions suggested by Anne Deering, Robert Dilts, and Julian Russell (2002) as a means for leaders to create a future state for an organization:

- If a time traveler from 25 years in the future could give you the answer to one question, what would it be?

- If you were looking back 10 years from now and telling the tale of the organization's greatest success, what would the story be and why?

- If you were looking back 10 years from now and telling the tale of the organization's greatest failure, what would the story be and why?

- What does the organization need to forget? What must it always remember?

- What are the most important strategic decisions we will have to make as an organization?

- What will prevent us from succeeding? What are the greatest risks and dangers?

- If you had the power to do one thing for the organization, what would it be, and why?

The 1-2-4-All exercise took about 12 minutes and engaged the audience as participants in generating questions, ideas, and suggestions for future directions of the organization. Participants broke into small groups, discussed and prioritized a prompt for two minutes, and then moved to a new group to address a new prompt. Participants engaged in a lively conversation about what is possible, included everyone, and tapped into know-how and imagination. Most importantly, participants (members of the organization) own the ideas, so no buy-in strategy is needed later on.

Wicked Questions: Revealing Entangled Challenges and Possibilities Not Readily Obvious

Wicked Questions is another provocative example of using Liberating Structures. A think tank of leaders in the Quality and Safety Education for Nurses (QSEN) project used Wicked Questions to consider how this loosely constructed group could achieve sustainability, remain current and relevant, and deliver resources to continue to improve quality and safety in nursing education and practice. The following sidebar is an exemplar of the session of Wicked Questions.

WICKED QUESTIONS IN ACTION

Shirley Moore, PhD, RN, FAAN and
Mary A. Dolansky, RN, PhD, Director, QSEN Institute
Frances Payne Bolton School of Nursing Case Western Reserve University

The Quality and Safety Education for Nurses (QSEN) Steering Team from Case Western Reserve University School of Nursing held a think tank as a part of the annual QSEN National Forum with key leaders to consider future directions and influences. Recognizing all groups and movements undergo periodic change, as QSEN approaches 10 years, having a conversation to maintain relevancy and sustainability can help determine continued sources of support, engagement, and influence. The session was shaped using the Wicked Question exercise from Liberating Structures (www.liberatingstructures.com/4-wicked-questions/). The group was divided into four tables. Each person would read the question and follow the format of another Liberating Structure, 1-2-All:

- *1 minute: Each person silently reflects on the question to collect his or her thoughts.*

- *2 minutes: Discuss in pairs.*

- *10 minutes: Engage in whole table discussion.*

- *20 minutes: Tables report key thoughts to the entire group.*

Wicked Questions highlight a pair of opposites or paradoxes at play regarding a particular issue or situation. In this case, it was in regard to academic-practice partnerships. A Wicked Question stimulates discussion of the tension that

continues

underlies our work together when a pair of opposites are true at the same time. This discussion can reveal innovative strategies for producing change.

The Wicked Questions for this session were:

1. *If both nursing practice and academic organizations have considerable knowledge regarding how to improve systems, how is it that we don't apply that knowledge to improve our academic-practice partnership systems?*

2. *Assurance of basic competency is a major mission of academia. Delivery of highest quality care is the mission of healthcare delivery organizations. How do these differences in mission play out in our academic-practice partnerships on a daily basis?*

3. *Given that a purpose of academic training for nurses is to help them to conceptualize and give ideal care, how do they learn to give/alter that care within the resource constraints of practice environments?*

4. *If a key feature of successful partnerships is that any partner should feel free to challenge an assertion or raise a concern, how is it that the avoidance of open disagreement is a key normative feature of relationships between nursing practice leaders and academic faculty?*

Leadership as Reflective Practice

The purpose of engaging members of an organization in futures work is not to predict the future but to envision desirable futures and avoid or prevent tragic ones. When leadership teams gather ideas from futures-thinking tools, such as Liberating Structures, they have a launching pad for moving forward. They can move forward with these ideas by discerning logical consequences of trends, stimulating strategic conversations about preferred visions, and considering the value of an integrally informed future.

Beyond this, leadership teams (boards of directors, in this illustration) must become a reflective community of interpretation where they talk seriously about members' feedback and consider it in light of the organizational purpose. "A board's capacity for retrospective sense making–acting then thinking, making sense of past events to produce new meanings" (Chait, Ryan, & Taylor, 2005,

p. 1) relies on effective governance and is key to strategic visioning for the future. Models and assessments that can help board members reflect on the organization's past to create new meanings include Robert Dilts' Logical Levels of Assessment and Reflection Guide (Dilts, 2014), the Purpose-To-Practice Liberating Structure process (Lipmanowicz & McCandless, 2013), and Ecocyle lessons (Hurst, 2012).

REFLECTIVE COMMUNITY OF INTERPRETATION
Working with a team to bring knowledge and wisdom to bear on feedback from others.

Dilts' Logical Levels of Assessment and Reflection Guide

Dilts' Logical Levels of Assessment and Reflection Guide (1996a, b) directs leaders of an organization to consider different levels of leadership (micro, macro, meta) and different levels of change (environment, behaviors, capabilities, beliefs and values, identity, organizational mission, and vision) through reflective questioning (see Table 17.1). *Microlevel leadership* requires attention to task, relationship, behavior, and environmental opportunities and limitations. *Macrolevel leadership* comprises attention to path-finding, culture-building, and sensitivity to beliefs, values, and roles. *Metalevel leadership* requires higher-level attention and mindfulness to issues of identity, mission, and vision. Leaders who work toward alignment of all three levels contribute to the greater good of the organization and those they serve.

The following questions typify the alignment guide and uncover the change an organization is attempting to influence.

- **From an environmental perspective:** What is the external context around strategic planning?

- **From a behavioral perspective:** What specifically must the board of directors do, or what behaviors must it develop to support realization of the strategic plan?

- **From capabilities:** How will the board organize itself to accomplish goals and behaviors? What skill sets are needed?

- **From the perspective of belief and values:** What motivates the board toward aspiration and renewal?

- **From identity:** Who will the board be if it engages those particular beliefs, values, capabilities, and behaviors?

- **From organizational mission:** What does the organization contribute to the larger system or greater universe in which it operates?

- **From vision:** How does clarity about the desired greater purpose influence the identity, mission, values, beliefs, capabilities, behaviors, and environment in which the board and organization finds itself? (See Table 17.1.)

Table 17.1: Dilts' Logical Levels of Assessment and Reflection Guide

Levels of Leadership	Levels of Change	Types of Questions for Reflective Learning
Micro	Environment, behavior, and capability	Where? When? What? How?
Macro	Beliefs, values, and role identity	Why? Who?
Meta	Mission and vision	Who? What else?

These questions get to the core of different levels of change; they influence and help board members to identify and address issues at all levels. Each level of change involves progressively more of the organization. Each level involves different types of interactions that incorporate information from the level above it. Effective leadership addresses issues at all levels.

Purpose-To-Practice Liberating Structure

The Purpose-To-Practice (Lipmanowicz & McCandless, 2013) Liberating Structure enables board members to generate a shared purpose, detailed at www.liberatingstructures.com/33-purpose-to-practice-p2p/. To clarify the organization's purpose, each board member should answer the following question: "Why is the work important to you and the larger community?" The next step is, as a group, to compare, sift, sort, and amplify the top ideas. Then, integrate themes and finalize the ideas for purpose.

Then, repeat this exercise by addressing questions (shown in Figure 17.1) for the following additional elements, which help to achieve the newly defined organizational purpose: principles, participants, structure, and practices. By using these five elements together, board members clarify how they can organize themselves to adapt in creative ways and scale-up for success.

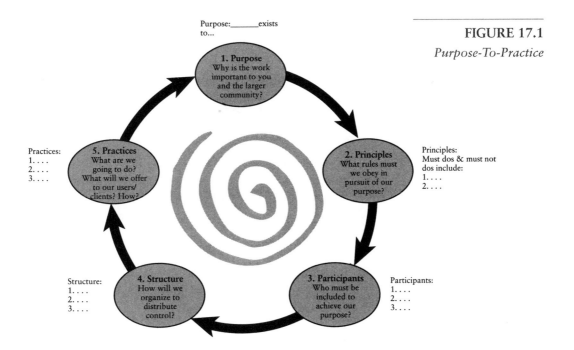

FIGURE 17.1

Purpose-To-Practice

For example, through formal facilitation (Pesut, 2014), one organizational board recently applied the Purpose-To-Practice process to begin to illuminate key components of transformations. Using Dilts' Logical Levels of Assessment and Reflection Guide, board members identified the need for and components of a new mission that was a more accurate reflection of the current activities of members. The board further applied the Purpose-To-Practice process using the Ecocyle activity (described in the next section), which helped recognize that the organizational structure had met maturity. This discovery was consistent with recommendations received from members during their 1-2-4-All Liberating Structures exercise and further confirmed the need for a new organizational direction. Finally, through engaging in the Purpose-To-Practice liberating structure activity, it became clear what a new structure might look like.

THE BACK STORY OF QSEN: LEADERSHIP THAT CHANGED NURSING EDUCATION

Gwen Sherwood, PhD, RN, FAAN, ANEF

Reflecting on the models and frameworks presented in the chapter leads me to recall the story of the Quality and Safety Education for Nursing (QSEN) project funded from 2005–2012 by the Robert Wood Johnson Foundation. Linda Cronenwett at the University of North Carolina–Chapel Hill School of Nursing is the thought leader who pulled the pieces together (Cronenwett, 2012; Cronenwett et al., 2007), who developed the vision of how nursing could begin to craft a response to the Institute of Medicine Quality Chasm series (IOM, 1999, 2001, 2003). The 2003 Health Professions Education: A Bridge to Quality provided a blueprint with a competency framework for all health professionals if we are to improve healthcare delivery systems: patient-centered care, teamwork and collaboration, evidence-based practice, quality improvement, safety, and informatics. Many were asking, "How do we define these competencies in nursing? What will be the vision?"

Looking back, I can see that in fact the development of QSEN followed the Purpose-To-Practice model (P2P) (shown earlier in Figure 17.1) and will share the story within that framework.

1. Purpose: Why is the work important to you and the larger community?

In thinking about developing quality and safety competencies for nursing, we were quick to recall the startling data revealed in the 1999 IOM report, To Err is Human. We were all struck by the numbers;

where did such events occur? How could this many people be dying in our hospitals without our realizing the collective impact? Now that the data had been released, we could not turn back. We had to act, and now the IOM provided a way forward with the 2003 report on health professions education. Ethically, we cannot ignore this imperative: We had to tackle the problem. Linda's idea was to invite an expert panel of national experts in each of the competencies and pedagogical experts who could help to drive the change we knew we needed. Knowing we would need policy changes, leaders from key organizations, including physicians, were invited to participate in an Advisory Council. The purpose of QSEN was to reform nursing professional identity to include a focus on quality and safety to be able to lead and work in redesigned healthcare systems.

2. *Principles: What rules must we obey in pursuit of our purpose?*

   We agreed we would meet together about twice per year; we committed to being present, engaged, and participative. Our work would be mostly completed using online and telephone communication. When we met, we agreed to have no long lectures. We would use theory bursts followed by table top discussions. Each session was carefully planned for small groups so that the people with the content knowledge were appropriately assigned. We would all respect diverse views, listen to each other, engage in the sessions, and complete all assignments in a timely manner.

3. *Participants: Who must be included to achieve our purpose?*

   I have already described the direct project participants for the National Expert Panel and Advisory Council. However, the project was about all of nursing, so it was important to include a broad diversity of nurses. First, the project distributed an electronic survey to all BSN Schools of Nursing and ADN programs in North Carolina for a baseline of what schools already had in the curriculum to address the six competencies. Then, Linda led nine focus groups with nursing faculty at national meetings of nurses and nurse educators (Cronenwett, 2012). The focus groups revealed more detailed information and confirmed the need for extending the QSEN project to include faculty development and pilot projects (Cronenwett, Sherwood, & Gelmon, 2009).

4. *Structure: How will we organize to distribute control?*

   This poses an interesting question because the power paradox helps us to realize that to increase power, we need to let go. Three

continues

strategies tell the story of how QSEN was restructured. First, QSEN was funded for Phase 2 to launch a Pilot School Learning Collaborative of early adopters to test the change. These 15 schools were competitively selected, based on projects they would complete in the coming year (Cronenwett, Sherwood, & Gelmon, 2009). These schools became the launching pad for the initial spread of the competencies. A second power distribution was the selection of 40 early adopters who were named QSEN Facilitators who would be available to other schools to help integrate the six competencies into their curriculum. The third power distribution was to offer free global access to QSEN materials on a robust website (http://qsen.org/), which offers multiple types of resource material.

5. **Practices: What are we going to do? What will we offer to our users/ clients? How?**

The generous funding of the Robert Wood Johnson Foundation made it possible to follow a basic tenet of QSEN: free access of all our products. The website was built with peer-reviewed teaching strategies, annotated bibliography, teaching modules, videos, and presentations. The goal was to provide faculty and others the resources needed to integrate the QSEN competencies into their curriculum. We initiated the annual QSEN National Forum; collaborated with the American Association of Colleges of Nursing, which offered regional faculty development workshops; and worked with publishers to integrate QSEN competencies and teaching strategies into textbooks. As the grant phase completed, QSEN transitioned to a new home at Case Western Reserve University School of Nursing to be able to maintain sustainability.

Ecocyle

The Ecocyle (Lipmanowicz & McCandless, 2013) is another tool that organizational leaders can use to make sense of and honor the past, as well as produce new meanings and guide the future. Lessons from the Ecocyle include:

- Change is continuous along the cycle.

- Renewal requires creative destruction.

- Need for crisis (root word "to sift").

- Need for firebreaks (don't burn everything).

- Balance in activities is the key to long-term survival and adaptability.

- Create conditions for renewal and more "births" (Pesut, 2014).

Ecocyle planning encourages "leaders to focus on creative destruction and renewal in addition to typical themes regarding growth and efficiency" (Lipmanowicz & McCandless, 2013, p. 295). See Figure 17.2.

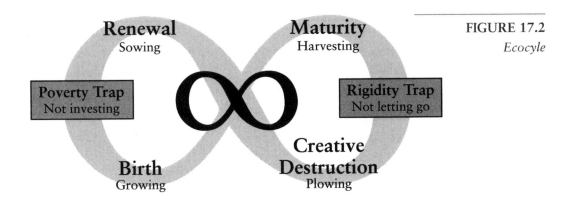

FIGURE 17.2

Ecocyle

The Ecocycle begins with birth (growing) and moves toward maturity (harvesting). When maturity has been reached, the cycle moves toward creative destruction (plowing) and creates space for renewal (sowing). In contrast, the conventional cycle includes birth, growth, and maturity but does not allow for creative destruction or renewal. These later cycles are often neglected; yet, without creative destruction, there is little opportunity for leaders to envision new options and create new opportunities. Traps leaders often fall into are not letting go of something after it has reached maturity (*rigidity trap*) and not funding new innovations (*poverty trap*). Using this cycle to consider where different aspects of an organization lie along the Ecocyle can unearth what immediately can be done to move one important element forward in an organization.

REFLECTING ON … ECOCYLE PLANNING

- *What new benefits, services, programs, and technologies are your members seeking?*

- *What aspects of your organization (committees, structures, and services) have reached maturity?*

- *What does your organization need to let go of to make space for something new?*

- *What aspects of your organization would benefit from renewal? How can you change a structure, an activity, a service, or a program to revitalize your group?*

The Partnership of Leaders and Followers: Ongoing Engagement and Honoring of Members

While leaders of an organization sift, sort, and work through the process of organizational transformation, it is essential to keep members informed and engaged along the way. Consistent, continual, and transparent communication is essential, whether face to face or virtual through electronic means.

In the preceding example, the key to the communication from the board was messaging that the organizational transformations the board had identified through its own work were based on and the result of the generative work the members had done through the 1-2-4-All Liberating Structure exercise. All messaging to members, regardless of communication vehicle (email, newsletter, website, verbal, print) consistently related the proposed organizational transformations to recommendations generated from members themselves.

In addition to traditional communication methods, the board engaged members by appointing a task force to study a proposed change to a membership benefit that had deep roots in the organization. The task force ultimately recommended the termination of the benefit, which the board approved. In communicating this action to members, the messaging recognized and honored members' longtime relationship with this benefit, and then reiterated the decision in part reflected the generative work of members.

The next step in engaging and honoring members was through more generative work—a survey to garner members' input on their vision of a new benefit approved by the board. The board valued their feedback—what they knew, believed, and valued—and used it as a foundation for defining and shaping the next iteration of the membership benefit. Clear messaging was that while the past was put to rest, the future was in the hands of members.

According to Chait and colleagues (2005), many nonprofit boards confront problems of purpose over performance and require leadership over management. Seen in this light, the board is a crucial and generative source of leadership for the organization. A board with a defined purpose is more engaged and able to work more meaningfully and partner with members around shared goals. *Partnered* or *collaborative leadership*—where the board values and relies on members' generative work as a basis of its own futures-thinking and visioning—will increase buy-in, minimize fear often associated with change, and lead to more productive outcomes in creating a preferred future.

To ensure the success of this process, it is important that board members attend meetings, participate in sense-making activities, engage in dialogue, provide feedback, and work through differences by helping to negotiate conflicts. Pesut (2007) states that polarities exist in every situation: Tensions exist between fear and aspiration, scarcity and abundance, greater purpose and deepest fear, and slow death and deep change. Managing polarities (Johnson, 1996) requires supporting organizational dialogue as members uncover the multiple dimensions—the upsides and downsides—of each stance.

Polarity management contributes to successful organizational leadership by seeking to understand all sides of an issue or stance. Johnson (1996) likens polarity management to breathing and asserts that leaders are charged to help organizations breathe. Thus, when leadership teams take time to unpack polarities with one another and members, they work toward solutions for all.

For example, consider the polarity of tradition and innovation. Members of each camp have a position they wish to advance. Often, the tradition bearers want to maintain the status quo, whereas the innovators want change. Each stance has some upsides and downsides. When both stances are considered in light of the purpose of the organization, it makes explicit the deepest fears of both, and then there is room for dialogue. Wesorick (2014) offers insights and suggestions about the use of polarity management skills for fostering interprofessional dialogue and reflection.

Final Reflections

The purpose of this chapter was to promote thoughtful consideration and reflection on organizational leadership where members are engaged as partners in creating a sustainable future. The value of leader self-knowledge and building teams with complementary versus similar strengths was emphasized. An exploration of the evolving trends within organizations as well as what it will take to prosper moving forward was addressed. Specific activities aimed at engaging members in generative thinking and sense-making were outlined to support futures-thinking and ensure an organization's prosperous future. Partnered-collaborative leadership emphasized incorporating members' generative work into futures-thinking and visions, along with the need for ongoing communication and clear messaging. Finally, through questions, readers were invited to reflect on ways to engage members and bring new life and new connections to their organizations to ensure a viable future.

Successfully engaging members as partners in organizational change requires leaders who know how to reflect on and cultivate their strengths while simultaneously empowering others to build and act upon their own. Partnered-collaborative leadership that emphasizes the importance of process-centric thinking through reflection, generative work, futures-thinking, visioning, ongoing communication, and clear messaging is essential to creating flexible, responsive, and viable organizations. As new opportunities for organizational innovation arise, leaders and teams who work together and value each member's strengths, contributions, and creativity will be well situated to thrive. It is by reflecting on what we have learned from past experiences that we can engage in creative thinking for sustaining the future through continual change and transformation.

References

Chait, R. P., Ryan, W. P., & Taylor, B. E. (2005). *Governance as leadership*. Hoboken, NJ: John Wiley & Sons.

Coerver, H., & Byers, M. (2011). *Race for relevance: 5 radical changes for associations*. Washington, DC: ASAE: The Center for Association Leadership.

Cronenwett, L., Sherwood, G., Barnsteiner, J., Disch, J., Johnson, J., Mitchell, P., … Warren, J. (2007). Quality and safety education for nurses. *Nursing Outlook, 55*(3), 122–131.

Cronenwett, L., Sherwood, G., & Gelmon, S. (2009). Improving quality and safety education: The QSEN Learning Collaborative. *Nursing Outlook, 57*(6), 304–312.

Cronenwett, L. (2012). A national initiative: Quality and Safety Education for Nurses (QSEN). In G. Sherwood, & J. Barnsteiner (Eds.), *Quality and safety in nursing: A competency approach to improving outcomes* (pp. 49–64). Hoboken, NJ: Wiley-Blackwell.

Deering, A., Dilts, R., & Russell, J. (2002). *Alpha leadership: Tools for business leaders who want more from life*. New York, NY: John Wiley & Sons.

Dilts, R. (1996a). *The new leadership paradigm*. Capitola, CA: Meta Publications.

Dilts, R. (1996b). *Visionary leadership*. Capitola, CA: Meta Publications.

Hurst, D. (2012). *The Ecocycle: A mental model for understanding complex systems. Leading forth: Strategy, leadership and change*. Retrieved from www.davidkhurst. com/the-ecocycle-a-mental-model-for-understanding-complex-systems-2/

Institute of Medicine (IOM). (1999). *To err is human: Building a safer health system*. Washington, DC: National Academies Press.

Institute of Medicine (IOM). (2001). *Crossing the quality chasm: A new health system for the 21st century*. Washington, DC: National Academies Press.

Institute of Medicine (2003). *Health professions education. A bridge to quality*. Washington, DC: National Academies Press.

Johnson, B. (1996). *Polarity management: Identifying and managing unsolvable problems.* Amherst, MA: HRD Press.

Lipmanowicz, H., & McCandless, K. (2013). *The surprising power of Liberating Structures: Simple rules to unleash a culture of innovation.* Seattle, WA: Liberating Structures Press.

Miller, R. (2011). Futures literacy: Embracing complexity and using the future. *Ethos, 10,* 23–28 .Retrieved from www.rielmiller.com/images/v03_ETHOS_issue10_riel_miller__v3.5_PRE_PUB_author_copy.pdf

Pesut, D. (2000). Looking forward: Being and becoming a futurist. In F. Bower (Ed.), *Nurses taking the lead: Personal qualities of effective leadership.* Philadelphia, PA: W. B. Saunders.

Pesut, D. (2014). *Creating desired futures.* International Society of Psychiatric Nurses 16th Annual Meeting, Greenville, SC, March 29, 2014.

Pesut, D. J., & Pesut, E. Z. (2010). Future forces affecting 21st century health professions education: Mastering the knowledge, skills, and abilities to support 21st century learning. In L. Caputi (Ed.), *Teaching nursing: The art and science,* Second Edition (Vol. 1) (pp. 198–228). Glen Ellyn, IL: College of Dupage Press.

Pesut, P. (2007). Leadership: How to achieve success in nursing organizations. In C. O'Lynn, & R. Tranbarger (Eds.), *Men in nursing: History, challenges, and opportunities.* New York, NY: Springer Publishing Co.

Pesut, D., & Thompson, S. (2015). Building academic cultures with reflective practice in mind: Leadership agility and transformational learning. In G. Sherwood, & S. Horton-Deutsch (Eds.). *Transforming organizations using principles of QSEN and reflective practice.* Indianapolis, IN: Sigma Theta Tau International.

Rath, T., & Conchie, B. (2008). *StrengthsFinder 2.0: Strengths-based leadership. Great leaders, teams and why people follow.* New York, NY: Gallup Press.

Sherwood, G., & Horton-Deutsch, S. (2012). *Reflective practice: Transforming education and improving outcomes.* Indianapolis, IN: Sigma Theta Tau International.

Wesorick, B. L. (2014). Polarity thinking: An essential skill for those leading interprofessional integration. *Journal of Interprofessional Healthcare, 1*(1). Retrieved from www.jihonline.org/jih/vol1/iss1/12

Appendix A
DEAL Model
Reflection Assignment

Assignment:
DEAL Experience Critical Reflection Paper

DEAL (Ash & Clayton, 2009)—Describe, Examine, and Articulate Learning— is not your typical academic paper; it is a critical self-reflection and examination and should be written in first person. It is an academic paper in that you are expected to demonstrate critical thinking and research (provide citations). You may want to refer to Paul and Elder's (2006; 2009) intellectual standards for critical thinking and use research (provide citations) on the topic. Therefore, your personal/professional experience as well as academic content should inform your reflection. Your paper should include three distinct sections (subheadings) and be written in APA format (current edition).

You will reflect upon this paper twice. The second iteration will be informed by your learning experiences in this course.

Iteration 1

I. Describe

Think of a personal (self, family member, or friend) or professional experience with addiction. Write the narrative/story of the experience. This content should be a thick description of the experience. A *thick description* is "[el]describing a phenomenon in sufficient detail so that one can begin to evaluate the extent to which the conclusions drawn are transferable to other times, settings, situations, and people" ("Thick description," 2008).

> One of the key terms in Clifford Geertz's anthropological theory is that of "thick description." Following Ryle, Geertz holds that anthropology's task is that of explaining cultures through thick description, which specifies many details, conceptual structures and meanings, and which is opposed to "thin description," which is a factual account without any interpretation. "Thin description" for Geertz is not only an insufficient account of an aspect of a culture: It is also a misleading one. According to Geertz, an ethnographer must present a thick description that is composed not only of facts but also of commentary, interpretation, and interpretations of those comments and interpretations. His task is to extract meaning structures that make up a culture; and for this, Geertz believes that a factual account will not suffice for these meaning structures are complexly layered atop and into each other so that each fact might be subjected to intercrossing interpretations which ethnography should study. ("Clifford Geertz's 'Thick Summary' Explained," 2012)

Now give the experience a name. The name should reflect the experience. For example, Jane might name her narrative of her mother's addiction to benzodiazepines "Mother Disappeared."

Name of the experience: _____

II. Examine (To look closely for the purpose of learning)

In fair detail, answer the following questions. Where you see a blank, insert the name you gave the experience. The purpose of this exercise is to externalize the experience for examination purposes as well as deconstruct (critique dominant understandings of a particular topic: in this example, you are looking at addiction).

1. If _____ could talk to me, what would it say to me? (Jane's sentence might read: If *Mother Disappeared* could talk to me, what would it say?)

2. What are the main themes related to _____ embedded in the narrative?

3. What does _____ have you thinking about addiction? About mental health?

4. What does _____ have you doing about or in relation to addiction?

5. Does _____ encourage particular ethics/values about addiction?

Now, reflect on your answers and write a reflective summary statement.

III. Articulate Learning

To begin, respond to the following questions:

- *What did I learn? About myself? Addiction? What I thought I thought?*

- *How did I learn it?* (Be specific. It is not sufficient to merely state, "I reflected or wrote.")

Next, think about what it is with regard to the assignment, afterward conversation, reflection, and so on that prompted your learning:

- *Why does it matter?* (Personally and professionally)

- *What will I do in the future, in light of it?* (Personally and professionally; be specific.)

Iteration 2
(At the end of the semester, as a part of your final exam)

Read, review, and reflect on you first paper in light of your ways of knowing and understanding addiction that you have learned in this course. For example, in light of your learning from readings and reflecting on class discussions, re-write your paper —this time with additional scholarship that reflects you learning during the course. Again, this should be a scholarly endeavor that includes critical thinking, creative problem-solving, and research.

DEAL Model Critical Thinking Standards

Intellectual Standard for Critical Thinking (http://www.criticalthinking.org)	Description	Checking Your Critical Thinking Skills
Relevance	Are all my statements relevant to the question at hand? Does what I'm saying connect to my central point?	How does this relate to the issue being discussed? How does this help me deal with the issue being discussed?
Accuracy	Are all my statements and all of my information factually correct and/or supported with evidence?	How do I know this? Is this true? How could I check on this to validate?
Precision	Are all my statements discussed in enough detail? More exact in identifying specifics in my examples?	Could I be more specific? Could I give more details?
Clarity	Do I expand on ideas, express ideas in another way, and provide examples or illustrations where appropriate?	Did I give an example? Is it clear what I mean by this? Could I elaborate further?
Depth	Do I explain the reasons behind my conclusions? Do I anticipate and answer the questions that my reasoning raises, and/or acknowledge the complexity of the issue?	Why is this so? What are some of the complexities here? What would it take for this to happen?
Breadth	Am I considering alternative points of view? Have I thought about how someone else might have interpreted the situation?	Would this look the same from the perspective of my client? Someone else? Is there another way to interpret this?
Logic	Does my line of reasoning make sense? Do my conclusions follow from the facts and/or my earlier statements?	Does what I said at the beginning fit with what I concluded at the end? Do my conclusions match the evidence?
Significance	Do my conclusions or goals represent a major issues raised by my reflection on experience?	Is this the most important issue on which to focus? Is this the most significant problem?

References

Ash, S. L., & Clayton, P. H. (2009). Generating, deepening, and documenting learning: The power of critical reflection in applied learning. *Journal of Applied Learning in Higher Education, 1*(Fall), 25–48.

"Clifford Geertz's 'Thick Summary' Explained." (2012). Retrieved from http://culturalstudiesnow.blogspot.com/2012/05/clifford-geertzs-thick-description.html

Paul, R., & Elder, L. (2006). *Critical thinking: Tools for taking charge of your learning and your life* (2nd ed.). Columbus, OH: Pearson/Prentice Hall.

Paul, R., & Elder, L. (2009). *The miniature guide to critical thinking. The foundation for critical thinking.* Santa Rosa, CA: Foundations for Critical Thinking. Retrieved from www.criticalthinking.org

Thick description. (2008). Retrieved from http://www.qualres.org/HomeThic-3697.html

Index

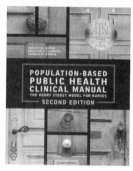
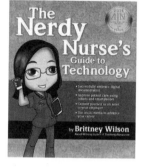
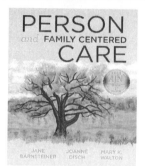
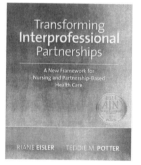
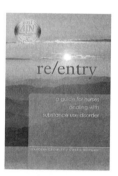
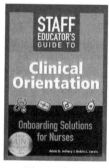
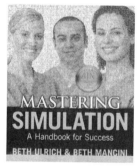

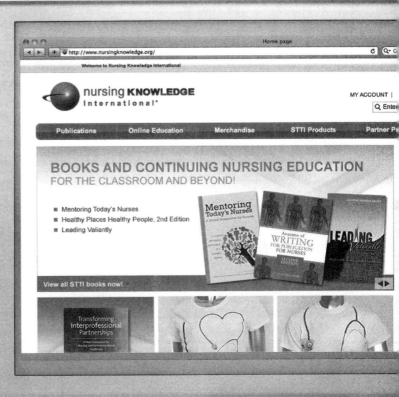

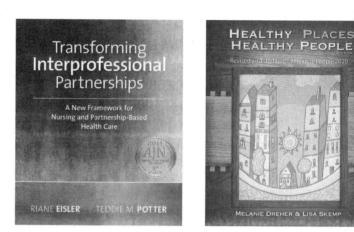
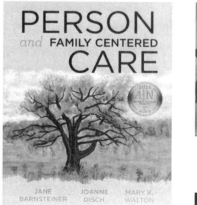
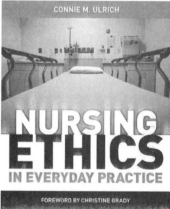